Diabetic Macular Edema

Sandeep Saxena • Gemmy Cheung
Timothy Y. Y. Lai • Srinivas R. Sadda
Editors

Diabetic Macular Edema

Springer

Editors
Sandeep Saxena
Department of Ophthalmology
King George's Medical University
Lucknow, India

Gemmy Cheung
Duke-NUS Medical School
National University of Singapore
Singapore, Singapore

Timothy Y. Y. Lai
Dept of Ophthalmology & Visual Sciences
Chinese University of Hong Kong
Kowloon, Hong Kong

Srinivas R. Sadda
Doheny Eye Institute
University of California
Los Angeles, CA, USA

ISBN 978-981-19-7306-2 ISBN 978-981-19-7307-9 (eBook)
https://doi.org/10.1007/978-981-19-7307-9

This Springer imprint is published by the registered company Springer Nature Singapore Pte Ltd.
The registered company address is: 152 Beach Road, #21-01/04 Gateway East, Singapore 189721, Singapore

Foreword

There is clearly a global epidemic of alarming proportion in developed countries and currently worsening in underdeveloped countries as rates of obesity continue to rise and are complicated by other medical diseases. This combined disorder or "Diabesity" has ocular complications that can lead to a state of severe vision loss. It is the number one leading cause of blindness where medical care is available worldwide. The problem is multidisciplinary with involvement of the heart, the brain, the peripheral circulation, the kidneys, and the ocular state. Well known to the general public and to physicians who care for such patients are the retinal manifestations. These are most dramatic as expressed secondary to perfusion and permeability abnormalities, most conspicuously the proliferation of vessels that tend to bleed, produce scarring in the vitreous to detach the retina, and infarct the circulation to a point of no return. Yet, examination of diabetic retinopathy will find patients suffering more from edema of the macula, producing central vision loss, or so-called legal blindness, the inability to see the large letters on a vision testing chart or less than 20/200 to ophthalmologists and optometrists familiar with eye care vision testing. There is a well-known distinction between the diabetes that produces severe detachment and total loss of vision versus this standard of legal blindness. Yet, there is no textbook available currently to focus on this latter dreaded complication. Unlike most diseases associated with severe vision loss, there are treatments based on evaluations of the state of the eye with multimodal imaging, with medications and/or interventional surgery, to benefit these patients.

Dr. Sandeep Saxena is joined by Dr. Gemmy Chung, Dr. Timothy Lai, and Dr. Srinivas Sadda to assemble a detailed study and description of the various parameters related to diabetic macular edema. Then they review current available treatment modalities based on clinical trials and their clinical knowledge and experience. The result is a comprehensive text to focus on this manifestation, its evaluation, and the related management considerations. Such a compilation of material has never been assembled before in the past. A review of the Table of Contents by readers is rewarded with a critical evaluation and treatment survey of typical and unusual case presentations for diabetic macular edema. The overall result is a familiarity with complex and challenging issues by readers and a useful approach to managing patients with diabetic macular edema with all of its realities and ambiguities. For me, an observer for more than a half century, this text is a new starting point in the study of a worldwide epidemic, armed with new developments in genetics, multimodal imaging, and novel forms of therapy. This book will serve now and in the future as a rational guide to those who are devoted to the study and the treatment of diabetic macular edema: scientists, clinicians, and patients alike. Readers will be obliged to begin with the early introductory chapters and extend their critical reading through to the elderly state where management of eye care is complicated further by cataract and glaucoma formation, and even age-related degeneration and all of its consequences.

Congratulations to the authors for assembling this comprehensive text which will be welcomed by eye care physicians and ancillary personnel, now and in the future, in their quest to manage diabetic patients with better preventative care and novel forms of interventional therapy.

Larry A. Yannuzzi

College of Physicians and Surgeons
Columbia University
New York, NY, USA

The Macula Foundation, Inc
The LuEsther T. Mertz Retinal Research Center
New York, NY, USA

Preface

The incidence of diabetes mellitus continues to grow worldwide, with the number of people with the disease expected to rise to 300 million by 2025. Diabetic retinopathy (DR) is a sight-threatening complication of diabetes mellitus. DR is the most frequent cause of blindness among adults aged 20–75 years. It is the leading cause of preventable blindness in adults of working age. The potential risk of blindness in an individual with diabetes is 2.5 times higher than that of an individual without diabetes. The prevalence of DR directly correlates with the duration of diabetes, ranging from 30% in people with <5 years of diabetes to 80% in people with more than 15 years of diabetes.

Diabetic macular edema results from blood retinal barrier breakdown and is associated with visual loss. This decrease in visual acuity is the most common cause of qualitative as well as quantitative reduction in health-related quality of life. Identification of disease in its early stages and timely intervention is crucial to improve visual outcome. Medical and surgical intervention for diabetic macular edema is improving constantly.

This book *Diabetic Macular Edema* is perhaps the first-ever effort to present state-of-the-art information on the subject. This book comprises 20 chapters and presents up-to-date knowledge on the diagnostic, medical, laser, and surgical aspects of the disease. Chapters have been presented in a lucid manner for a better understanding. Chapters have a global authorship and are well supported by black and white and color figures.

We are sure that this book will be useful for general ophthalmologists, resident doctors, retinal physicians, and fellows in training.

Lucknow, India — Sandeep Saxena
Singapore, Singapore — Gemmy Cheung
Kowloon, Hong Kong — Timothy Y. Y. Lai
Los Angeles, CA, USA — Srinivas R. Sadda

Contents

About the Editors

Sandeep Saxena is chief of retina service, Department of Ophthalmology, King George's Medical University, Lucknow, India. He completed two 1-year fellowships at Eye Institute, St Louis University and Barnes Retina Institute, St Louis, USA, and New York-Presbyterian Hospital of Columbia and Cornell, New York, USA. He is DAAD fellow, Bonn, Germany, and has been a visiting fellow to Harvard and Oxford. He has been a visiting professor to several universities across the globe. He has over 150 publications in indexed journals, 25 textbooks, and 4 classification systems to his credit. He has designed an instrument: Saxena Retina Grid-520 & 428, Ocular Instruments, USA.

Gemmy Cheung is currently professor, Duke-NUS Medical School, National University of Singapore, and head of the medical retina department, Singapore National Eye Center. She also heads the Retina Research Group at the Singapore Eye Research Institute. She has published more than 10 book chapters and has completed a number of clinical trials in antivascular endothelial growth factor therapies in the capacity of principal investigator. Prof. Cheung has received a number of prestigious awards, including the APAO Outstanding Service in Prevention of Blindness Award (2013), the APAO Nakajima Award (2014) and Achievement Award (2017), the Young Investigator Award (Macula Society 2017), the AAO Achievement Award (2017), AAO Secretariat Award (2018), as well as the APVRS Constable lectureship in 2018.

Timothy Y. Y. Lai is currently a clinical professor (honorary) of the Department of Ophthalmology and Visual Sciences, The Chinese University of Hong Kong, and director of the 2010 Retina and Macula Centre, Hong Kong. His clinical and research interests lie in the medical and surgical management of retinal diseases, particularly polypoidal choroidal vasculopathy, choroidal neovascularization, central serous chorioretinopathy, myopic maculopathy, diabetic retinopathy, visual electrophysiology, and genetics of retinal diseases and uveitis. Prof. Lai has published more than 250 papers in international peer-reviewed journals and has a Scopus h-factor of 53. He has received a number of international awards including the Nakajima Award of the Asia-Pacific Academy of Ophthalmology, Senior Achievement Award of the American Academy of Ophthalmology, and Achievement Award of the Asia-Pacific Academy of Ophthalmology. Prof. Lai serves on the editorial boards of various international ophthalmic journals including *Retina*, *Eye*, *Clinical and Experimental Ophthalmology*, *Ophthalmologica*, and *Asia-Pacific Journal of Ophthalmology*, and was former editor-in-chief of the *Hong Kong Journal of Ophthalmology*. His other leadership roles include vice president of the Asia-Pacific Vitreo-Retina Society, and section chair of the International Ocular Inflammation Society.

Srinivas R. Sadda, MD is professor of ophthalmology at the University of California—Los Angeles (UCLA). He received his MD from Johns Hopkins University, where he also completed ophthalmology residency and neuro-ophthalmology and medical retina fellowships (Wilmer Eye Institute). Dr. Sadda's major research interests include retinal image analysis, advanced retinal imaging technologies, and clinical trial endpoint design. He has more than

600 peer-reviewed publications and 20 book chapters and has given over 450 presentations worldwide. Dr. Sadda also serves as an editor-in-chief of *Graefe's* and is an editorial board member of *Ophthalmic Surgery, Lasers & Imaging, Retina, Ophthalmology Retina, Ophthalmology Science*, and *Ophthalmology*. Among Dr. Sadda's awards and honors are a Research to Prevent Blindness Physician-Scientist Award, a Senior Honor Award from the American Society of Retina Specialists, an Achievement Award and a Secretariat Award from the American Academy of Ophthalmology, John H. Zumberge Research and Innovation Award, the Macula Society Young Investigator Award, Asia-Pacific Academy of Ophthalmology (APAO) Achievement Award, the Macula Society Paul Henkind Lecture and Award, and American Society of Retina Specialists Young Investigator Award. He is also a gold fellow and trustee (retina) for the Association for Research in Vision and Ophthalmology. He has been named to the Best Doctors of America list for several consecutive years.

Diabetic Macular Edema: An Introduction

1

Yuen Yew Sen and Jagjit Singh Gilhotra

1.1 Diabetic Macular Edema: Introduction

In 2015, the Global Burden of Disease report estimated that the prevalence of diabetes rose from approximately 333 million persons in 2005 to approximately 435 million persons in 2015, an increase of 30.6% [1], underscoring the increasing burden of this disease. In a separate study [2] examining the global prevalence of diabetic retinopathy, 35% of people with diabetes had some form of diabetic retinopathy; 7% had proliferative diabetic retinopathy, 7% had diabetic macular edema, and 10% were affected by these vision-threatening stages. Table 1.1 outlines the ETDRS definitions for background retinopathy.

For DME, the landmark ETDRS [3] definition of macular edema (CSME: Clinically Significant Macular Edema) took into account both edema affecting the fovea and edema threatening the fovea (Figs. 1.1 and 1.2). Left alone, 33% of 221 eyes in the ETDRS with center-involved DME developed "moderate visual loss," defined as a 15 or more letter decrease in visual acuity over a 3-year period [4].

The pathophysiology underlying the visual loss in diabetic macular edema is thought to be due to breakdown in the blood–retinal barrier with resultant abnormal leakage of fluid and macromolecules such as lipoproteins from retinal capillaries into the extravascular space [5]. Hyperglycemia is thought to be the strongest risk factor contributing to the

Table 1.1 ETDRS definition for background retinopathy [3]

Background Retinopathy
(ETDRS Classification; Early Treatment of Diabetic Retinopathy Study)

Non proliferative diabetic retinopathy (NPDR)

- Mild NPDR
  - o At least 1 microaneurysm, but not enough to qualify as moderate NPDR
- Moderate NPDR
  - o Extensive intraretinal hemorrhages and/or microaneurysms, cotton wool spots, venous beading but not enough to qualify as severe NPDR
- Severe NPDR
  - o Defined as '4-2-1' rule as any one of the following
    - i. Intraretinal hemorrhages and/or microaneurysms in all 4 quadrants
    - ii. Venous beading in at least 2 quadrants
    - iii. IRMA (Intraretinal microvascular abnormalities) in at least 1 quadrant

Proliferative diabetic retinopathy (PDR)

- Presence of new vessels on the disc (NVD)
- Presence of new vessels elsewhere (NVE)

Y. Y. Sen
National University Health System, Singapore, Singapore

J. S. Gilhotra (✉)
University of Adelaide, Adelaide, SA, Australia

S. Saxena et al. (eds.), *Diabetic Macular Edema*, https://doi.org/10.1007/978-981-19-7307-9_1

pathogenesis of DME. It is believed to lead to increased oxidative stress, inflammation, and vascular dysfunction with resultant upregulation of growth factors and cytokines, such as VEGF, angiopoietins, tumor necrosis factor, interleukins, and matric metalloproteinases, which contribute to the breakdown of the blood–retinal barrier and the development of DME [5]. It is important to realize it is a complex of factors and not simply a VEGF-driven disease.

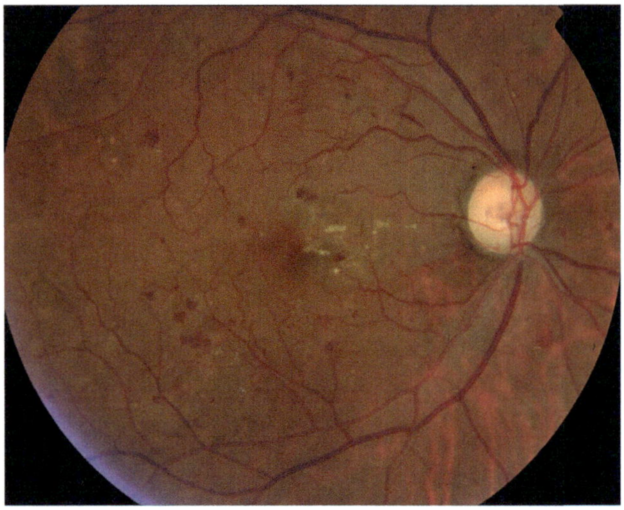

Fig. 1.1 Example of CSME with hard exudates and edema within 500 µm of the fovea

There is also a concern that vitreomacular traction (Fig. 1.3), or the vitreous itself, may play a role in increased retinal vascular permeability. Removal of the vitreous or relief of vitreomacular traction with vitrectomy and membrane peeling may be followed by substantial resolution of macular edema and corresponding improvement in visual acuity. However, this treatment may be applicated to only a small subset of eyes that have a visually significant component of vitreomacular traction or ERM exacerbating the edema. The DRCR [6] investigated the same issue and concluded that most patients showed improvement of the retinal thickening but improvement of visual acuity by 10 letters occurred in only 38% of patients. This disconnect between changes in OCT and visual acuity was quite stark. The correlation between changes in OCT central subfield thickness from baseline to 6 months and changes in visual acuity during this time was −0.31. Except for cases with very large decreases in central subfield thickness (>350 µm), a given decrease in OCT was associated with a wide range of changes in visual acuity [6].

In the ETDRS [4], it was demonstrated that moderate visual loss, defined as a doubling of the visual angle, can be reduced by 50% or more by focal/grid laser photocoagulation. Unfortunately, the original ETDRS treatment regimen may require laser burn placement close to the fovea, which, over time, may develop into areas of progressive RPE and retinal atrophy larger than the original laser spot size with encroachment onto the fovea (Fig. 1.4).

Fig. 1.2 CSME definition [3]

Clinically Significant Macular Edema (CSME) Definition (ETDRS 1985)
One of the following:

- Thickening within 500um of the fovea
- Hard exudates within 500um of the fovea with associated retinal thickening
- Area of retinal thickening of 1 disc area in size, any part of which is within 1 disc diameter of the fovea

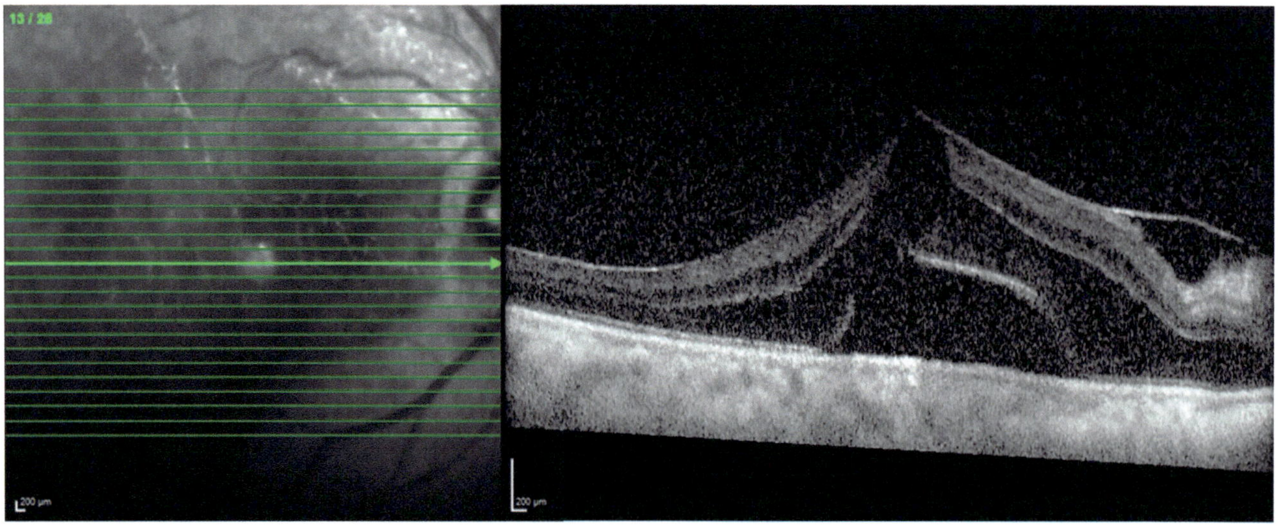

Fig. 1.3 Vitreomacular traction

However, over the last 20 years, the advent of anti-VEGF [7–9] and corticosteroid therapy [10] has increased the options available for the management of diabetic macular edema and given patients therapeutic options with higher chances of improving vision compared to laser alone [11]. Anti-VEGF options are varied with bevacizumab, ranibizumab, and aflibercept being investigated in DRCR Protocol T [11]. Newer agents in the pipeline include brolucizumab (targeting VEGF-A) and faricimab. Faricimab is a bispecific antibody that targets two distinct pathways, VEGF-A and angiopoietin-2 (Ang-2), and recently obtained FDA approval for use in DME.

The threshold for treatment also shifted away from the traditional classification of CSME to looking at purely edema affecting the fovea. In the DRCR network group of studies, center involving DME was taken as the main clinical definition of DME in making a decision to treat (Figs. 1.5 and 1.6).

Simultaneously, for non-center involving DME, DRCR modified the ETDRS focal/grid treatment [12] (M-ETDRS) to utilize less intense laser burns, greater spacing, directly targeting microaneurysms and avoiding the perifoveal vasculature within at least 500 μm of the center of the macula. This M-ETDRS focal/grid laser technique was shown by DRCR to be comparable to results in similar eyes in ETDRS [13] and, as such, is the standard laser technique adopted in the DRCR.net studies.

The diagnostic classification has also changed since the time of the ETDRS in the 1980s. In the ETDRS, CSME was assessed using stereo contact lens biomicroscopy or stereophotography [4] as OCT was not available at the time. Since then, OCT has emerged as a crucial tool in assessing the severity of DME in recent clinical trials, including those carried out by the DRCR network with a shift in focus toward differentiating patients into center-involving vs. non-center-involving DME. Center-involved DME in the DRCR was defined as OCT subfoveal thickness of 250 μm or more on the Zeiss Stratus or the equivalent on spectral domain OCT based on gender-specific cut-offs in DRCR [11].

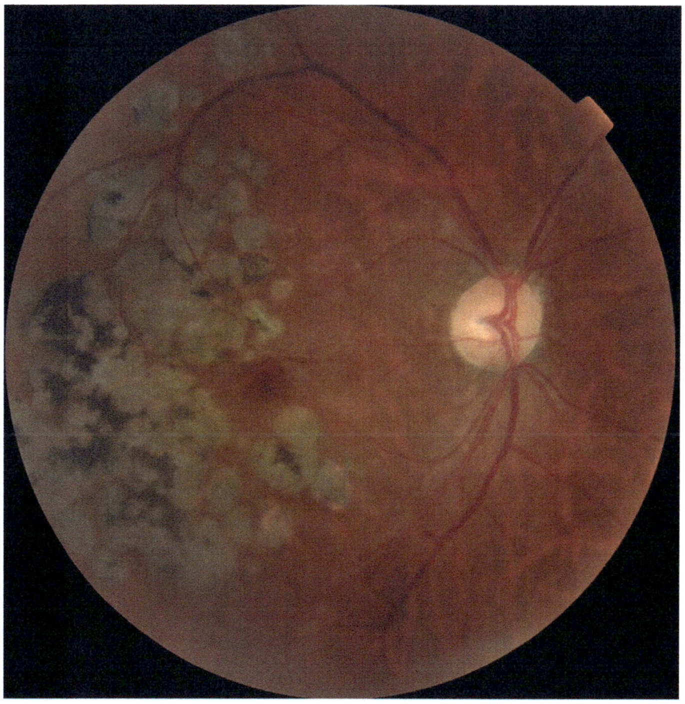

Fig. 1.4 Focal laser scars with enlargement and gradual creep threatening the fovea

Fig. 1.5 DRCR OCT criteria for DME [11]

DRCR OCT Criteria For Retinal Thickening From DME

- Central subfield thickness on OCT more than/equal to 250um on Zeiss Stratus or the equivalent on spectral domain OCTs.

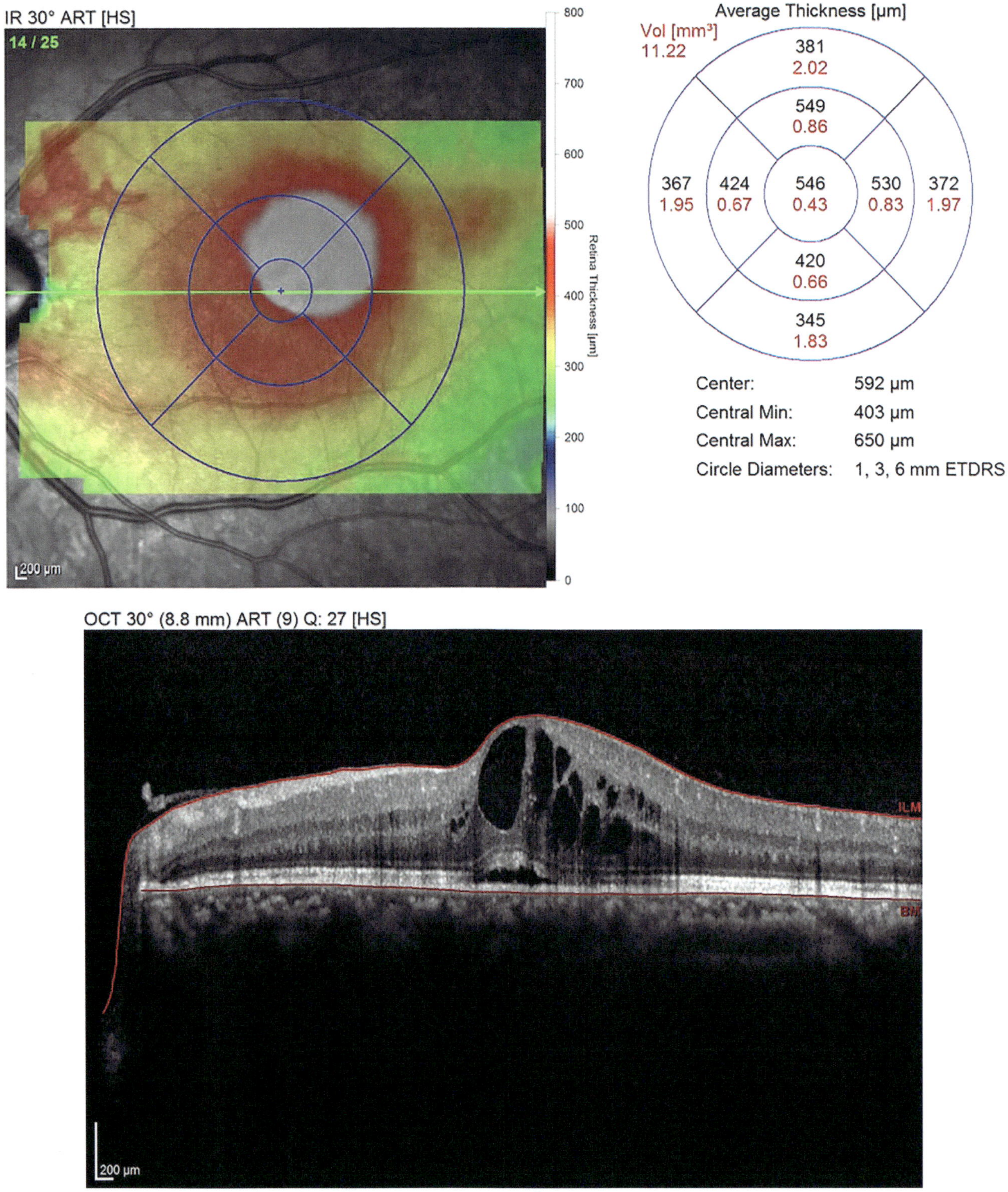

Fig. 1.6 Center involving DME with a subfoveal thickness of 546 µm

Visual acuity has also been taken into account with DRCR stratifying treatment strategies for DME patients with good VA [14] (20/25 or better) vs. poor VA (20/32 to 20/320) [11]. A differentiation has also been made for patients with worse baseline VA of 20/50 to 20/320 in DRCR protocol T [11], where aflibercept had superior 2-year VA outcomes compared with bevacizumab, but the superiority of aflibercept over ranibizumab, noted at 1 year, was no longer identified.

In summary, our evaluation and management of DME has evolved significantly since the landmark ETDRS studies in the 1980s. With the advent of newer imaging modalities (OCT) and better therapeutic agents (intravitreal anti-VEGF and steroids), our options for managing DME has improved significantly, affording our patients a greater chance of visual improvement.

References

1. Vos T, Allen C, Arora M, et al. Global, regional, and national incidence, prevalence, and years lived with disability for 310 diseases and injuries, 1990–2015: a systematic analysis for the Global Burden of Disease Study 2015. Lancet. 2016;388(10053):1545–602. https://doi.org/10.1016/S0140-6736(16)31678-6.
2. Yau JWY, Rogers SL, Kawasaki R, et al. Global prevalence and major risk factors of diabetic retinopathy. Diabetes Care. 2012;35(3):556–64. https://doi.org/10.2337/dc11-1909.
3. Photocoagulation for diabetic macular edema: early treatment diabetic retinopathy study report number 1 early treatment diabetic retinopathy study research group. Arch Ophthalmol. 1985;103(12):1796–806. https://doi.org/10.1001/archopht.1985.01050120030015.
4. Photocoagulation for diabetic macular edema: early treatment diabetic retinopathy study report no. 4. The early treatment diabetic retinopathy study research group. Int Ophthalmol Clin. 1987;27(4):265–72. https://doi.org/10.1097/00004397-198702740-00006.
5. Das A, McGuire PG, Rangasamy S. Diabetic macular edema: pathophysiology and novel therapeutic targets. Ophthalmology. 2015;122(7):1375–94. https://doi.org/10.1016/J.OPHTHA.2015.03.024.
6. Network DRCR. Vitrectomy outcomes in eyes with diabetic macular edema and vitreomacular traction. Ophthalmology. 2010;117(6):1087. https://doi.org/10.1016/J.OPHTHA.2009.10.040.
7. Soheilian M, Garfami KH, Ramezani A, Yaseri M, Peyman GA. Two-year results of a randomized trial of intravitreal bevacizumab alone or combined with triamcinolone versus laser in diabetic macular edema. Retina. 2012;32(2):314–21. https://doi.org/10.1097/IAE.0b013e31822f55de.
8. Nguyen QD, Brown DM, Marcus DM, et al. Ranibizumab for diabetic macular edema: results from 2 phase iii randomized trials: RISE and RIDE. Ophthalmology. 2012;119(4):789–801. https://doi.org/10.1016/j.ophtha.2011.12.039.
9. Heier JS, Brown DM, Chong V, et al. Intravitreal Aflibercept (VEGF trap-eye) in wet age-related macular degeneration. Ophthalmology. 2012;119(12):2537–48. https://doi.org/10.1016/j.ophtha.2012.09.006.
10. Ip MS, Bressler SB, Antoszyk AN, et al. A randomized trial comparing intravitreal triamcinolone and focal/grid photocoagulation for diabetic macular edema baseline features. Retina. 2008;28(7):919–30. https://doi.org/10.1097/IAE.0b013e31818144a7.
11. Wells JA, Glassman AR, Ayala AR, et al. Aflibercept, bevacizumab, or ranibizumab for diabetic macular edema two-year results from a comparative effectiveness randomized clinical trial. Ophthalmology. 2016;123(6):1351–9. https://doi.org/10.1016/j.ophtha.2016.02.022.
12. Fong DS, Strauber SF, Aiello LP, et al. Comparison of the modified early treatment diabetic retinopathy study and mild macular grid laser photocoagulation strategies for diabetic macular edema. Arch Ophthalmol. 2007;125(4):469–80. https://doi.org/10.1001/ARCHOPHT.125.4.469.
13. Beck RW, Edwards AR, Aiello LP, et al. Three-year follow-up of a randomized trial comparing focal/grid photocoagulation and intravitreal triamcinolone for diabetic macular edema. Arch Ophthalmol. 2009;127(3):245–51. https://doi.org/10.1001/ARCHOPHTHALMOL.2008.610.
14. Baker CW, Glassman AR, Beaulieu WT, et al. Effect of initial management with aflibercept vs laser photocoagulation vs observation on vision loss among patients with diabetic macular edema involving the center of the macula and good visual acuity: a randomized clinical trial. JAMA. 2019;321(19):1880–94. https://doi.org/10.1001/JAMA.2019.5790.

Pathophysiology of Diabetic Macular Edema

2

Andrea P. Cabrera, Emma L. Wolinsky, Rushi N. Mankad, Finny Monickaraj, and Arup Das

2.1 Introduction

Diabetic macular edema (DME), a complication of diabetic retinopathy (DR), is the most common cause of vision loss among diabetics [1, 2]. According to the International Diabetes Federation (IDF), the number of retinopathy cases is estimated to reach 191 million by 2030 [3]. With 537 million people currently living with diabetes, the urgency to understand, treat and help prevent this disease is highlighted. Thus, in this chapter we focus on the pathophysiology underlying DME and examine the blood–retinal barrier (BRB), key molecules involved in its alteration, and current clinical trials targeting these novel molecules in this vision-threatening phenotype.

2.2 Pathophysiology of Diabetic Macular Edema

Hyperglycemia is the strongest risk factor contributing to the pathogenesis of DME, as evidenced by large prospective clinical studies [4–6]. Though the exact pathways and mechanisms underlying this disease remain to be fully elucidated, it is recognized that the hyperglycemia-induced pathogenesis of DR is related to four major biochemical pathways: (1) polyol, (2) advanced glycation end products, (3) protein kinase C (PKC), and (4) hexosamine [7, 8]. All of these pathways lead to increased oxidative stress and upregulation of pro-inflammatory cytokines and growth factors, which together with matrix metalloproteinases (MMPs) contribute to vascular dysfunction and breakdown of the blood–retinal barrier (BRB) (Fig. 2.1). The persistent hyperglycemic, pro-inflammatory environment, degeneration of the endothelium and pericytes, and the inability to restore vascular homeostasis lead to the clinical manifestations seen in DME.

2.2.1 Alteration of Blood–Retinal Barrier

The blood–retinal barrier (BRB), separating the inner and outer retina, is a physiological barrier that tightly regulates fluid and electrolyte balance in the surrounding tissue. The outer BRB is formed by the highly specialized retinal pigment epithelial (RPE) cells, located adjacent to the choriocapillaris [9]. The inner BRB is formed by tight junctions between retinal capillary endothelial cells (ECs) and underlying basement membrane, surrounding pericytes and Müller cells [10]. The unique structural organization of the retinal microvasculature is primarily responsible for the regulation of vascular permeability within this tissue. Thus, an intact BRB is essential in maintaining normal visual function through these processes. Junctional modification and changes in permeability can take place through nonproteolytic mechanisms involving biochemical modification of junction proteins or through physical interactions with the cell cytoskeleton [11–14]. Diabetes-induced BRB alterations described in both diabetic animal models and humans include (1) breakdown of cell–cell junctions between endothelial cells, (2) pericyte loss, and (3) basement membrane thickening, as shown in Fig. 2.2. Loss of cell-to-cell junctions in the

A. P. Cabrera · E. L. Wolinsky · R. N. Mankad
Department of Ophthalmology, University of New Mexico School of Medicine, Albuquerque, NM, USA
e-mail: apcabrera@salud.unm.edu; EWolinsky@salud.unm.edu; RMankad@salud.unm.edu

F. Monickaraj
Department of Ophthalmology, University of New Mexico School of Medicine, Albuquerque, NM, USA

New Mexico VA Health Care System, Albuquerque, NM, USA
e-mail: FMonickaraj@salud.unm.edu

A. Das (✉)
Department of Ophthalmology, University of New Mexico School of Medicine, Albuquerque, NM, USA

New Mexico VA Health Care System, Albuquerque, NM, USA

Department of Cell Biology and Physiology, University of New Mexico School of Medicine, Albuquerque, NM, USA
e-mail: adas@unm.edu

S. Saxena et al. (eds.), *Diabetic Macular Edema*, https://doi.org/10.1007/978-981-19-7307-9_2

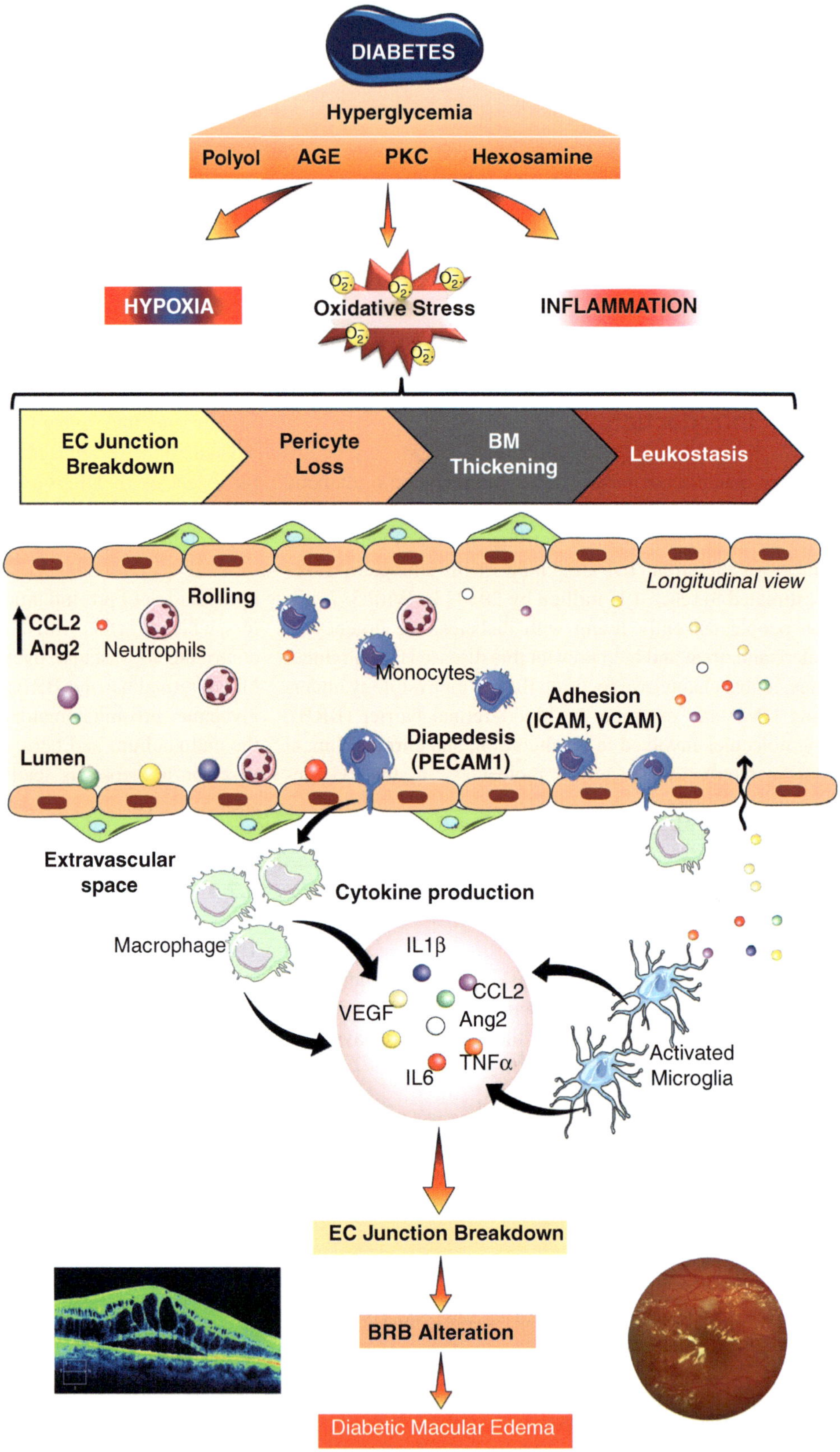

Fig. 2.1 Pathophysiology of diabetic macular edema (DME). Hyperglycemia in diabetes activates different biochemical pathways that lead to increased hypoxia, reactive oxygen species (ROS) formation, and release of various pro-inflammatory growth factors and cytokines. The oxidative stress in diabetes leads to pericyte loss and basement membrane (BM) thickening. Increased CCL2 and Ang2 leads to increased leukocyte adhesion (leukostasis), rolling, extravasation into the surrounding tissues (diapedesis), influx of monocytes into the retina and increased production of cytokines including VEGF, TNFα, IL6, IL1b, and Ang2. The activation of macrophages serves to amplify cytokine production, enabling the activation of resident microglia, further fueling the pro-inflammatory environment. All these cytokines act on the endothelial cell–cell junctions resulting in the breakdown of the blood–retinal barrier (BRB) and increased retinal vascular permeability that leads to plasma "leakage," the clinical manifestation of DME. *AGE* advanced glycation end-products, *PKC* protein kinase C, *EC* endothelial cell, *BM* basement membrane, *Ang2* angiopoietin-2, *CCL2* chemokine (C-C motif) ligand 2, *ICAM* intercellular adhesion molecule, *VCAM* vascular cell adhesion molecule, *PECAM1* platelet endothelial cell adhesion molecule-1, *IL1β* interleukin-1β, *IL6* interleukin-6, *TNFα* tumor necrosis factor-α, *VEGF* vascular endothelial growth factor, *BRB* blood–retinal barrier, *DME* diabetic macular edema

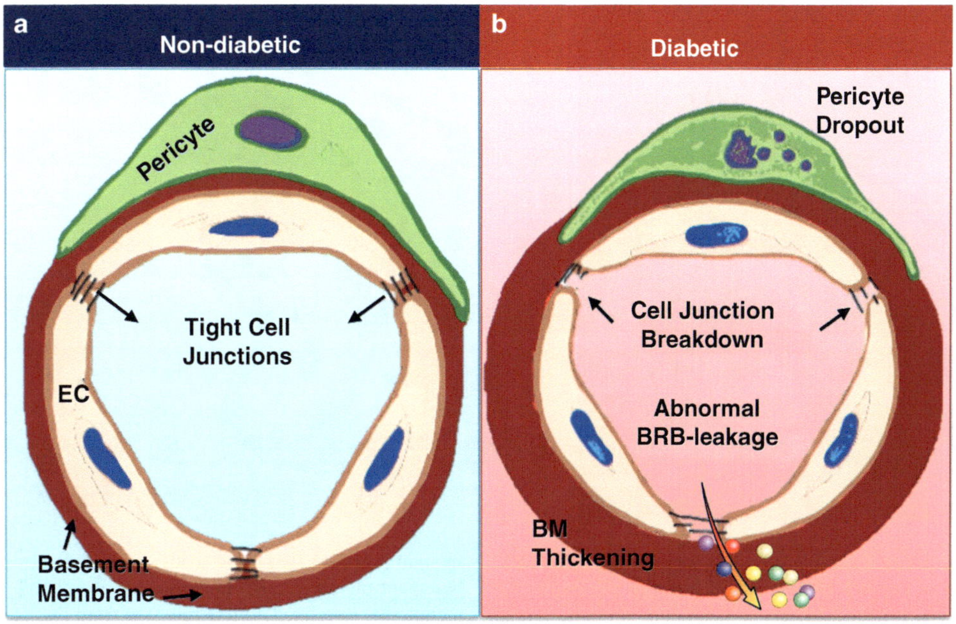

Fig. 2.2 Alteration of the blood–retinal barrier (BRB) in diabetes mellitus. (**a**) The blood–retinal barrier (BRB) is formed by a highly regulated interaction between pericytes, endothelial cells (EC), and surrounding basement membrane (BM). Astrocytes and microglia with long processes (not pictured) also surround the capillaries, maintaining the normal homeostasis for neuronal signaling and synaptic transmission. (**b**) In diabetes, hyperglycemia induces BRB alterations including pericyte dropout, cell junction breakdown, and basement membrane thickening, resulting in increased permeability and altered BRB. *EC* endothelial cell, *BM* basement membrane

endothelium results in the leakage of red blood cells, plasma, and lipid into the retina [15].

2.2.2 Outer Blood–Retinal Barrier

The *retinal pigment epithelial cells (RPE)* form a highly specialized tissue layer responsible for (1) nutrient, ion, and water exchange, (2) light absorption, (3) clearance of metabolic waste, and (4) secretion of growth factors essential for retinal health [9, 16]. In addition to being a source of local complement protein production, the single-cell RPE tissue layer forms a highly selective barrier [17]. The permeability of this outer BRB component is regulated by cell–cell interactions among neighboring conditions in the retina which in turn leads to the overexpression of vascular endothelial growth factor (VEGF) by RPE [18]. This secretion of VEGF by RPE further alters the retinal vasculature.

2.2.3 Inner Blood–Retinal Barrier

The inner BRB is formed at the level of the retinal capillaries and is comprised of endothelial cells, pericytes, and basement membrane as shown in Fig. 2.3.

(a) *Endothelial Cells* (ECs) form a tight monolayer in which individual ECs are joined to each other by tight junctional complexes and adherens junctions. In animal models of diabetes, the disruption cell–cell junctions occurs through a decrease in occludin and VE-cadherin expression [11, 16, 19, 20]. Intravitreal injection of vascular endothelial growth factor (VEGF) has been shown in animal models to result in increased phosphorylation of occludin and zona occludin [12]. In addition to the breakdown of the cell–cell junctions, capillary ECs, together with pericytes, also undergo apoptosis, ultimately forming acellular capillaries, an advanced lesion seen in DR [13].

Tight junction proteins are made up of a complex array of interacting proteins, which together help generate and regulate the permeability of the BRB [11, 21]. Endothelial cells contribute to the function of the BRB through the formation of specialized intercellular junctions including adherens and tight junctions. Vascular endothelial (VE)-cadherin, a member of the cadherin family, is an integral endothelial adhesion protein providing a molecular link between neighboring cells and anchorage point between the plasma membrane and the actin cytoskeleton through its interactions with the cytoplasmic proteins β- and γ-catenin [22, 23]. VE-cadherin also plays a role in the regulation of a variety of endothelial cell behaviors including motility, morphogenesis, responsiveness to growth factors, and cell survival [24, 25]. The integrity of the adherens junctions between adjacent endothelial cells is thought to be critical for normal barrier function.

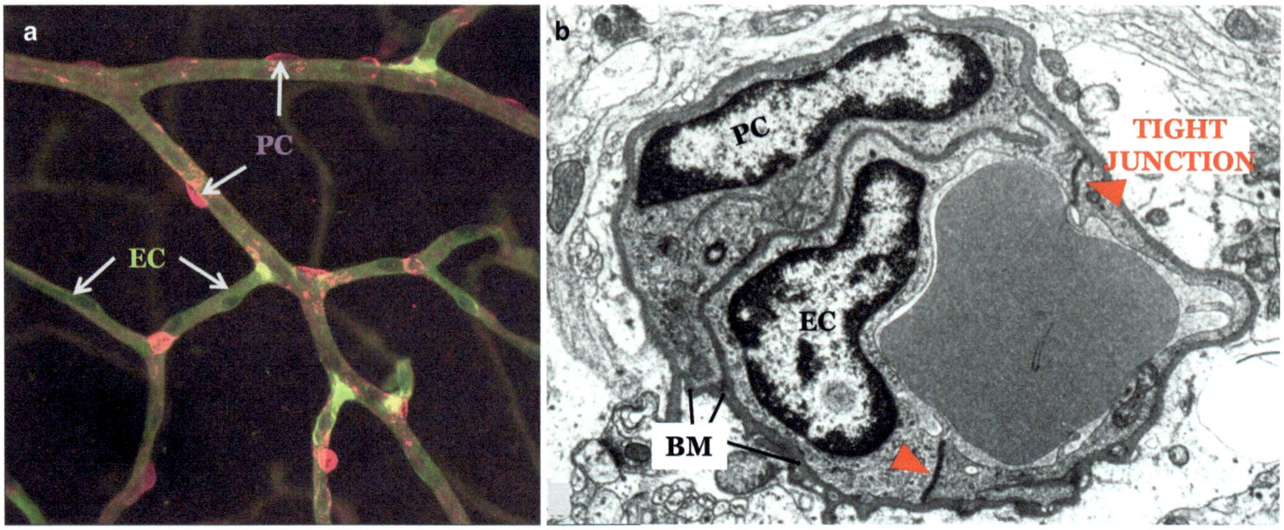

Fig. 2.3 Tight junction proteins Regulate the Permeability of the BRB. (**a**) En face confocal capture of interaction between pericytes and underlying endothelial cells and basement membrane in mouse retinal capillaries. (**b**) Transmission electron microcopy cross-sectional view of a monkey retinal capillary showing endothelial cells joined together by tight junctions (red arrowheads), surrounded by pericytes and a thin basement membrane. *PC* pericyte, *EC* endothelial cell, *BM* basement membrane. Reprinted with permission from Das et al. Ophthalmology. 2015;122:1375–1394

N-cadherin mediates adhesion, recognition, and signaling between pericytes and endothelial cells. This pericyte–EC interaction can be induced by stimulation of the sphingosine 1-phosphate (S1P) receptor on endothelial cells, which has been shown to induce N-cadherin trafficking to the cell surface and promote cell–cell interactions [21, 26]. The mechanisms that regulate the interaction of pericytes and endothelial cells in the retinal microvasculature, and the factors involved in the local regulation of microvascular permeability in the retina have not been well-characterized.

(b) *Basement membrane*: The basement membrane underlies a single-cell layer of endothelial cells on their abluminal side, while also completely enclosing pericytes. In addition to providing structural support, the basement membrane is a regulator of cell proliferation and differentiation and serves as a filtration barrier [27]. In DR, increased thickening of the capillary basement membrane occurs due to increased collagen IV and laminin [28, 29]. However, it is unclear how basement membrane thickening increases diffusion of molecules and results in the plasma "leakage" observed in DME. An alteration of the molecular structure of the basement membrane or the distribution of negatively charged heparin sulfate proteoglycan molecules likely contributes to the increased porosity of this barrier in diabetes [29].

(c) *Pericytes* are contractile smooth muscle cells overlying capillary endothelium which regulate retinal capillary blood flow and help maintain the integrity of the BRB [30]. In tandem with endothelial cells, pericytes also play a central role in vascular development and angiogenesis through their expression of platelet-derived growth factor receptor-beta (PDGFRβ), which enables their recruitment by platelet-derived growth factor (PDGF) secreted by the endothelium [31, 32]. In the formation of capillaries, pericyte arrival coincides with the production of basement membrane components by the endothelium. Pericyte-EC contact results in the activation of transforming growth factor-β (TGF-β), which also serves to regulate endothelial cell proliferation [33, 34]. Pericyte-EC survival and vascular stabilization is further promoted by the production of angiopoietin-1 (Ang-1) by perivascular cells that competes with endothelial cell produced angiopoietin-2 (Ang-2) for binding to the Tie-2 receptor [35]. In diabetes, these functions are lost as pericyte dropout occurs. Alterations in PDGFRβ in early diabetes may affect pericyte viability, leading to pericyte loss [7]. Under normal conditions,

PDGFRβ promotes proliferation and migration of pericytes. Animal studies have shown mice deficient in PDGFRβ lead to pericyte loss and microaneurysm formation, as also seen in diabetic persons [36]. Pericyte loss as seen in diabetic retinopathy results in focal endothelial cell proliferation and likely contributes to the formation of microaneurysms in the weakened wall of retinal capillaries.

The neurovascular unit consists of Müller cells, astrocytes, ganglion cells, amacrine cells, retinal vascular endothelial cells, and pericytes. Of note, is the role of Müller cells, which help form an extensive network of villi that intimately surround the neighboring vessels in addition to releasing factors that induce the formation of tight junctions in these vessels [37]. In diabetes, dysfunctional Müller cells likely affect this barrier property. Although diabetic retinopathy is considered primarily a vascular phenomenon with alteration to the BRB, recent work suggests that the pathology lies in alteration of the neurovascular unit [38].

The neuronal dysfunction in diabetic retinopathy is attributed to biochemical changes, including impaired glutamate metabolism, loss of synapses and dendrites, and ganglion cell apoptosis [39, 40]. The visual functional changes (loss of color and contrast sensitivity, abnormal electroretinogram [oscillatory potential], and visual field defects) preceding the appearance of vascular lesion seen in early DR may be explained by these neuronal changes.

Photoreceptors: Photoreceptors are the most abundant cells in the retina in addition to being the most metabolically active [40]. Known for their light-sensing properties, photoreceptors have increasingly become recognized for their role in the vascular dysfunction associated with DR. Their contribution was highlighted in animal studies where diabetic mice lacking photoreceptors did not experience a decrease in retinal microvasculature density normally seen in diabetes [41]. More recent studies have shown that photoreceptors inhibit diabetes-induced increases in superoxide and inflammatory proteins in the retina [42].

Clinical observations also point to a central role for photoreceptors in DR pathogenesis. In a case series of diabetic patients with retinitis pigmentosa, a disease characterized by the progressive degeneration of photoreceptors, none showed signs of retinopathy despite long duration of diabetes [43]. Such a clinical observation points to the fact that retinitis pigmentosa, by an unknown mechanism, protects against the development of diabetic retinopathy.

Immune cells are known to play an important role in the pathogenesis of DR [44]. However, their role in DME has yet to be fully elucidated. Schroder et al., first described leukostasis in the retinal vasculature as an important phenomenon for the increased neutrophil and monocytes previously shown to be associated with retinal vascular abnormalities in diabetic rat models [45]. Herein we highlight, microglia, macrophages, and neutrophils for their contributing roles in the development of DR.

Microglia are resident cells that mediate immune response in the retina. Their immune surveillant behavior includes the constant sensing of their environment by extending and retracting their processes in addition to phagocytosis of cell debris [46, 47]. Microglia also produce local complement proteins and regulators. Under normal conditions, these resident cells remain inactivate [48, 49]. However, diabetes-induced changes lead to low-level activation. In animal models of diabetes, increased number of activated microglia can be observed shortly after the onset of diabetes, coinciding with the decrease in the number of neuronal cells [50].

Macrophages are activated monocytes that differentiate into macrophages upon transversing endothelium. Important mediators of inflammation and tissue remodeling, they secrete cytokines and growth factors implicated in DR pathogenesis including VEGF, Ang-2, TNF-α, ILs, MMP-2, and MMP-9 [51, 52]. Activation leads to increased leukocyte–endothelial interactions, termed leukostasis, which may further stimulate cytokine production and induce cell death [53, 54].

Our own observations demonstrate monocyte/macrophage trafficking into the extravascular retinal tissues in wild-type diabetic animals in comparison with control non-diabetic animals (Fig. 2.4) [55]. The increased monocyte trafficking into the retina in early diabetes seems to be regulated by the levels of monocyte chemoattractant protein (MCP)-1 also known as "chemokine ligand 2 (CCL2)." Gene expression array results indicate that MCP-1 is remarkably upregulated (16-fold) compared with other angiogenic factors such as VEGF, Ang-2, and TNF-α [55].

Neutrophils are circulating leukocytes who surveil for signs of microbial infections, in addition to trapping and killing invading pathogens. Elevated numbers of neutrophils have been described in retinal and choroidal vessels of human diabetic subjects and diabetic monkeys [45, 56]. Though diabetic conditions cause a reduction in phagocytosis and bactericidal activity, neutrophils from type 1 and type 2 diabetes (T1D and T2D) patients are more active in comparison to those from healthy controls as evidenced by increased production of proinflammatory cytokines and expression of adhesion molecules [57–59]. Our recent work shows that the chemokine CXCL1 is elevated in retinal tissues in diabetic animals resulting in neutrophil recruitment and cytokine production leading to alteration of the BRB [60].

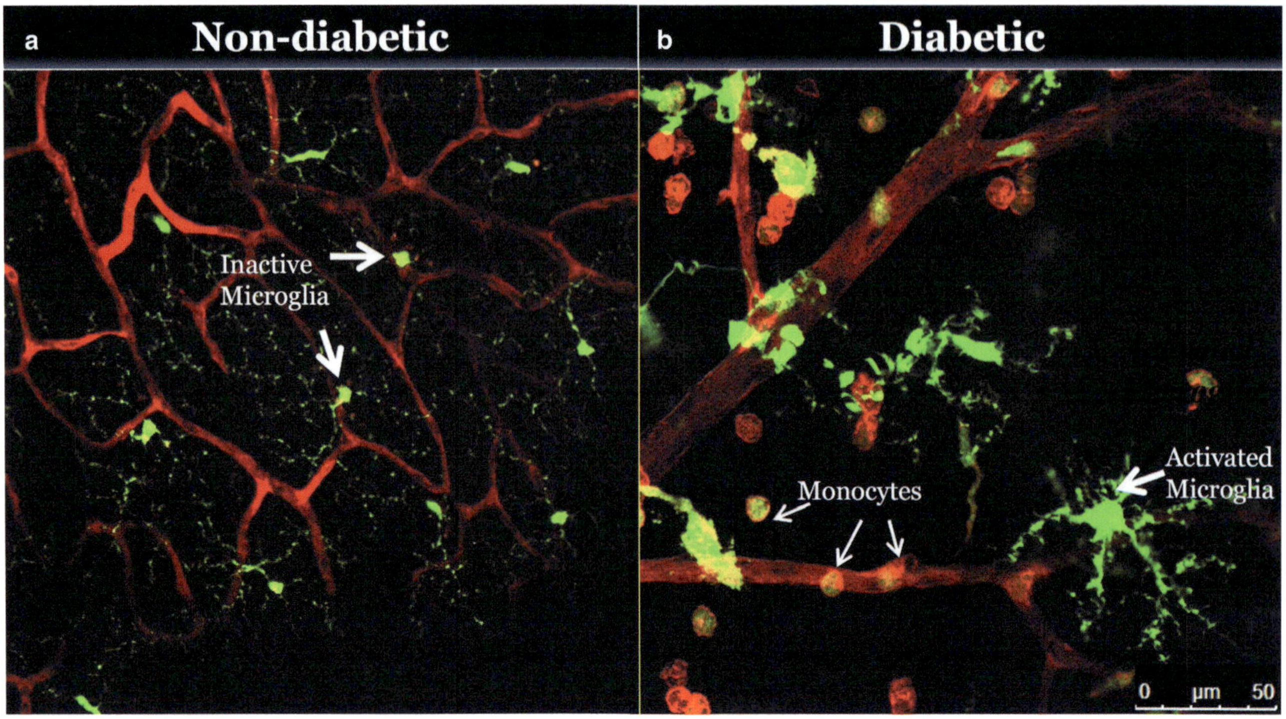

Fig. 2.4 Diabetes increases monocyte/macrophage infiltration and activates retinal microglia. Representative confocal images of retinal whole mounts from Cx3cr1-GFP$^+$ mice counterstained with TRITC-labeled GS-IB4 isolectin (red) for blood vessel and activated monocyte/macrophage identification. (**a**) Normal nondiabetic mice reveal GFP$^+$ retinal microglia (green) uniformly distributed with long, ramified processes. (**b**) High magnification image of the retina from a 4-week diabetic animal demonstrates co-localization of GFP$^+$/isolectin$^+$ in several monocytes/macrophages in the extravascular space closely associated with the outer surface of retinal capillaries. Activated GFP$^+$ microglial cells exhibit ameboid, round morphology with ramified processes. (Reprinted with permission from Rangasamy S et al. PloS one. 2014; 9(10):e108508)

2.3 Mechanisms of Disease

2.3.1 Oxidative Stress

The metabolic demand of the retina makes it a susceptible environment for the accumulation of oxygen-derived free radicals [61]. Collectively known as reactive oxygen species (ROS), these metabolic byproducts are generally cytotoxic to tissues. Under physiological conditions, ROS produced during normal metabolic processes are eliminated but, in disease states, this clearance mechanism becomes dysregulated. The imbalance between accumulation and clearance of ROS, termed oxidative stress, has been shown to cause DNA damage, disrupt cellular homeostasis, and further amplify ROS production [62]. In diabetes, oxidative stress upregulates expression of various proinflammatory proteins such as VEGF, angiopoietins, tumor necrosis factor (TNF), interleukins (ILs), and matrix metalloproteinases (MMPs), all of which are implicated in the breakdown of the BRB [63, 64]. Thus, we highlight some of the biochemical pathways shown to induce oxidative stress in DR for their involvement in the pathogenesis of this disease.

(a) *Polyol pathway* is a metabolic pathway in which glucose is reduced to sorbitol and then converted to fructose. Aldose reductase (AR), the first enzyme involved in this pathway, has low affinity to glucose at normal concentrations; however, in diabetes, increasing amounts of glucose are converted to sorbitol by AR [65]. The presence of sorbitol and AR have been observed at the site of diabetic lesions in human tissues and organs, providing the evidence implicating polyol pathway as a mechanism to help explain hyperglycemia-induced microvascular complications [66, 67]. Inhibition of aldose reductase, the rate-limiting enzyme, has been shown to prevent retinopathy-like lesions in diabetic rodent models [68, 69]. However, clinical trials targeting this pathway have not been successful [70].
(b) *Advanced glycation end products (AGEs)* are a heterogeneous group of highly glycosylated proteins implicated in the alteration of several pathways underlying DR pathogenesis [71, 72]. Changes in the function of the retinal vasculature and the progression of retinopathy may be mediated by the presence of AGEs. In vitro studies have demonstrated that the response of cells to stimu-

lation with AGEs is mediated by the receptor for AGEs (RAGEs) found on the endothelial cell surface [73, 74]. Results suggest a novel role for MMPs in altering BRB function by modifying the endothelial cell surface presentation of VE-cadherin following AGE stimulation. However, a better understanding of the downstream mechanisms mediated by AGE and RAGE leading to the pathophysiological phenomena seen in retinopathy warrant further study.

(c) *Protein kinase C (PKC)* is a phosphorylating enzyme implicated in vascular alterations including increases in permeability, contractility, extracellular matrix synthesis, in addition to leukocyte adhesion and cytokine amplification [75–77]. PKC activation has also been shown to contribute to pericyte dropout [78]. In animal models, increased PKC b-isoform activity has been shown to diminish the integrity of the BRB as well as inducing neovascularization [79]. The involvement of this enzyme in the early vascular dysfunction seen in DR has made PKC a potential target for therapeutic inhibition.

PKC inhibition has generated great interest as a potential target to suppress the BRB-altering processes observed in retinopathy. The Diabetic Macular Edema Study, a multicenter, randomized, double-masked, parallel, placebo-controlled clinical trial evaluated the effect of three doses of orally administered ruboxistaurin mesylate (Eli Lilly, Indianapolis, IN), a PKCb-isozyme-selective inhibitor on the progression of DME [80]. The delay in progression to the primary outcome (progression to sight-threatening DME or application of focal/grid photocoagulation for DME) was not statistically significant, failing to prevent progression of this disease.

(d) *Hexosamine pathway* is activated under hyperglycemic conditions by the conversion of glucose to glucose-6-phosphate, to fructose-6-phosphate [80]. Fructose-6-phosphate is then converted to N-acetyl glucosamine-6-phosphate by the enzyme glutamine fructose-6-phosphate amidotransferase. In diabetes, the rapid metabolism of glucosamine-6-phosphate leads to the formation of uridine diphosphate N-acetylglucosamine (UDP-GlcNAc), implicated in apoptosis of retinal neurons and endothelial cells [81]. Hexosamine has been found to be increased in retinal tissues of humans and rats with diabetes [82]. In vitro and in vivo studies have demonstrated the role of hexosamine pathway in insulin resistance, and stimulation of growth factor synthesis [81, 83].

2.3.2 Mitochondrial Alterations

Mitochondrial health is governed by biochemical and epigenetic changes. In diabetes, the constant metabolic demand of the retina, coupled with the hyperglycemic environment, leads to an increased accumulation of ROS, resulting in mitochondrial alterations [63, 84]. More recently, studies have highlighted the role of mitochondrial morphology changes in DR [85]. Ultrastructure observations show hyperglycemic-induced alterations including breakdown of cristae, impaired membrane integrity, cytochrome C leakage, and compromised function of the electron transport chain [86, 87]. Cytosolic ROS-producing enzymes, NADPH oxidases, are also activated, further fueling ROS damage to mitochondrial integrity. Increased ROS production has also been shown to result in the activation of metalloproteinase 9 (MMP-9), which with the help of heat shock proteins, is translocated inside the mitochondria and further aids the breakdown of mitochondrial membranes and initiation of the apoptotic process [88]. In vitro models have demonstrated that hyperglycemic conditions cause increased mitochondrial fragmentation, which in turn contributes to apoptotic death in retinal vascular and Müller cells [84].

2.3.3 Vascular Dysfunction

(a) *Integrins* constitute a class of proteins that serve as cell surface receptors to extracellular matrix and immunoglobulin molecules. By the interaction with growth factor receptors, they are able to regulate cell function [89]. The process of leukostasis that is enhanced in diabetic retinopathy is dependent on specific integrins particularly containing the beta 2 chain [90].

ALG-1001 is an integrin antagonist (Luminate, Allegro Ophthalmics, LLC, San Juan Capistrano, CA) blocking all integrin a-b combinations rather than subunits, shown to be effective in patients with DME [91]. Clinical trials showed that after three monthly intravitreal injections of ALG-1001 there was significant visual improvement and reduction of CRT. In addition to targeting integrin receptors involved in cell signaling and cell adhesion, this drug has the added advantage of inducing posterior vitreous detachment and vitreolysis.

(b) *NOTCH3* is a receptor enriched in vascular smooth muscle cells and pericytes. In the retina, *Notch3* genetic deficiency results in progressive loss of pericytes, pointing to its critical role in vascular development, stability, and cell survival [92, 93]. In DR, diabetes-induced pericyte dropout has been shown to precede endothelial cell dysfunction and contribute to BRB alterations; however, the underlying molecular mechanisms are poorly understood [94]. Despite the clinical relevance of NOTCH3 in the survival of retinal pericytes, this pathway remains largely uncharacterized. Our own transcriptomic studies demonstrate a role for this stabilizing receptor in the alteration of BRB, where Notch3 downregulation leads to increased expression of inflammatory and autophagy genes, decreased PDGFRβ expression and increased permeability (Fig. 2.5) [95].

(c) *Sphingosine 1-phosphate (S1P)* is a bioactive lipid, able to illicit response from a variety of signaling pathways involved with cell proliferation, differentiation, and migration as well as inflammation and angiogenesis [26, 96, 97]. Tightly regulated by the balance between synthesis by sphingosine kinases and degradation, S1P is secreted by platelets, monocytes, endothelial, and smooth muscle cells (including pericytes). In addition to being able to regulate immune response, S1P is also known for its role in regulating vascular integrity and as such is implicated in the alteration of the BRB associated with DR pathogenesis.

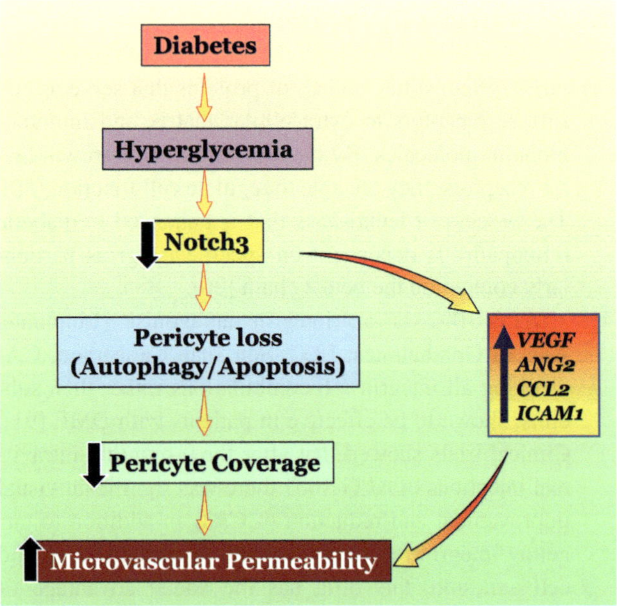

Fig. 2.5 Role of Notch3 in the alteration of the BRB. In diabetic animal models, hyperglycemia leads to the downregulation of Notch3 in retinal pericytes. The loss of this stabilizing receptor leads to pericyte loss (apoptosis/autophagy) and increased expression of pro-inflammatory genes (VEGF, ANG2, CCL2, ICAM1). The resulting decreased pericyte coverage simultaneously leads to increased microvascular permeability and further upregulation of pro-inflammatory genes. *VEGF* vascular endothelial growth factor; *ANG2* angiopoietin-2, *CCL2* chemokine (C-C motif) ligand 2, *ICAM1* intercellular adhesion molecule-1. (Reprinted with permission from Rangasamy S.et al. Exp. Eye. Res. 2020; 195:108043)

Demonstrated in animal models, our previous studies have shown hyperglycemia-induced low expression of S1P in the retina. In vitro, we have shown the increased mRNA expression of tight junction proteins, N- and VE-cadherin, on endothelium within hours upon addition of purified S1P [21]. This bioactive lipid also altered endothelial monolayer resistance within minutes after its addition. This rapid cellular response, occurring as a result of the reorganization of actin cytoskeletal proteins and the formation of focal adhesion-adherens junction complexes, coincided with an increase in endothelial integrity as measured by electrical impedance. Taken together, our studies suggest that the initial formation and long-term maintenance of increased endothelial resistance are dependent on the S1P-induced N- and VE-cadherin expression which may function solely for the purpose of maintaining normal endothelial cell–pericyte interactions. As such, S1P may be key for its potential benefit in the maintenance of the blood–retinal barrier in DR.

2.4 Inflammation

Many features of inflammation, such as complement activation, upregulation of cytokines, macrophage infiltration, microglial activation, increased vascular permeability, and tissue edema have been described in both humans and animal models of diabetic retinopathy (Fig. 2.6) [98–101]. An early event in inflammatory cascade is the activation of vascular endothelial cells, a process which also aids in the recruitment of leukocytes to tissues via chemokines. Consistently observed in DR: (1) increased expression of endothelial adhesion molecules such as ICAM1, VCAM1, PECAM-1, P-Selectin, etc., (2) adhesion of leukocytes to the endothelium, (3) release of inflammatory cytokines, growth and vascular permeability factors, (4) alteration of adherens and tight junctional proteins (e.g., VE-Cadherin, ZO-1, Claudin, etc.), and (5) infiltration of leukocytes (diapedesis) into the retina, these features consistently implicate inflammation in the breakdown of the BRB [102]. Herein, we focus on key inflammatory molecules for their direct involvement in DR pathogenesis and their therapeutic potential.

2.4.1 Molecules Involved and Therapeutic Potential

The involvement of growth factors and cytokines in the pathogenesis of DR was confirmed with early proteomic studies in which the vitreous of eyes from diabetics, and more so those with retinopathy, expressed increased levels of these molecules [100, 101]. The first studies confirmed the

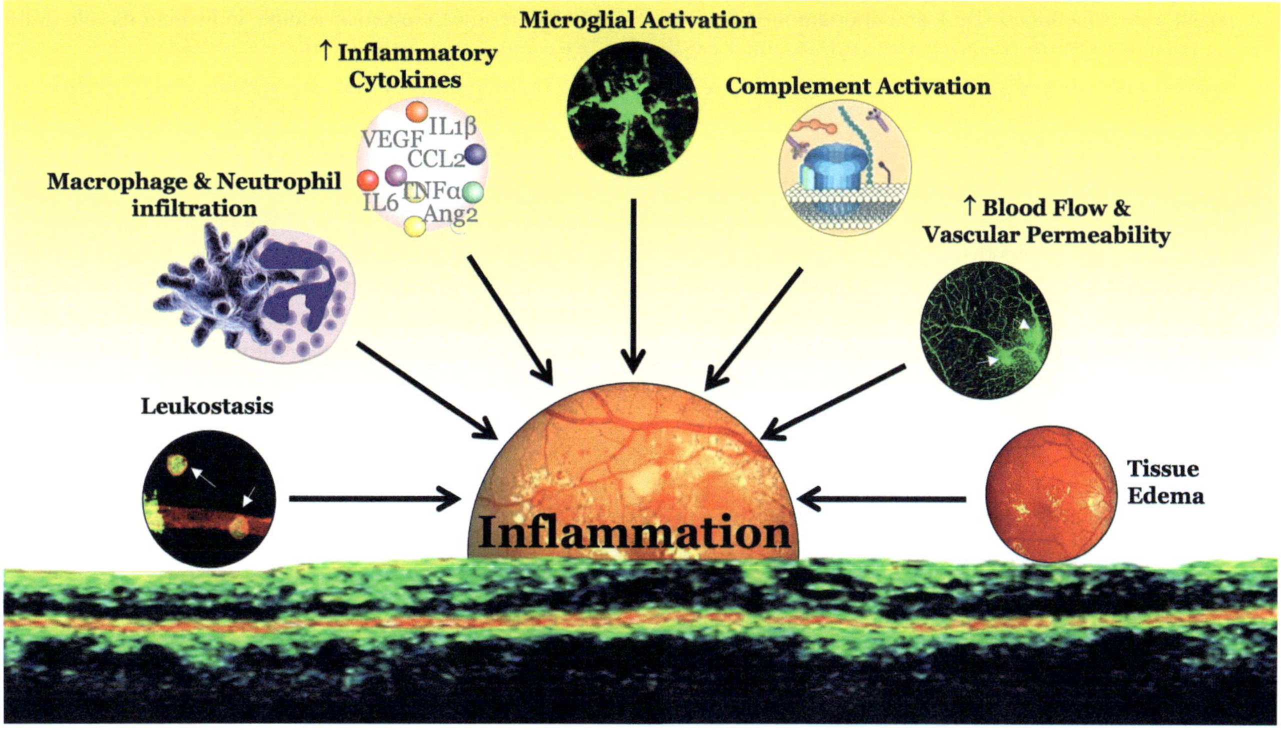

Fig. 2.6 All hallmarks of inflammation are seen in DME. Leukostasis, macrophage and neutrophil infiltration, upregulation of cytokines, microglial activation, complement activation, increased blood flow, vascular hyperpermeability, and tissue edema have all been reported in animal models of diabetic retinopathy and human DR. These hallmarks of inflammation are consistently linked to blood–retinal barrier alterations observed in DME

role of vascular endothelial growth factor (VEGF), which has held its central role in this disease. Since then, proteomic technology has evolved significantly, and finer refinement of growth factor and cytokines involved in the pathogenesis of DR have been made. To date being the only other potent angiogenic/vasopermeability factor to successfully reach phase 3 clinical trials, angiopoietin-2 (Ang-2) is the most recently discovered. Herein, we highlight VEGF and Ang-2, among many others, for their therapeutic potential in restoring the BRB.

2.4.2 Growth Factors

(a) *Vascular endothelial growth factor (VEGF)*: VEGF is a potent vasoactive cytokine known to cause increased vascular permeability by affecting endothelial tight junction proteins. By inducing the phosphorylation of VE-cadherin, occludin, and ZO-1, VEGF causes a disruption of the BRB and results in plasma "leakage," leading to the clinical manifestation of retinal edema [102–104]. In DME, VEGF levels are significantly elevated when compared with non-diabetic eye conditions [105]. VEGF has also been shown to stimulate increased leukostasis in the microvessels of the retina [106]. Thus, currently intravitreal anti-VEGF therapy is the accepted first-line of treatment in DME.

Major randomized clinical trials have consistently demonstrated the efficacy of intravitreal anti-VEGF injections in the treatment of center-involving DME compared to laser photocoagulation treatment [107–109]. However, the response to anti-VEGF drugs in the treatment of DME is widely variable with only 27–38% of patients responding well (>15 letters of vision improvement after 2 years). Currently, there are variety of drugs, administered by intravitreal injection, that target the VEGF molecule. Direct inhibitors include anti-VEGF aptamer pegaptanib (Macugen; OSI Pharmaceuticals, Long Island, NY), monoclonal antibody fragment ranibizumab (Lucentis; Genentech, South San Francisco, CA), full-length antibody bevacizumab (Avastin; Genentech), and single chain antibody fragment, Brolucizumab (Beovu, Novartis, Basel, Switzerland). Other anti-VEGF molecular targets include soluble VEGF receptor analogs, VEGF-Trap (Regeneron, Tarrytown, NY), and small interfering RNAs bevasiranib (Opko Health, Miami, FL) and rapamycin (Sirolimus, MacuSight, Union City, CA).

(b) *Angiopoietin-2* (Ang-2): Angiopoietins represent another family of inflammatory growth factors, binding to the receptor tyrosine kinase Tie2, an important modulator of angiogenesis [35]. The secretion of angiopoietin-1 (Ang-1) in normal quiescent vessels serves as a stabilizing factor by maintaining contacts between neighboring endothelial cells (ECs) and between pericyte-ECs (Fig. 2.7) [110, 111]. Ang-2 is thought to antagonize the action of Ang-1, resulting in vessel destabilization. Work by Pfister et al. has reported that Ang-2 can induce subtle changes in pericyte attachment and migration on specific regions of the capillary network, which may govern EC behavior [112]. The vitreous levels of Ang-2 have been shown to be significantly elevated in patients with clinically significant macular edema, indicating its role in the alteration of the BRB [104].

In the retinas of diabetic animals, Ang-2 expression is increased and coincides with the decrease in the barrier properties of the endothelium. Our own in vitro studies have shown Ang-2 induces loss of VE-cadherin mediated through the phosphorylation mechanism [113]. A more recent study shows Ang-2 promotes monocyte adhesion by sensitizing endothelial cells to TNF-α and modulates the TNF-α-induced expression of endothelial cell adhesion molecule, ICAM-1 [114]. This finding identified Ang-2 as an autocrine regulator

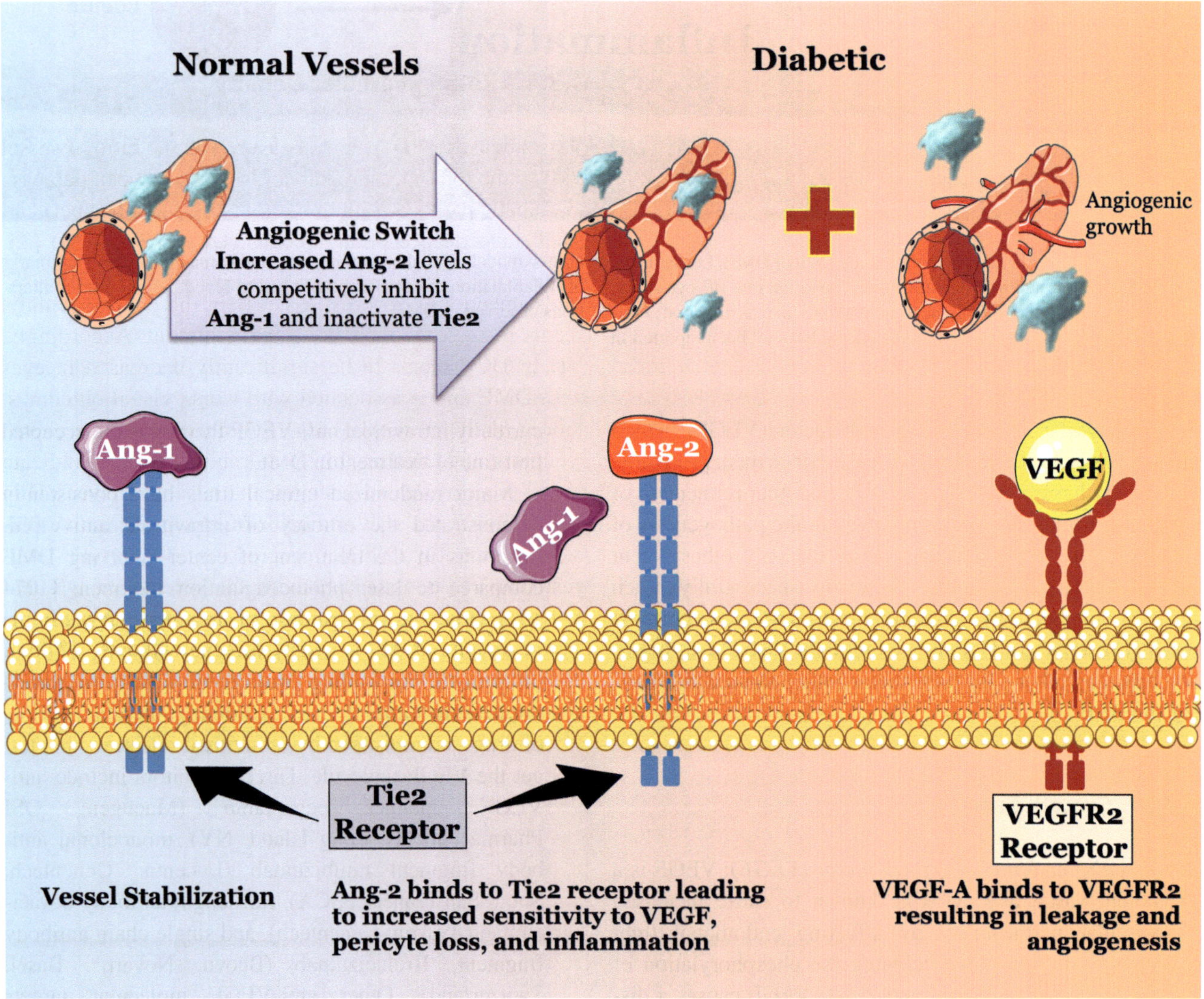

Fig. 2.7 Angiopoietins and VEGF are key drivers of angiogenesis, permeability, and microvascular inflammation. In healthy vasculature, the inhibitory molecule Ang-1 binds to the receptor Tie2, necessary for the maintenance of stable vasculature. In diabetes, Ang-2 levels increase, competitively inhibit Ang-1, and bind Tie2 receptor. The binding of Ang-2 to Tie2 leads to increased VEGF sensitivity, pericyte loss, inflammation. At the same time, VEGF simultaneously binds to VEGF2 receptor, causing increased permeability and vessel sprouting. *Ang-1* angiopoietin-2, *Ang-2* angiopoietin-2, *Tie2* Tyrosine-protein kinase receptor 2, *VEGF* vascular endothelial growth factor, *VEGFR2* vascular endothelial growth factor receptor 2

of endothelial cell inflammatory responses. Thus, Ang-2 appears to serve as an important therapeutic target in DME.

The therapeutic role of Ang-2 in diabetic retinopathy was pointed to by experiments showing that intravitreal injection of stabilizing factor, Ang-1, in diabetic animals prevented retinal vascular leakage [110]. Because Ang-2 is antagonistic to Ang-1, Ang-2 offers therapeutic potential. Studies from our lab where the first to show increased Ang-2 levels in the retina during angiogenesis which can be inhibited by a Tie-2 antagonist (Fig. 2.8) [115]. Currently in phase 3 clinical trials, Faricimab (Vabysmo, Genentech) is a bispecific antibody targeting Ang-2 and VEGF. Recently approved by the US FDA for both DME and wet ARMD patients, the YOSEMITE and RHINE trials showed that intravitreal injections of facricimab achieved dosing intervals of 16 weeks in 50% patients, and 12 weeks in 75% patients [116, 117]. The average vision gain with intravitreal faricimab was non-inferior to intravitreal aflibercept therapy [118].

(c) *Insulin-like growth factor-1 (IGF-1)*: Intraocular insulin-like growth factor-1 (IGF-1), but not systemic IGF-1, has been found to contribute to BRB breakdown and increase retinal vascular permeability [119]. On the basis of this rationale, an open label study of Teprotumumab (Genmab, Princeton, NJ), an IGF-1 receptor blocker given by intravenous infusion, examined the safety and efficacy of this drug in patients with DME [120].

(d) *Erythropoietin*: Because hypoxia-induced VEGF production is involved in the pathogenesis of diabetic retinopathy, increasing the oxygen tension in tissue by administration of erythropoietin is an attractive approach to treatment of DME. Erythropoietin also acts as a neuroprotective, antioxidant, and antiapoptotic factor. In a case series, Friedman et al. published the results of erythropoietin use in anemic azotemic diabetic subjects who had improvement of macular edema [121]. In another case series, intravitreal injection of erythropoietin in patients with chronic DME resulted in improved visual acuity and clearing of hard exudates [122].

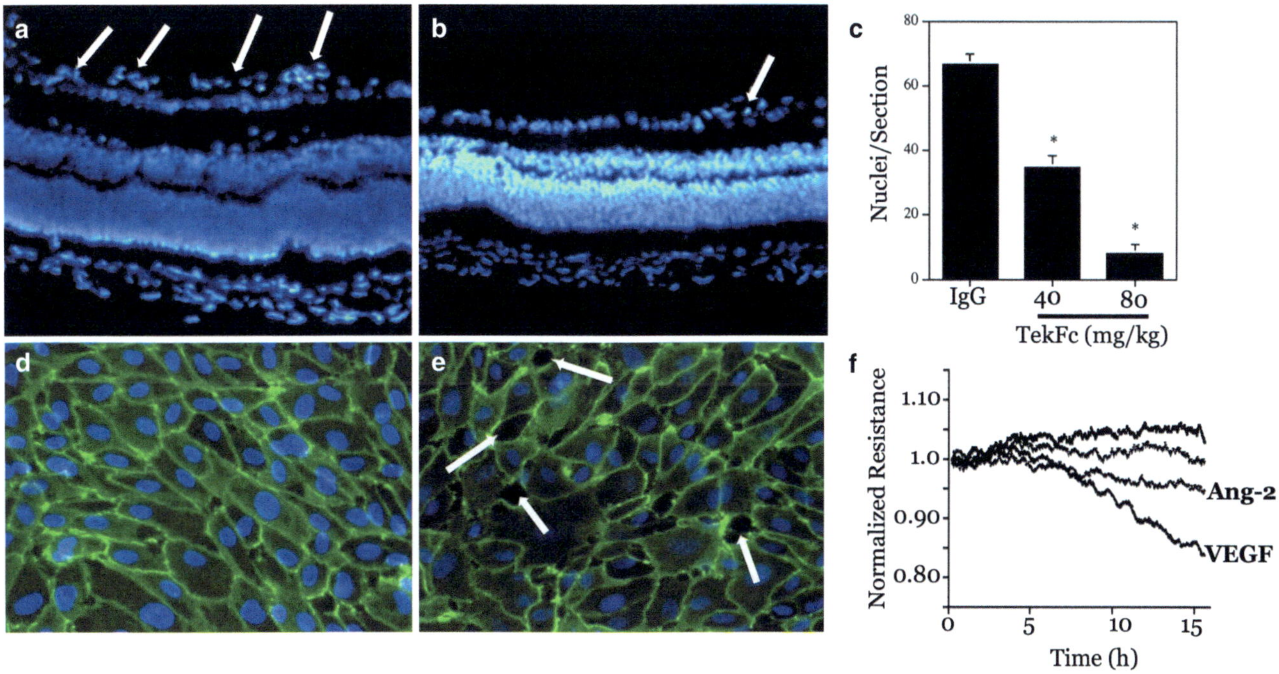

Fig. 2.8 Ang-2 alters the endothelial cell function. (**a**) Representative mouse retinal sections from oxygen-treated day-17 animals receiving intraperitoneal injection of 80 mg/kg IgG on days 12–16 reveal numerous capillary tufts (angiogenesis) as seen on the vitreal side of the inner limiting membrane (*arrows*). (**b**) Animals receiving 80 mg/kg intraperitoneal injection of muTek delta Fc on days 12–16 demonstrate significant decrease in the number of capillary tufts on the vitreal side of the inner limiting membrane (*arrow*). (**c**) Quantitative analysis of neovascularization in animals treated with 40 or 80 mg/kg muTek delta Fc demonstrated 46% and 87% inhibition of neovascularization, respectively. Values reported are mean ± SEM for $n = 5$ animals (40 sections/animal) for each treatment group. $*p < 0.01$. Representative images of VE-cadherin staining in (**d**) untreated or (**e**) Ang-2-treated (200 ng/mL) human retinal endothelial cells (HRECs) showing disruption of the monolayer as evident by the discontinuous VE-cadherin staining along cell borders and the presence of gaps between adjacent cells (arrows). (**f**) Representative electrical impedance measurements reveal decreased endothelial barrier resistance in HRECs treated with Ang-2 of VEGF. (Reprinted with permission from Das A, et al. Lab Invest. 2003; 83:1637-45 (**a–c**) and Rangasamy S, et al. Invest Ophthalmol Vis Sci. 2011; 52:3784-91)

2.4.3 Cytokines and Chemokines

(a) *Tumor necrosis factor*: TNF-α is a crucial mediator of retinal leukostasis and a potent chemoattractant that directly aids in the upregulation of adhesion molecules. In diabetic rats, the TNF-α inhibitor etanercept (Enbrel, Amgen, Thousand Oaks, CA) has been shown to reduce leukocyte adhesion and retinal ICAM-1 expression, suppressing BRB breakdown [123]. A double-blind, randomized, placebo-controlled crossover study of 11 patients with DME (persisting after two sessions of laser treatment) showed significantly improved visual acuity and reduction in retinal thickness with intravenous TNF-α inhibitor infliximab (5 mg/kg) (Janssen Biotech, Horsham, PA) [124]. Larger clinical trials for longer periods are needed to confirm the efficacy of systemic anti-TNF drugs for treatment of DME.

(b) *Interleukins* (ILs) are a family of 18 cytokines known for their role in the activation and differentiation of immune cells, in addition to modulating proliferation, maturation, migration, and adhesion [54]. They are secreted rapidly and briefly in response to a stimulus. ILs have both paracrine and autocrine function, and dual, antagonistic pro-inflammatory, and anti-inflammatory properties. In DR, elevated levels of IL-1β, IL-6, and IL-8 are detected in the vitreous [125, 126]. This increase in ILs is also present in the retinas of diabetic rats [127].

Intravitreal administration of an antibody against human IL-6, EBI-029 (Eleven Biotherapeutics, Cambridge, MA), potently inhibits IL-6 cis and trans-signaling and has been effective in an animal model of choroidal neovascularization. Further development of EBI-029 as a therapy for DME is in progress [128].

(c) *Proteases* have been demonstrated to have a role in the modification of endothelial intercellular junctions and alterations of monolayer permeability [11, 129]. Furthermore, several studies have reported the secretion of proteases from cells including macrophages, found in elevated levels in the plasma of patients with diabetes [130, 131].

Matrix metalloproteinases (MMPs) are zinc-dependent proteinases capable of degrading structural components of the extracellular matrix (ECM) in addition to non-ECM proteins. There is increasing evidence implicating MMPs as major regulators of innate and acquired immunity [132]. Furthermore, studies in knockout mice have shown that MMPs play an important role in acute as well as chronic inflammation [133, 134]. Proteolytic alteration of chemokines by MMPs is important for its activation. Several members of the CCL/monocyte chemoattractant protein (MCP) family of chemokines are cleaved by MMPs rendering them proactive molecules that amplify the pro-inflammatory response. Increased endothelial permeability may involve the production and activation of MMPs [135–137].

The role of these proteinases in the maintenance of systemic vessel integrity and remodeling has been well documented in animal models of vascular morphogenesis and angiogenesis [138–140]. In animal model of diabetes, both MMP-2 and MMP-9 are elevated in the retina. Notably, proteomic studies have shown MMP-9 to be increased in the vitreous of eyes with DR compared to those without [141, 142]. Our work has previously reported the upregulation of MMPs in the diabetic retina and their possible role in the proteolytic breakdown of junctional proteins essential for maintaining the integrity of the BRB [129]. More specifically, the increased retinal vascular permeability observed in diabetic animals coinciding with the decrease of cell–cell junctional protein VE-cadherin could be dampened using by inhibiting MMPs [11]. These observations suggest a possible mechanism by which diabetes contributes to BRB breakdown through the proteolytic degradation of VE-cadherin, and thus indicate a role for extracellular proteinases in the alteration of the BRB associated with DR.

(d) *Cathepsin D (CD)* is a macrophage-derived, aspartyl protease known to play a role in EC–pericyte interactions. Its function in the degradation of proteins and activator of inactive precursors proteins has made it an attractive candidate to warrant further examination for its potential to induce BRB alterations. Indeed, previous studies have demonstrated a role for proteases in the modification of endothelial intercellular junctions, which *in vitro* results in monolayer hyperpermeability [143, 144]. Our own study has shown CD to be elevated in the serum of DME patients when compared to nondiabetic and diabetic patients without retinal complications [145].

Our studies in diabetic animal models have detected this protease in the retina [146]. In vitro, exposure to CD causes disruption of endothelial junctional proteins via an increase in Rho/ROCK-dependent cell contractility. That Rho/ROCK-dependent EC contractility mediates permeability was confirmed when ROCK inhibition prevented the CD-induced changes in EC barrier integrity. More recently, Rho inhibitors have appeared on the market for the treatment of glaucoma: Ripasudil (K-115), clinically approved in Japan and Netarsudil (AR-13503) in the United States [147].

(e) *Chemokine Ligand 2 (CCL2)/Monocyte Chemotactic Protein-1 (MCP-1):* The chemokine ligand 2 (CCL2), also known as monocyte chemotactic protein-1 (MCP-1), is considered to play an important role in vascular inflammation because it induces leukocyte recruitment and activation [148, 149]. Induced by hyperglycemia,

CCL2/MCP-1 is generated by retinal vascular endothelial cells, pigmented epithelial cells, and Müller's glial cells [150]. Found in elevated amounts in the vitreous of patients with diabetic retinopathy, CCL2 is another molecule implicated in the breakdown of the BRB [151]. Furthermore, CCL2 gene polymorphism has been indicated as a potential risk factor for this disease [152, 153]. Studies from our laboratory have indicated that a genetic knockout of the *CCL2* gene in diabetic mice prevents BRB alteration [149]. Our preliminary animal studies indicate that selective inhibition of the *CCL2* gene can prevent the alteration of the BRB in diabetes by significantly reducing retinal vascular leakage in the retina and monocyte infiltration after induction of diabetes [55].

The ligation of the MCP-1 with its receptor C-C chemokine receptor type 2 (CCR2) mediates its effects. Thus, inhibition of this chemokine pathway via its receptor offers a novel approach to target the early leukocyte influx and monocyte trafficking as shown by our group [154]. Systemic use of CCR2 inhibitors is in current clinical trials targeting several inflammatory diseases like atherosclerosis, multiple sclerosis, rheumatoid arthritis, and systemic lupus erythematosus [155]. However, CCR2/5 inhibitor PF-04634817 (Pfizer, Brooklyn, NY) was shown to be inferior to monthly ranibizumab injections in the treatment of DME [156]. The reasons for modest improvement with this oral drug could be due to short duration of treatment, lack of bioavailability of the drug in the retina, and route of administration by oral route.

(f) *Kallikrein-Kinin*: Vitreous proteomics in advanced stages of diabetic retinopathy have shown increased levels of plasma kallikrein-kinin system components, including plasma kallikrein, coagulation factor XII, and high-molecular-weight kininogen [157]. Preclinical studies in diabetic rats have reported activation of the intraocular kallikrein-kinin system, and administration of plasma kallikrein inhibitors and B1R antagonists to diabetic rats suppresses retinal vascular leakage and inflammation. The first trial evaluating the efficacy of plasma kallikrein inhibitors in DME failed to meet the primary endpoint in phase 2 trials (KVD001; KalVista Pharmaceuticals, Porton Down, UK) [158].

2.5 Pharmacotherapies in Diabetic Macular Edema

Although vitreous VEGF levels are generally elevated in DME compared to nondiabetics, many DME patients have very high or very low levels of VEGF [105]. The varying levels of this growth factor make DME appear to be a heterogenous disease. In the treatment of DME, anti-VEGF therapy still remains the gold standard. However, the macular edema does not always resolve with anti-VEGF treatment as demonstrated by large clinical trials [107–109]. More than 35% of DME patients do not achieve ≥10-letter improvement in vision and more than 55% do not achieve ≥15-letter improvement after 2 years of anti-VEGF therapy. Proteomics studies of DR, and more specifically DME, have consistently pointed to the involvement of various proinflammatory cytokines and growth factors beyond VEGF involved in the pathogenesis of this disease [100, 105]. It is possible that poor responders to anti-VEGF treatment may have too low or too high VEGF accompanied by other inflammatory cytokines like Ang-2 and IL-6.

Large-scale clinical trials have demonstrated the efficacy of intravitreal anti-inflammatory therapies (steroids) in the treatment of DME. Known to suppress a number of proinflammatory transcription factors including NF-κB via glucocorticoid receptors, these therapies also inhibit inflammatory cytokine production, leukostasis, and phosphorylation of cell-junction proteins. Steroids importantly target pathways independent from VEGF involved in the pathogenesis of DME. Steroid therapies have shown to improve vision and reduce central retinal thickness. However, because of side effects, the use of intravitreal steroid therapies in clinical practice is currently reserved as the second line of therapy in those who poorly respond to intravitreal anti-VEGF therapy (after 4–6 monthly injections).

Sustained-release steroids were developed in effort to decrease the number of injections a DME patient may require. The *dexamethasone implant* (Ozurdex; Allergan, Inc.) is a biodegradable copolymer that releases dexamethasone over a 6-month period. Safety and efficacy of Ozurdex have been evaluated in multiple phase II studies, the implant being effective in decreasing vascular leakage and improving vision. In the Macular Edema: Assessment of Implantable Dexamethasone in Diabetes (MEAD) Study, dexamethasone intravitreal implant resulted in visual improvement of >15 letters in 22% patients (0.7 mg) and 18% (0.35 mg) compared with 12% in the sham group [159]. Cataract formation was seen in up to 68% of treated patients, and increases in IOP could be managed with medication, or no therapy. On the other hand, the Fluocinolone Acetonide for Macular Edema (FAME) study, a randomized, multicenter, trial, demonstrated the efficacy of the non-biodegradable fluocinolone acetonide microimplant (Iluvien, Alimera Sciences). This new generation flucinolone acetonide implant containing 190 μg of drug and releasing 0.2 μg of drug per day, provided substantial benefit of visual improvement in patients with DME. Intravitreal inserts of fluocinolone acetonide (releasing 0.2 and 0.5 mg/day). However, almost all patients receiving fluocinolone acetonide formed cataracts [160].

2.6 Strategies for the Future: Current Clinical Trials in DME

On average, it takes more than 10 years for a Phase I trial to progress to regulatory approval. While treatments for diabetic retinopathy (DR) and diabetic macular edema (DME) have made significant advances, treatment modalities with better efficacy and longer durability are still needed. Many ongoing trials aim to validate new treatment options ranging from new drugs to advances in dosing or administration of established pharmaceuticals to entirely new modalities. Herein, we highlight a variety of clinical trials currently in different phases that if successful will further maximize the efficacy and duration of action of novel drugs in the treatment of DME (Table 2.1).

1. Anti-VEGF agents with longer duration of action

   KSI-301: A novel anti-VEGF biopolymer conjugate, KSI-301 (Kodiak Sciences Inc., Palo Alto, CA), has been developed to have higher affinity for VEGF-A with longer duration of action. The phase 3 GLEAM and GLIMMER trials are evaluating the efficacy of this anti-VEGF agent in treatment-naïve DME patients [161, 162]. This agent can be used once every 2–6 months after three loading monthly doses. About 84% patients with DME patients were on a 4-month or longer intervals at the end of the first year of the trial.

   AXT-107: An intravitreal self-assembling gel depot has been developed as a potential yearly dosed injection, and thus can reduce the treatment burden of monthly injections. The AXT-107 drug (Asclepix Therapeutics, Baltimore, Maryland) inhibits both VEGF-A and VEGF-C in addition to activating Tie2 receptors. A Phase 2 trial (CONGO) using AXT-107 is evaluating safety and bioactivity in DME patients [163].
2. Anti-inflammatory agents

   Redox effector factor-1 (Ref-1): Ref-1 is a master regulator extensively studied for its role in DNA repair and reduction-oxidation signaling. Critical in the regulation of transcription factors, Ref-1 has been shown to be involved in several pathways related to inflammation and angiogenesis, specifically through NF-kB and HIF-1α. A Phase 2 clinical trial ZETA-1 using an oral Ref-1 inhibitor APX3330 (Ocuphire Pharma Inc., Farmington Hills, MI) is ongoing to evaluate its efficacy in DME [164]. If successful, APX3330 would provide the first oral treatment option for DR, potentially to be used in combination with currently approved drugs such as the intravitreal anti-VEGF agents.
3. Anti-apoptotic, neuroprotective agent

   Erythropoietin: Intraocular EPO levels have been demonstrated to be elevated in DME patients, and its overexpression in mice results in increased retinal vascular permeability. A Phase 2 trial with an intravitreal EPO inhibitor LKA651 (Novartis, Basel, Switzerland) is ongoing in patients with center-involving DME [165].
4. Anti-endothelial dysfunction agents

   Rho/ROCK signaling: The Rho kinase/ROCK signaling pathway is implicated in cell proliferation, migration (angiogenesis), leukostasis, and macrophage infiltration (inflammation). A Phase 1 study using a ROCK inhibitor AR-13503 (Aerie Pharma., Bedminster, NJ) as an intra-

Table 2.1 Current clinical trials in DME. Ongoing trials validating new treatment modalities ranging from new drug developments to advances in dosing or administration of established pharmaceuticals [161–169]

Development	Phase 3	Phase 2	Phase 2	Phase 2	Phase 1	Phase 1	Phase 2	Phase 2
Treatment	Intravitreal injection	Intravitreal injection	Small- molecule oral tablet	Intravitreal injection	Implant	Oral capsule	Intravitreal injection	Intravitreal injection
Target	Anti-VEGF antibody biopolymer conjugate	Derived from a cryptic peptide within collagen IV, inhibits VEGF-A and VEGF-C and activates Tie2	Redox factor-1 (Ref-1) inhibition; can potentially reduce proinflammatory and hypoxic signaling	Erythropoietin inhibitor	Active metabolite of netarsudil and inhibitor of Rho kinase (ROCK) and Protein kinase C (PKC)	Inhibitor of vascular leakage and inflammation as shown in various animal models	Bicyclic peptide inhibitor targeting plasma kallikrein	AAV8 vector containing a transgene for anti-VEGF fab
Mechanism	Anti-angiogenic	Anti-angiogenic	Anti-inflammatory	Anti-apoptotic	Endothelial dysfunction blocker	Endothelial dysfunction blocker	Endothelial dysfunction blocker	Gene therapy
Drug	KSI-301	AXT107	APX3330	LKA651	AR-13503	CU06-1004	THR-149	RGX-314

vitreal implant alone or in combination with aflibercept is being evaluated in patients with DME [166].

cAMP/cortactin pathway: The cAMP/cortactin pathway is critical in maintaining endothelial cell junctions in the blood–retinal barrier. A novel modulator of this pathway CU06-1004 (Curacle Co. Ltd., South Korea) enhances survival of endothelial cells and stabilizes endothelial cell junctions, while also inhibiting VEGF, IL-1b, and MCP-1. A Phase 1 trial using oral CU06-1004 is currently being evaluated to assess the safety and tolerability of single and multiple ascending oral doses in patients with DME [167].

Plasma Kallikrein-kinin (PKal-kinin): THR-149 (Oxurion, Leuven, Belgium) is an inhibitor of the plasma kallikrein-kinin (PKal-kinin) system shown to prevent the induction of retinal vascular permeability, inflammation, and angiogenesis in preclinical studies. Phase 1 data has demonstrated THR-149 resulting in a mean BCVA gain of 6.1 letters at the 3-month endpoint. Currently in Phase 2 trials, the KALAHARI study is evaluating the efficacy of THR-149 in patients who have not previously responded to anti-VEGF in the treatment of DME [168].

5. Gene therapy

Anti-VEGF: A novel, one-time subretinal injection of the NAV AAV8 vector containing a gene encoding for a monoclonal antibody neutralizing VEGF has been recently developed (RGX-314; RegenXbio Inc., Rockville, MD). The Phase 2 trial, ALTITUDE, using suprachoroidal delivery of this vector, is currently ongoing in diabetic retinopathy patients [169].

2.7 Conclusion

The last 10 years have represented a period of intensified molecular research exploring the full therapeutic potential of anti-VEGF drugs. However, the suboptimal treatment response demonstrated by large trials in DME and other diseases (cancer- and age-related macular degeneration) highlights the need to establish novel therapeutic targets that can help alleviate the burden of this vision-threatening condition. Data consistently point to inflammation as a key driver underlying the pathogenesis of DME. With the involvement of several inflammatory molecules and the response to anti-VEGF drugs being variable, novel approaches such as the ones in current trials offer promising strategies to overcome the burden of intravitreal injections. Though the success of anti-VEGF drugs is not to be overshadowed, DME is a disease involving more than this vasopermeability factor alone. Thus, highlighting the role of the various inflammatory mediators, offers a step toward establishing more disease-encompassing treatments. Also, genomics may play a role in the variable response to anti-VEGF drugs in DME. Our ongoing study, the Diabetic Retinopathy Genomics (DRGen) Study, uses the next-generation technology for whole-exome sequencing to examine the contribution of rare and common variants related to pro-inflammatory pathways underlying DME pathogenesis [170].

Acknowledgments The work reported in this chapter was supported by the National Institutes of Health under award number NIH R01 EY 028606-01-A1 and VA Merit Review award number 1I01BX005348-01A1.

None of the authors have any financial/conflicting interests to disclose.

References

1. Centers for Disease Control and Prevention. Diabetes and vision loss. Atlanta: Department of Health and Human Services, Centers for Disease Control and Prevention; 2021. https://www.cdc.gov/diabetes/managing/diabetes-vision-loss.html.
2. Services USDoHaH. Diabetic retinopathy data and statistics. National Institutes of Health, National Institute of Mental Health; 2021.
3. Federation ID. IDF diabetes atlas. Brussels: International Diabetes Federation; 2021.
4. Lee R, Wong TY, Sabanayagam C. Epidemiology of diabetic retinopathy, diabetic macular edema and related vision loss. Eye Vis. 2015;2:17.
5. Ding J, Wong TY. Current epidemiology of diabetic retinopathy and diabetic macular edema. Curr Diab Rep. 2012;12:346–54.
6. Yau JW, Rogers SL, Kawasaki R, et al. Global prevalence and major risk factors of diabetic retinopathy. Diabetes Care. 2012;35:556–64.
7. Frank RN. Etiologic mechanisms in diabetic retinopathy. In: Ryan SJ, Schachat AP, editors. Retina. St. Louis: Elsevier Mosby; 2001.
8. Ola MS, Nawaz MI, Siddiquei MM, Al-Amro S, Abu El-Asrar AM. Recent advances in understanding the biochemical and molecular mechanism of diabetic retinopathy. J Diabetes Complicat. 2012;26:56–64.
9. Simó R, Villarroel M, Corraliza L, Hernández C, Garcia-Ramírez M. The retinal pigment epithelium: something more than a constituent of the blood-retinal barrier–implications for the pathogenesis of diabetic retinopathy. J Biomed Biotechnol. 2010;2010:190724.
10. Díaz-Coránguez M, Ramos C, Antonetti DA. The inner blood-retinal barrier: cellular basis and development. Vis Res. 2017;139:123–37.
11. Navaratna D, McGuire PG, Menicucci G, Das A. Proteolytic degradation of VE-cadherin alters the blood-retinal barrier in diabetes. Diabetes. 2007;56:2380–7.
12. Antonetti DA, Barber AJ, Hollinger LA, Wolpert EB, Gardner TW. Vascular endothelial growth factor induces rapid phosphorylation of tight junction proteins occludin and zonula occluden 1. A potential mechanism for vascular permeability in diabetic retinopathy and tumors. J Biol Chem. 1999;274:23463–7.
13. Mizutani M, Kern TS, Lorenzi M. Accelerated death of retinal microvascular cells in human and experimental diabetic retinopathy. J Clin Invest. 1996;97:2883–90.
14. Kuwabara T, Cogan DG. Retinal vascular patterns. VI. Mural cells of the retinal capillaries. Arch Ophthalmol. 1963;69:492–502.
15. Frank RN. Diabetic retinopathy. N Engl J Med. 2004;350:48–58.

16. Fuhrmann S, Zou C, Levine EM. Retinal pigment epithelium development, plasticity, and tissue homeostasis. Exp Eye Res. 2014;123:141–50.
17. Li Y, Song D, Song Y, et al. Iron-induced local complement component 3 (C3) up-regulation via non-canonical transforming growth factor (TGF)-β signaling in the retinal pigment epithelium. J Biol Chem. 2015;290:11918–34.
18. Boulton M, Foreman D, Williams G, McLeod D. VEGF localisation in diabetic retinopathy. Br J Ophthalmol. 1998;82:561–8.
19. Rangasamy SSR, McGuire PG, Das A. Diabetic macular edema: molecular mechanisms. In: Friberg T, editor. Therapy for ocular angiogenesis. Philadelphia: Wolters Kluwer; 2011. p. 88–99.
20. Antonetti DA, Barber AJ, Khin S, Lieth E, Tarbell JM, Gardner TW. Vascular permeability in experimental diabetes is associated with reduced endothelial occludin content: vascular endothelial growth factor decreases occludin in retinal endothelial cells. Penn State Retina Research Group. Diabetes. 1998;47:1953–9.
21. McGuire PG, Rangasamy S, Maestas J, Das A. Pericyte-derived sphingosine 1-phosphate induces the expression of adhesion proteins and modulates the retinal endothelial cell barrier. Arterioscler Thromb Vasc Biol. 2011;31:e107–15.
22. Vestweber D, Winderlich M, Cagna G, Nottebaum AF. Cell adhesion dynamics at endothelial junctions: VE-cadherin as a major player. Trends Cell Biol. 2009;19:8–15.
23. Dejana E, Bazzoni G, Lampugnani MG. Vascular endothelial (VE)-cadherin: only an intercellular glue? Exp Cell Res. 1999;252:13–9.
24. Luo Y, Radice GL. N-cadherin acts upstream of VE-cadherin in controlling vascular morphogenesis. J Cell Biol. 2005;169:29–34.
25. Sauteur L, Krudewig A, Herwig L, et al. Cdh5/VE-cadherin promotes endothelial cell interface elongation via cortical actin polymerization during angiogenic sprouting. Cell Rep. 2014;9:504–13.
26. Paik JH, Skoura A, Chae SS, et al. Sphingosine 1-phosphate receptor regulation of N-cadherin mediates vascular stabilization. Genes Dev. 2004;18:2392–403.
27. Kruegel J, Miosge N. Basement membrane components are key players in specialized extracellular matrices. Cell Mol Life Sci. 2010;67:2879–95.
28. Das A, Frank RN, Zhang NL, Turczyn TJ. Ultrastructural localization of extracellular matrix components in human retinal vessels and Bruch's membrane. Arch Ophthalmol. 1990;108:421–9.
29. Das A, Frank RN, Zhang NL, Samadani E. Increases in collagen type IV and laminin in galactose-induced retinal capillary basement membrane thickening–prevention by an aldose reductase inhibitor. Exp Eye Res. 1990;50:269–80.
30. Bandopadhyay R, Orte C, Lawrenson JG, Reid AR, De Silva S, Allt G. Contractile proteins in pericytes at the blood-brain and blood-retinal barriers. J Neurocytol. 2001;30:35–44.
31. Park DY, Lee J, Kim J, et al. Plastic roles of pericytes in the blood-retinal barrier. Nat Commun. 2017;8:15296.
32. Klaassen I, Van Noorden CJ, Schlingemann RO. Molecular basis of the inner blood-retinal barrier and its breakdown in diabetic macular edema and other pathological conditions. Prog Retin Eye Res. 2013;34:19–48.
33. Stratman AN, Malotte KM, Mahan RD, Davis MJ, Davis GE. Pericyte recruitment during vasculogenic tube assembly stimulates endothelial basement membrane matrix formation. Blood. 2009;114:5091–101.
34. Antonelli-Orlidge A, Saunders KB, Smith SR, D'Amore PA. An activated form of transforming growth factor beta is produced by cocultures of endothelial cells and pericytes. Proc Natl Acad Sci U S A. 1989;86:4544–8.
35. Maisonpierre PC, Suri C, Jones PF, et al. Angiopoietin-2, a natural antagonist for Tie2 that disrupts in vivo angiogenesis. Science. 1997;277:55–60.
36. Lindahl P, Johansson BR, Levéen P, Betsholtz C. Pericyte loss and microaneurysm formation in PDGF-B-deficient mice. Science. 1997;277:242–5.
37. Wang J, Xu X, Elliott MH, Zhu M, Le YZ. Müller cell-derived VEGF is essential for diabetes-induced retinal inflammation and vascular leakage. Diabetes. 2010;59:2297–305.
38. Antonetti DA, Klein R, Gardner TW. Diabetic retinopathy. N Engl J Med. 2012;366:1227–39.
39. Barber AJ, Gardner TW, Abcouwer SF. The significance of vascular and neural apoptosis to the pathology of diabetic retinopathy. Invest Ophthalmol Vis Sci. 2011;52:1156–63.
40. Kern TS, Berkowitz BA. Photoreceptors in diabetic retinopathy. J Diabetes Investig. 2015;6:371–80.
41. de Gooyer TE, Stevenson KA, Humphries P, Simpson DA, Gardiner TA, Stitt AW. Retinopathy is reduced during experimental diabetes in a mouse model of outer retinal degeneration. Invest Ophthalmol Vis Sci. 2006;47:5561–8.
42. Du Y, Veenstra A, Palczewski K, Kern TS. Photoreceptor cells are major contributors to diabetes-induced oxidative stress and local inflammation in the retina. Proc Natl Acad Sci U S A. 2013;110:16586–91.
43. Arden GB. The absence of diabetic retinopathy in patients with retinitis pigmentosa: implications for pathophysiology and possible treatment. Br J Ophthalmol. 2001;85:366–70.
44. Vinores SA, Gadegbeku C, Campochiaro PA, Green WR. Immunohistochemical localization of blood-retinal barrier breakdown in human diabetics. Am J Pathol. 1989;134:231–5.
45. Kim SY, Johnson MA, McLeod DS, Alexander T, Hansen BC, Lutty GA. Neutrophils are associated with capillary closure in spontaneously diabetic monkey retinas. Diabetes. 2005;54:1534–42.
46. Nimmerjahn A, Kirchhoff F, Helmchen F. Resting microglial cells are highly dynamic surveillants of brain parenchyma in vivo. Science. 2005;308:1314–8.
47. Hanisch UK, Kettenmann H. Microglia: active sensor and versatile effector cells in the normal and pathologic brain. Nat Neurosci. 2007;10:1387–94.
48. Chen M, Forrester JV, Xu H. Synthesis of complement factor H by retinal pigment epithelial cells is down-regulated by oxidized photoreceptor outer segments. Exp Eye Res. 2007;84:635–45.
49. Xu H, Chen M, Mayer EJ, Forrester JV, Dick AD. Turnover of resident retinal microglia in the normal adult mouse. Glia. 2007;55:1189–98.
50. Zeng HY, Green WR, Tso MO. Microglial activation in human diabetic retinopathy. Arch Ophthalmol. 2008;126:227–32.
51. Kakehashi A, Inoda S, Mameuda C, et al. Relationship among VEGF, VEGF receptor, AGEs, and macrophages in proliferative diabetic retinopathy. Diabetes Res Clin Pract. 2008;79:438–45.
52. Rodero MP, Khosrotehrani K. Skin wound healing modulation by macrophages. Int J Clin Exp Pathol. 2010;3:643–53.
53. Chibber R, Ben-Mahmud BM, Chibber S, Kohner EM. Leukocytes in diabetic retinopathy. Curr Diabetes Rev. 2007;3:3–14.
54. Kern TS. Contributions of inflammatory processes to the development of the early stages of diabetic retinopathy. Exp Diabetes Res. 2007;2007:95103.
55. Rangasamy S, McGuire PG, Franco Nitta C, Monickaraj F, Oruganti SR, Das A. Chemokine mediated monocyte trafficking into the retina: role of inflammation in alteration of the blood-retinal barrier in diabetic retinopathy. PLoS One. 2014;9:e108508.
56. McLeod DS, Lefer DJ, Merges C, Lutty GA. Enhanced expression of intracellular adhesion molecule-1 and P-selectin in the diabetic human retina and choroid. Am J Pathol. 1995;147:642–53.
57. Bradshaw EM, Raddassi K, Elyaman W, et al. Monocytes from patients with type 1 diabetes spontaneously secrete proinflammatory cytokines inducing Th17 cells. J Immunol. 2009;183:4432–9.

58. Hatanaka E, Monteagudo PT, Marrocos MS, Campa A. Neutrophils and monocytes as potentially important sources of proinflammatory cytokines in diabetes. Clin Exp Immunol. 2006;146:443–7.
59. Xu H, Chen M. Diabetic retinopathy and dysregulated innate immunity. Vis Res. 2017;139:39–46.
60. Monickaraj FAG, Cabrera A, Das A. The chemokine CXCL1 contributes to vascular inflammation and disruption of tight-junctions associated with diabetic retinopathy. Invest Ophthalmol Vis Sci. 2021;62(68):3032.
61. Abcouwer SF, Gardner TW. Diabetic retinopathy: loss of neuroretinal adaptation to the diabetic metabolic environment. Ann N Y Acad Sci. 2014;1311:174–90.
62. Kowluru RA, Chan PS. Oxidative stress and diabetic retinopathy. Exp Diabetes Res. 2007;2007:43603.
63. Kowluru RA, Mishra M. Oxidative stress, mitochondrial damage and diabetic retinopathy. Biochim Biophys Acta. 2015;1852:2474–83.
64. Pan HZ, Zhang H, Chang D, Li H, Sui H. The change of oxidative stress products in diabetes mellitus and diabetic retinopathy. Br J Ophthalmol. 2008;92:548–51.
65. Lorenzi M. The polyol pathway as a mechanism for diabetic retinopathy: attractive, elusive, and resilient. Exp Diabetes Res. 2007;2007:61038.
66. Brownlee M. Biochemistry and molecular cell biology of diabetic complications. Nature. 2001;414:813–20.
67. Dvornik E, Simard-Duquesne N, Krami M, et al. Polyol accumulation in galactosemic and diabetic rats: control by an aldose reductase inhibitor. Science. 1973;182:1146–8.
68. Obrosova IG, Minchenko AG, Vasupuram R, et al. Aldose reductase inhibitor fidarestat prevents retinal oxidative stress and vascular endothelial growth factor overexpression in streptozotocin-diabetic rats. Diabetes. 2003;52:864–71.
69. Asnaghi V, Gerhardinger C, Hoehn T, Adeboje A, Lorenzi M. A role for the polyol pathway in the early neuroretinal apoptosis and glial changes induced by diabetes in the rat. Diabetes. 2003;52:506–11.
70. Sorbinil Retinopathy Trial Research Group. A randomized trial of sorbinil, an aldose reductase inhibitor, in diabetic retinopathy. Arch Ophthalmol. 1990;108:1234–44.
71. Stitt AW. AGEs and diabetic retinopathy. Invest Ophthalmol Vis Sci. 2010;51:4867–74.
72. Yamagishi S, Matsui T. Advanced glycation end products (AGEs), oxidative stress and diabetic retinopathy. Curr Pharm Biotechnol. 2011;12:362–8.
73. Zong H, Ward M, Stitt AW. AGEs, RAGE, and diabetic retinopathy. Curr Diab Rep. 2011;11:244–52.
74. Barile GR, Pachydaki SI, Tari SR, et al. The RAGE axis in early diabetic retinopathy. Invest Ophthalmol Vis Sci. 2005;46:2916–24.
75. Huang Q, Yuan Y. Interaction of PKC and NOS in signal transduction of microvascular hyperpermeability. Am J Phys. 1997;273:H2442–51.
76. Park JY, Takahara N, Gabriele A, et al. Induction of endothelin-1 expression by glucose: an effect of protein kinase C activation. Diabetes. 2000;49:1239–48.
77. Williams B, Gallacher B, Patel H, Orme C. Glucose-induced protein kinase C activation regulates vascular permeability factor mRNA expression and peptide production by human vascular smooth muscle cells in vitro. Diabetes. 1997;46:1497–503.
78. Pomero F, Allione A, Beltramo E, et al. Effects of protein kinase C inhibition and activation on proliferation and apoptosis of bovine retinal pericytes. Diabetologia. 2003;46:416–9.
79. Titchenell PM, Lin CM, Keil JM, Sundstrom JM, Smith CD, Antonetti DA. Novel atypical PKC inhibitors prevent vascular endothelial growth factor-induced blood-retinal barrier dysfunction. Biochem J. 2012;446:455–67.
80. Schleicher ED, Weigert C. Role of the hexosamine biosynthetic pathway in diabetic nephropathy. Kidney Int Suppl. 2000;77:S13–8.
81. Nakamura M, Barber AJ, Antonetti DA, et al. Excessive hexosamines block the neuroprotective effect of insulin and induce apoptosis in retinal neurons. J Biol Chem. 2001;276:43748–55.
82. Nerlich AG, Sauer U, Kolm-Litty V, Wagner E, Koch M, Schleicher ED. Expression of glutamine: fructose-6-phosphate amidotransferase in human tissues: evidence for high variability and distinct regulation in diabetes. Diabetes. 1998;47:170–8.
83. Kolm-Litty V, Sauer U, Nerlich A, Lehmann R, Schleicher ED. High glucose-induced transforming growth factor beta1 production is mediated by the hexosamine pathway in porcine glomerular mesangial cells. J Clin Invest. 1998;101:160–9.
84. Tien T, Zhang J, Muto T, Kim D, Sarthy VP, Roy S. High glucose induces mitochondrial dysfunction in retinal Müller cells: implications for diabetic retinopathy. Invest Ophthalmol Vis Sci. 2017;58:2915–21.
85. Trudeau K, Molina AJ, Guo W, Roy S. High glucose disrupts mitochondrial morphology in retinal endothelial cells: implications for diabetic retinopathy. Am J Pathol. 2010;177:447–55.
86. Zhong Q, Kowluru RA. Diabetic retinopathy and damage to mitochondrial structure and transport machinery. Invest Ophthalmol Vis Sci. 2011;52:8739–46.
87. Trudeau K, Muto T, Roy S. Downregulation of mitochondrial connexin 43 by high glucose triggers mitochondrial shape change and cytochrome C release in retinal endothelial cells. Invest Ophthalmol Vis Sci. 2012;53:6675–81.
88. Kowluru RA, Zhong Q, Santos JM. Matrix metalloproteinases in diabetic retinopathy: potential role of MMP-9. Expert Opin Investig Drugs. 2012;21:797–805.
89. Alam N, Goel HL, Zarif MJ, et al. The integrin-growth factor receptor duet. J Cell Physiol. 2007;213:649–53.
90. Barouch FC, Miyamoto K, Allport JR, et al. Integrin-mediated neutrophil adhesion and retinal leukostasis in diabetes. Invest Ophthalmol Vis Sci. 2000;41:1153–8.
91. AllegroOphthalmics. Allegro ophthalmics announces positive topline results from DEL MAR phase 2b trial Evaluating Luminate® in patients with diabetic macular edema. https://www.allegroeye.com/allegro-ophthalmics-announces-positive-topline-results-from-del-mar-phase-2b-trial-evaluating-luminate-in-patients-with-diabetic-macular-edema/.
92. Liu H, Zhang W, Kennard S, Caldwell RB, Lilly B. Notch3 is critical for proper angiogenesis and mural cell investment. Circ Res. 2010;107:860–70.
93. Kofler NM, Cuervo H, Uh MK, Murtomäki A, Kitajewski J. Combined deficiency of Notch1 and Notch3 causes pericyte dysfunction, models CADASIL, and results in arteriovenous malformations. Sci Rep. 2015;5:16449.
94. Engerman RL. Pathogenesis of diabetic retinopathy. Diabetes. 1989;38:1203–6.
95. Rangasamy S, Monickaraj F, Legendre C, et al. Transcriptomics analysis of pericytes from retinas of diabetic animals reveals novel genes and molecular pathways relevant to blood-retinal barrier alterations in diabetic retinopathy. Exp Eye Res. 2020;195:108043.
96. Olivera A, Spiegel S. Sphingosine-1-phosphate as second messenger in cell proliferation induced by PDGF and FCS mitogens. Nature. 1993;365:557–60.
97. Lee MJ, Van Brocklyn JR, Thangada S, et al. Sphingosine-1-phosphate as a ligand for the G protein-coupled receptor EDG-1. Science. 1998;279:1552–5.
98. Adamis AP, Berman AJ. Immunological mechanisms in the pathogenesis of diabetic retinopathy. Semin Immunopathol. 2008;30:65–84.

99. Antonetti DA, Barber AJ, Bronson SK, et al. Diabetic retinopathy: seeing beyond glucose-induced microvascular disease. Diabetes. 2006;55:2401–11.
100. Aiello LP, Avery RL, Arrigg PG, et al. Vascular endothelial growth factor in ocular fluid of patients with diabetic retinopathy and other retinal disorders. N Engl J Med. 1994;331:1480–7.
101. Adamis AP, Miller JW, Bernal MT, et al. Increased vascular endothelial growth factor levels in the vitreous of eyes with proliferative diabetic retinopathy. Am J Ophthalmol. 1994;118:445–50.
102. Rangasamy S, McGuire PG, Das A. Diabetic retinopathy and inflammation: novel therapeutic targets. Middle East Afr J Ophthalmol. 2012;19:52–9.
103. Haller JA, Qin H, Apte RS, et al. Vitrectomy outcomes in eyes with diabetic macular edema and vitreomacular traction. Ophthalmology. 2010;117:1087–93.e1083.
104. Ozaki H, Hayashi H, Vinores SA, Moromizato Y, Campochiaro PA, Oshima K. Intravitreal sustained release of VEGF causes retinal neovascularization in rabbits and breakdown of the blood-retinal barrier in rabbits and primates. Exp Eye Res. 1997;64:505–17.
105. Funatsu H, Noma H, Mimura T, Eguchi S, Hori S. Association of vitreous inflammatory factors with diabetic macular edema. Ophthalmology. 2009;116:73–9.
106. Miyamoto K, Khosrof S, Bursell SE, et al. Prevention of leukostasis and vascular leakage in streptozotocin-induced diabetic retinopathy via intercellular adhesion molecule-1 inhibition. Proc Natl Acad Sci U S A. 1999;96:10836–41.
107. Elman MJ, Qin H, Aiello LP, et al. Intravitreal ranibizumab for diabetic macular edema with prompt versus deferred laser treatment: three-year randomized trial results. Ophthalmology. 2012;119:2312–8.
108. Klein R, Klein BE, Moss SE, Cruickshanks KJ. The Wisconsin Epidemiologic Study of Diabetic Retinopathy. XV. The long-term incidence of macular edema. Ophthalmology. 1995;102:7–16.
109. White NH, Sun W, Cleary PA, et al. Effect of prior intensive therapy in type 1 diabetes on 10-year progression of retinopathy in the DCCT/EDIC: comparison of adults and adolescents. Diabetes. 2010;59:1244–53.
110. Joussen AM, Poulaki V, Tsujikawa A, et al. Suppression of diabetic retinopathy with angiopoietin-1. Am J Pathol. 2002;160:1683–93.
111. Shen J, Frye M, Lee BL, et al. Targeting VE-PTP activates TIE2 and stabilizes the ocular vasculature. J Clin Invest. 2014;124:4564–76.
112. Pfister F, Feng Y, vom Hagen F, et al. Pericyte migration: a novel mechanism of pericyte loss in experimental diabetic retinopathy. Diabetes. 2008;57:2495–502.
113. Rangasamy S, Srinivasan R, Maestas J, McGuire PG, Das A. A potential role for angiopoietin 2 in the regulation of the blood-retinal barrier in diabetic retinopathy. Invest Ophthalmol Vis Sci. 2011;52:3784–91.
114. Coffelt SB, Tal AO, Scholz A, et al. Angiopoietin-2 regulates gene expression in TIE2-expressing monocytes and augments their inherent proangiogenic functions. Cancer Res. 2010;70:5270–80.
115. Das A, Fanslow W, Cerretti D, Warren E, Talarico N, McGuire P. Angiopoietin/Tek interactions regulate mmp-9 expression and retinal neovascularization. Lab Investig. 2003;83:1637–45.
116. ClinicalTrials.gov. A study to evaluate the efficacy and safety of faricimab (RO6867461) in participants with diabetic macular edema (RHINE). NCT03622593. Bethesda: U.S. National Library of Medicine. https://clinicaltrials.gov/ct2/show/NCT03622593.
117. ClinicalTrials.gov. A study to evaluate the efficacy and safety of faricimab (RO6867461) in participants with diabetic macular edema (YOSEMITE). NCT03622580. Bethesda: U.S. National Library of Medicine. https://clinicaltrials.gov/ct2/show/NCT03622580.
118. Genentech I. FDA accepts application for Genentech's faricimab for the treatment of wet age-related macular degeneration (AMD) and diabetic macular edema (DME). Press release. 2021. https://www.gene.com/media/press-releases/14923/2021-07-28/fda-accepts-application-for-genentechs-f.
119. Haurigot V, Villacampa P, Ribera A, et al. Increased intraocular insulin-like growth factor-I triggers blood-retinal barrier breakdown. J Biol Chem. 2009;284:22961–9.
120. ClinicalTrials.gov. A phase 1, open-label study of teprotumumab in patients with diabetic macular edema (DME). NCT02103283. Bethesda: U.S. National Library of Medicine. http://clinicaltrials.gov/show/NCT02103283.
121. Friedman EA, Brown CD, Berman DH. Erythropoietin in diabetic macular edema and renal insufficiency. Am J Kidney Dis. 1995;26:202–8.
122. Li W, Sinclair SH, Xu GT. Effects of intravitreal erythropoietin therapy for patients with chronic and progressive diabetic macular edema. Ophthalmic Surg Lasers Imaging. 2010;41:18–25.
123. Joussen AM, Poulaki V, Mitsiades N, et al. Nonsteroidal anti-inflammatory drugs prevent early diabetic retinopathy via TNF-alpha suppression. FASEB J. 2002;16:438–40.
124. Sfikakis PP, Grigoropoulos V, Emfietzoglou I, et al. Infliximab for diabetic macular edema refractory to laser photocoagulation: a randomized, double-blind, placebo-controlled, crossover, 32-week study. Diabetes Care. 2010;33:1523–8.
125. Abu el Asrar AM, Maimone D, Morse PH, Gregory S, Reder AT. Cytokines in the vitreous of patients with proliferative diabetic retinopathy. Am J Ophthalmol. 1992;114:731–6.
126. Yuuki T, Kanda T, Kimura Y, et al. Inflammatory cytokines in vitreous fluid and serum of patients with diabetic vitreoretinopathy. J Diabetes Complicat. 2001;15:257–9.
127. Carmo A, Cunha-Vaz JG, Carvalho AP, Lopes MC. L-arginine transport in retinas from streptozotocin diabetic rats: correlation with the level of IL-1 beta and NO synthase activity. Vis Res. 1999;39:3817–23.
128. Schmidt MTA, Lowden P, Kovalchin J, Furfine ES. Optimized IL-6 blockade for the treatment of diabetic macular edema. Invest Ophthalmol Vis Sci. 2014;55:1062.
129. Giebel SJ, Menicucci G, McGuire PG, Das A. Matrix metalloproteinases in early diabetic retinopathy and their role in alteration of the blood-retinal barrier. Lab Investig. 2005;85:597–607.
130. Schröder S, Palinski W, Schmid-Schönbein GW. Activated monocytes and granulocytes, capillary nonperfusion, and neovascularization in diabetic retinopathy. Am J Pathol. 1991;139:81–100.
131. Omri S, Behar-Cohen F, de Kozak Y, et al. Microglia/macrophages migrate through retinal epithelium barrier by a transcellular route in diabetic retinopathy: role of PKCζ in the Goto Kakizaki rat model. Am J Pathol. 2011;179:942–53.
132. Parks WC, Wilson CL, López-Boado YS. Matrix metalloproteinases as modulators of inflammation and innate immunity. Nat Rev Immunol. 2004;4:617–29.
133. Nissinen L, Kähäri VM. Matrix metalloproteinases in inflammation. Biochim Biophys Acta. 1840;2014:2571–80.
134. Gutiérrez-Fernández A, Inada M, Balbín M, et al. Increased inflammation delays wound healing in mice deficient in collagenase-2 (MMP-8). FASEB J. 2007;21:2580–91.
135. Alexander JS, Elrod JW. Extracellular matrix, junctional integrity and matrix metalloproteinase interactions in endothelial permeability regulation. J Anat. 2002;200:561–74.
136. Mehta D, Malik AB. Signaling mechanisms regulating endothelial permeability. Physiol Rev. 2006;86:279–367.
137. Valable S, Montaner J, Bellail A, et al. VEGF-induced BBB permeability is associated with an MMP-9 activity increase in cerebral ischemia: both effects decreased by Ang-1. J Cereb Blood Flow Metab. 2005;25:1491–504.
138. Vacca A, Ribatti D, Iurlaro M, et al. Human lymphoblastoid cells produce extracellular matrix-degrading enzymes and induce endothelial cell proliferation, migration, morphogenesis, and angiogenesis. Int J Clin Lab Res. 1998;28:55–68.

139. Ghajar CM, George SC, Putnam AJ. Matrix metalloproteinase control of capillary morphogenesis. Crit Rev Eukaryot Gene Expr. 2008;18:251–78.
140. Davis GE, Senger DR. Endothelial extracellular matrix: biosynthesis, remodeling, and functions during vascular morphogenesis and neovessel stabilization. Circ Res. 2005;97:1093–107.
141. Loukovaara S, Robciuc A, Holopainen JM, et al. Ang-2 upregulation correlates with increased levels of MMP-9, VEGF, EPO and TGFβ1 in diabetic eyes undergoing vitrectomy. Acta Ophthalmol. 2013;91:531–9.
142. Abu El-Asrar AM, Mohammad G, Nawaz MI, et al. Relationship between vitreous levels of matrix metalloproteinases and vascular endothelial growth factor in proliferative diabetic retinopathy. PLoS One. 2013;8:e85857.
143. Benes P, Vetvicka V, Fusek M. Cathepsin D–many functions of one aspartic protease. Crit Rev Oncol Hematol. 2008;68:12–28.
144. Berchem G, Glondu M, Gleizes M, et al. Cathepsin-D affects multiple tumor progression steps in vivo: proliferation, angiogenesis and apoptosis. Oncogene. 2002;21:5951–5.
145. Monickaraj F, McGuire PG, Nitta CF, Ghosh K, Das A. Cathepsin D: an Mϕ-derived factor mediating increased endothelial cell permeability with implications for alteration of the blood-retinal barrier in diabetic retinopathy. FASEB J. 2016;30:1670–82.
146. Monickaraj F, McGuire P, Das A. Cathepsin D plays a role in endothelial-pericyte interactions during alteration of the blood-retinal barrier in diabetic retinopathy. FASEB J. 2018;32(5):2539–48.
147. Moshirfar M, Parker L, Birdsong OC, et al. Use of Rho kinase inhibitors in ophthalmology: a review of the literature. Med Hypothesis Discov Innov Ophthalmol. 2018;7:101–11.
148. Gregory JL, Morand EF, McKeown SJ, et al. Macrophage migration inhibitory factor induces macrophage recruitment via CC chemokine ligand 2. J Immunol. 2006;177:8072–9.
149. Das ARS, Maestas J, McGuire P. CC Chemokines play an important role in alteration of the blood-retinal barrier in diabetes. Invest Ophthalmol Vis Sci. 2011;52(14):997.
150. García-Ramallo E, Marques T, Prats N, Beleta J, Kunkel SL, Godessart N. Resident cell chemokine expression serves as the major mechanism for leukocyte recruitment during local inflammation. J Immunol. 2002;169:6467–73.
151. Bian ZM, Elner VM, Yoshida A, Kunkel SL, Elner SG. Signaling pathways for glycated human serum albumin-induced IL-8 and MCP-1 secretion in human RPE cells. Invest Ophthalmol Vis Sci. 2001;42:1660–8.
152. Chen M, Forrester JV, Xu H. Dysregulation in retinal para-inflammation and age-related retinal degeneration in CCL2 or CCR2 deficient mice. PLoS One. 2011;6:e22818.
153. Tuo J, Bojanowski CM, Zhou M, et al. Murine ccl2/cx3cr1 deficiency results in retinal lesions mimicking human age-related macular degeneration. Invest Ophthalmol Vis Sci. 2007;48:3827–36.
154. Monickaraj F, Oruganti SR, McGuire P, Das A. A potential novel therapeutic target in diabetic retinopathy: a chemokine receptor (CCR2/CCR5) inhibitor reduces retinal vascular leakage in an animal model. Graefes Arch Clin Exp Ophthalmol. 2021;259:93–100.
155. Xia M, Sui Z. Recent developments in CCR2 antagonists. Expert Opin Ther Pat. 2009;19:295–303.
156. Gale JD, Berger B, Gilbert S, et al. A CCR2/5 inhibitor, PF-04634817, is inferior to monthly ranibizumab in the treatment of diabetic macular edema. Invest Ophthalmol Vis Sci. 2018;59:2659–69.
157. Liu J, Feener EP. Plasma kallikrein-kinin system and diabetic retinopathy. Biol Chem. 2013;394:319–28.
158. Pharmaceuticals K. Kal Vista pharmaceuticals reports phase 2 clinical trial results in patients with diabetic macular edema. Press release. 2019. https://ir.kalvista.com/news-releases/news-release-details/kalvista-pharmaceuticals-reports-phase-2-clinical-trial-results. Accessed February 4, 2022.
159. Boyer DS, Yoon YH, Belfort R, et al. Three-year, randomized, sham-controlled trial of dexamethasone intravitreal implant in patients with diabetic macular edema. Ophthalmology. 2014;121:1904–14. Date accessed October 5, 2021
160. Campochiaro PA, Brown DM, Pearson A, et al. Sustained delivery fluocinolone acetonide vitreous inserts provide benefit for at least 3 years in patients with diabetic macular edema. Ophthalmology. 2012;119:2125–32.
161. ClinicalTrials.gov. A study to evaluate the efficacy, durability, and safety of KSI-301 compared to aflibercept in participants with diabetic macular edema (DME) (GLIMMER). NCT04603937. Bethesda: U.S. National Library of Medicine. https://clinicaltrials.gov/ct2/show/NCT04603937. Accessed October 5, 2021.
162. ClinicalTrials.gov. A trial to evaluate the efficacy, durability, and safety of KSI-301 compared to aflibercept in participants with diabetic macular edema (DME) (GLEAM). NCT04611152. Bethesda: U.S. National Library of Medicine. https://clinicaltrials.gov/ct2/show/NCT04611152. Accessed October 5, 2021.
163. ClinicalTrials.gov. Safety and bioactivity of AXT107 in subjects with diabetic macular edema (CONGO). NCT04697758. Bethesda: U.S. National Library of Medicine. https://clinicaltrials.gov/ct2/show/NCT04697758. Accessed October 5, 2021.
164. ClinicalTrials.gov. Study of the Safety and Efficacy of APX3330 in Diabetic Retinopathy (ZETA-1). NCT04692688. U.S. National Library of Medicine. https://clinicaltrials.gov/ct2/show/NCT04692688. Accessed October 5, 2021.
165. ClinicalTrials.gov. Multiple dose safety and efficacy of LKA651 in patients with diabetic macular edema. NCT03927690. Bethesda: U.S. National Library of Medicine. https://clinicaltrials.gov/ct2/show/NCT03927690. Accessed October 5, 2021.
166. ClinicalTrials.gov. A study assessing AR-13503 implant in subjects with nAMD or DME. NCT03835884. Bethesda: U.S. National Library of Medicine. https://clinicaltrials.gov/ct2/show/NCT03835884. Accessed October 5, 2021.
167. ClinicalTrials.gov. First-in-human study of CU06-1004 following single and multiple ascending doses in healthy volunteers. NCT04795037. Bethesda: U.S. National Library of Medicine. https://clinicaltrials.gov/ct2/show/NCT04795037. Accessed October 5, 2021.
168. ClinicalTrials.gov. A study to evaluate THR-149 treatment for diabetic macular oedema (KALAHARI). NCT04527107 Bethesda: U.S. National Library of Medicine. https://clinicaltrials.gov/ct2/show/NCT04527107. Accessed October 5, 2021.
169. ClinicalTrials.gov. RGX-314 gene therapy administered in the suprachoroidal space for participants with diabetic retinopathy (DR) without center involved-diabetic macular edema (CI-DME) (ALTITUDE). NCT04567550. Bethesda: U.S. National Library of Medicine. https://clinicaltrials.gov/ct2/show/NCT04567550. Accessed October 5, 2021.
170. Cabrera AP, Mankad RN, Marek L, et al. Genotypes and phenotypes: a search for influential genes in diabetic retinopathy. Int J Mol Sci. 2020;21(8):2712.

Optical Coherence Tomography Biomarkers in Diabetic Macular Edema

3

Sashwanthi Mohan, Garima, and Muna Bhende

3.1 Introduction

Diabetic retinopathy (DR) is one of the major micro vascular diseases usually affecting the population of working-age group and is due to long-term effects of diabetes that ultimately lead to vision-threatening complications [1]. Diabetic macular edema (DME) can occur at any stage of DR, but the risk increases with severity of DR. It is now considered as the most prevalent vision-threatening form of DR in developed countries, particularly among adults with type 2 diabetes [2]. The main event leading to DME is the structural damage to blood–retinal barrier. The two main molecular mediators responsible for DME are vascular endothelial growth factor (VEGF) and inflammatory cytokines [3].

Clinically, DME is identified by the presence of hard exudates, microaneurysms, dot and blot haemorrhages within 1 DD of the centre of the macula [4] (Fig. 3.1). Apart from clinical detection, there are numerous diagnostic modalities for detecting DME.

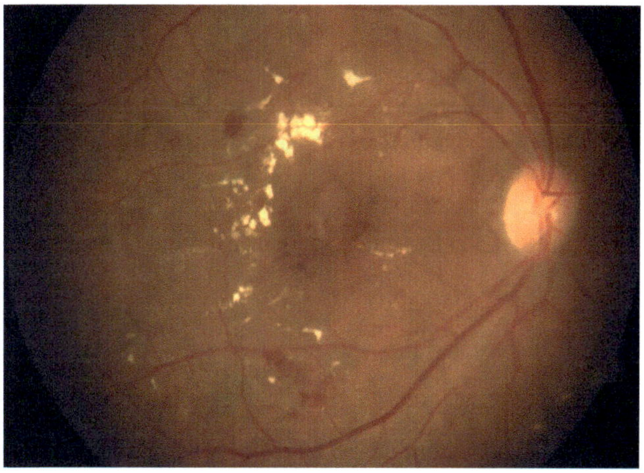

Fig. 3.1 Fundus photo of the right eye of a patient showing diabetic macular edema, i.e., hard exudates, microaneurysms, dot and blot haemorrhages within 1 DD of the centre of the macula

Fundus fluorescein angiography (FFA) has long been considered the gold standard in the study of retinal vasculature. Though not indicated for the diagnosis of DME, it can provide information that classifies DME into focal, diffuse or ischemic maculopathy [5]. Fundus autofluorescence being a non-invasive investigation can also be an aid in diagnosing DME as excess accumulation of lipofuscin pigment and depletion of luteal pigment at retinal pigment epithelium (RPE) leads to an increased FAF signal [6, 7]. OCT and OCT A have proved to be important tools inunderstanding the pathogenesis and management of DME. Both modalities carry an additional advantage of being non-invasive and hence easily repeatable should the need arise . Previously the only biomarker in detecting DME was increased foveal thickness on OCT (Fig. 3.2), but with ongoing research, it has been possible to identify various biomarkers that have both diagnostic and prognostic implications. These are changes within the retinal layers (outer and inner retina) and changes at the vitreomacular interface [8–10].

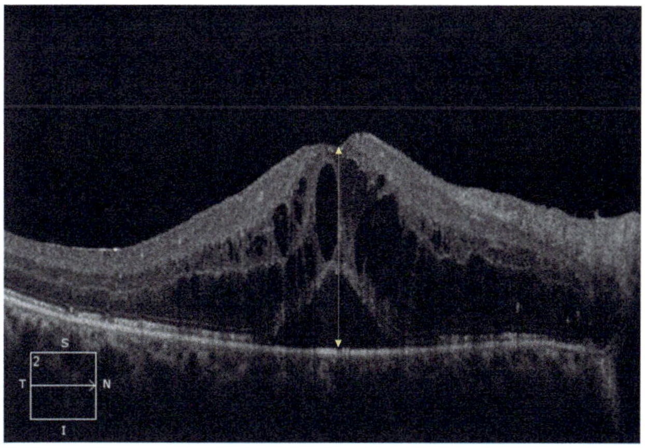

Fig. 3.2 OCT showing centre-involving diabetic macular edema (CI-DME) with increased foveal thickness

OCT angiography (OCT A) allows visualization of the retinochoroidal circulation and allows the separation of

S. Mohan · Garima · M. Bhende (✉)
Shri Bhagwan Mahavir Vitreoretinal Services, Medical Research Foundation, Chennai, India
e-mail: drmuna@snmail.org

S. Saxena et al. (eds.), *Diabetic Macular Edema*, https://doi.org/10.1007/978-981-19-7307-9_3

capillaries at three different levels. OCT A can identify microaneurysms, areas of capillary nonperfusion and neovascularization much before they are appreciated clinically [11].

3.2 OCT Biomarkers in Diabetic Macular Edema

Intravitreal anti-VEGF agents are now the first-line treatment for centre involving DME after the landmark RISE/RIDE trials and DRCR.net studies which showed a significant improvement in baseline visual acuity in over 60% of the cases [12]. Intravitreal steroid injections are more often used in patients who do not respond to anti-VEGF injections. OCT biomarkers serve as a useful tool for predicting functional and anatomical outcomes in response to these injections. Various biomarkers on OCT have been described to influence treatment and predict visual outcomes in DME.

3.3 Retinal Biomarkers

3.3.1 Retinal Thickness

Increased retinal thickness occurs due to edema caused by breakdown of the inner blood–retinal barrier and lipid extravasation in DME. Saxena et al. suggested three OCT biomarkers for DME—central subfield thickness (CST), cube average thickness (CAT) and cube volume (CV). CST measured on spectral domain-OCT (SD-OCT) is used to assess the retinal thickness and thus the degree of DME. It is measured in the central circle of 1 mm diameter on the circular ETDRS grid map. CAT refers to the overall average thickness of the tissue layers between ILM and the RPE over the entire 6 × 6 mm scanned area, the mean of thicknesses in nine sections. CV is defined as the overall average volume of the tissue layers between ILM-RPE over the same area. All the three biomarkers can independently predict severity of retinopathy and visual acuity [13]. However, in some other reports, CST is not found to be a reliable indicator of final visual acuity. This is because even if DME resolves, and retinal thickness decreases, permanent damage to the photoreceptors can cause poor visual acuity [14]. Cross-sectional area of retinal tissue between the plexiform layers in CME is found to be a better predictor of visual acuity than macular thickness [15].

3.3.2 Disorganization of Retinal Inner Layers

Disorganization of retinal inner layers (DRIL) is defined as the loss of boundaries between the ganglion cell layer, inner plexiform layer and outer nuclear and plexiform layers of the retina seen on OCT (Fig. 3.3). Cells in these layers are important for transmission of visual signals from photoreceptors to ganglion cells, and disorganization leads to abnormal visual processing. Hence, the integrity or lack of it can be of prognostic value in patients with DME. It is measured in OCT B scans at the central 1 mm retinal zone [14]. A 300 μm increase in DRIL at 4 months is found to be associated with a one line decrease in visual acuity at 8 months [16]. The change in DRIL extent is thus predictive of future visual outcomes. DRIL correlates strongly with visual acuity in centre involving-DME (CI-DME) and is associated with disruption of external limiting membrane (ELM) and ellipsoid zone (EZ) layers and the presence of epiretinal membrane (ERM) [16].

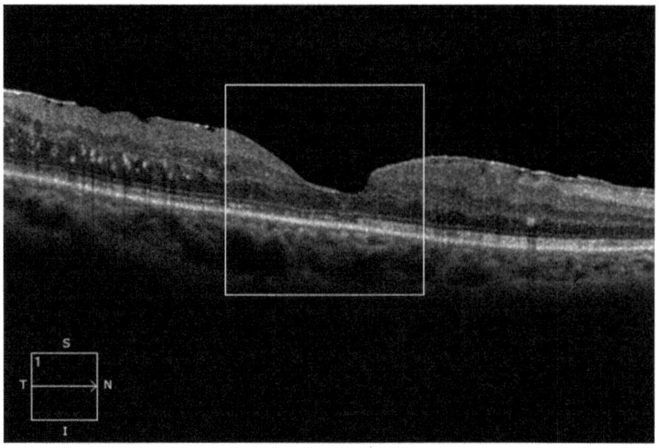

Fig. 3.3 OCT showing disorganization of the inner retinal layers (DRIL) in the central 1 mm

Nadri et al. studied the correlation between DRIL, macular thickness, EZ disruption and retinal nerve fibre layer (RNFL) thickness in DR using SD-OCT. DRIL was graded as 0 (absent) and 1 (present), and EZ was graded as 0 (intact), 1 (focal disruption) and 2 (global disruption). DRIL was found to be significantly associated with severity of DR. DRIL had a strong positive correlation with CST, CAT and grades of EZ disruption and a negative correlation with RNFL thickness [17].

3.3.3 Hyperreflective Retinal Foci and Hard Exudates

Three different types of hyperreflective retinal foci (HRF) are described according to their location, size and reflectivity [18].

1. <30 μm, similar reflectivity to the nerve fibre layer, absence of back shadowing, located in the inner and outer retina, associated with activated microglial cells

2. >30 μm, similar reflectivity to the RPE-Bruch membrane complex, presence of back shadowing, location in the outer retina, may represent hard exudates
3. >30 μm, similar reflectivity to the RPE-Bruch membrane complex, presence of back shadowing, location in the inner retina, may represent microaneurysms

Small HRFs <30 μm in diameter are said to be of inflammatory origin and serve as biomarkers on OCT [19] in eyes with DME. They are seen in conditions where inner blood–retinal barrier breakdown occurs leading to lipoprotein extravasation such as DME. Other theories of HRF origin are microglial proliferation or RPE migration (Fig. 3.4).

A strong correlation was found between hard exudates at baseline and HRF in every layer before and after treatment [20]. Various studies have shown a decrease in HRF after anti-VEGF or steroid therapy. Number as well as position of HRF is strongly predictive for final visual outcomes. Multiple HRF at baseline predicted a significant decrease in DME after anti-VEGF therapy [21]. HRF closer to the outer retina is predictive of increased EZ and ELM disruption, contributing to poorer visual outcomes [22].

HRF larger than 30 μm in the outer retina with back shadowing represents hard exudates. Hard exudates are lipoproteinaceous material that accumulate secondary to the breakdown of the inner blood retinal barrier [18]. Hard exudates in DME, especially when they are subfoveal, have been shown to respond better to intravitreal steroids compared to anti-VEGF therapy [23].

A meta-analysis concluded that there is a definite reduction in quantitative HRF following either intravitreal anti-VEGF or steroid therapy [24]. Eyes with treatment naïve DME showed a positive correlation between HRF and visual acuity gain and central macular thickness (CMT) reduction compared to eyes with refractory DME. The prompt response to intravitreal injections demonstrates that inflammation plays a major role in treatment naïve eyes when they present with HRF.

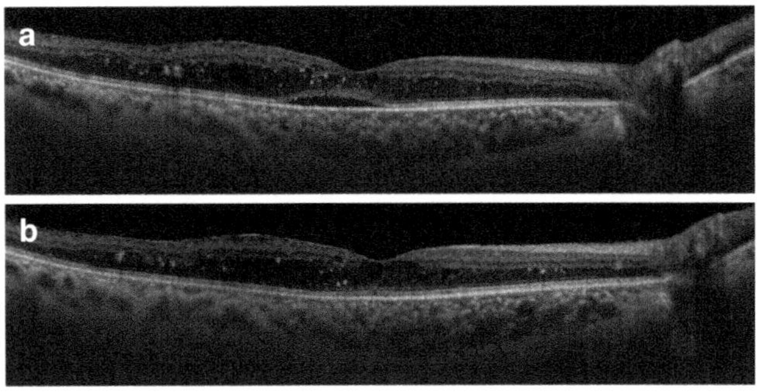

Fig. 3.4 OCT prior to anti-VEGF showing CI-DME with subretinal fluid and multiple HRFs and hard exudates (**a**) and OCT post anti-VEGF showing reduction in macular edema, resolution of subretinal fluid and reduction in number of HRFs and hard exudates (**b**)

3.3.4 Intraretinal Cystoid Spaces

Cysts in the outer nuclear layer (ONL) can damage photoreceptor cells and disrupt the inner segment—outer segment (IS/OS) junction, i.e., EZ thus affecting visual acuity permanently [25] (Fig. 3.5). The cysts can be classified based on size as small (<100 μm), large (101–200 μm) and giant (>200 μm). Larger cysts are associated with poorer visual prognosis as they affect the outer nuclear layer and damage the IS/OS junction. Size of the cyst also correlates with severity of macular ischemia [26]. Anti-VEGF treatment, by decreasing the permeability of the inner blood–retinal barrier, can decrease the number and size of ONL cysts leading to better visual acuity [27].

3.3.5 Pearl Necklace Sign

This refers to hyperreflective dots in a contiguous ring around the inner wall of cystoid spaces in the retina seen on OCT. This sign is believed to be a precursor to development of hard exudates in exudative maculopathies such as DME. Subfoveal location of this sign may cause irreversible damage to the photoreceptors in that area, contributing to poor visual outcomes (Fig. 3.6).

3.3.6 Bridging Retinal Processes

Bridging retinal processes seen between cystic cavities are found to be associated with better visual acuity after treatment with bevacizumab injection [28]. These processes are believed to consist of Muller and bipolar cells which help in transmitting visual impulses to the optic nerve axons. Eyes with absence of bridging retinal processes are shown to have a poor prognosis post treatment with development of foveal atrophy (Fig. 3.7).

3.3.7 Subfoveal Neurosensory Detachment

Subfoveal neurosensory detachment [29] (SND) in DME is seen as a hyporeflective area beneath the neurosensory retina on OCT and has a prevalence of 15–30% in eyes with DME [30–32] (Fig. 3.4). An increase in inflammatory cytokine, interleukin-6 is associated with SND in DME. SND is secondary to the migration of fluid from the intra-retinal cystoid spaces or directly from the choroidal circulation to the subretinal space [33]. RESTORE and RISE/RIDE studies have shown a protective role of SND with better visual gains in eyes with SND. These eyes also respond better to anti-VEGF ranibizumab therapy [34]. VIVID-DME and VISTA-DME studies also showed that greater treatment effect of intravit-

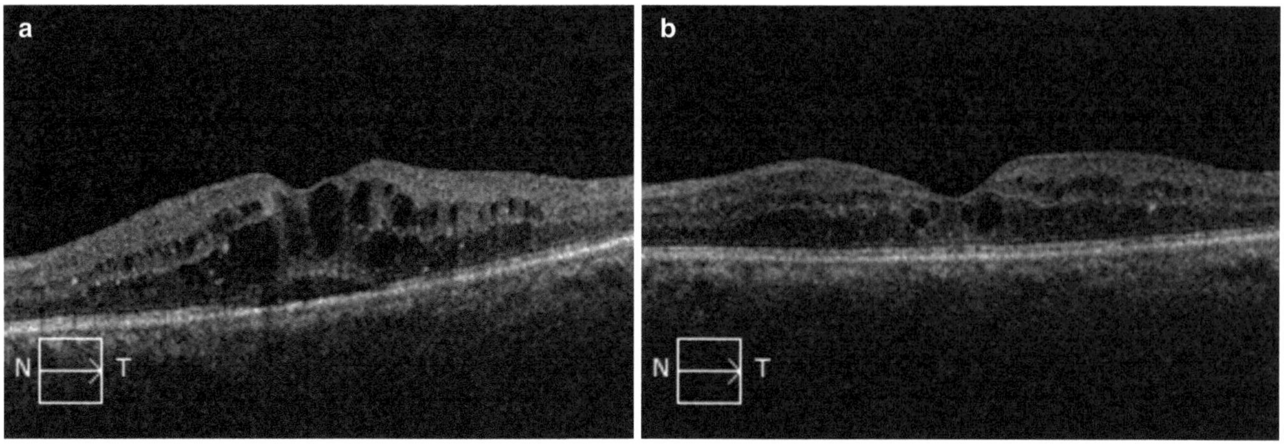

Fig. 3.5 OCT prior to anti-VEGF showing diabetic macular edema with intraretinal cystoid spaces and subretinal fluid (**a**) and OCT post anti-VEGF injection showing decrease in size and number of intraretinal cystoid spaces and resolution of subretinal fluid (**b**)

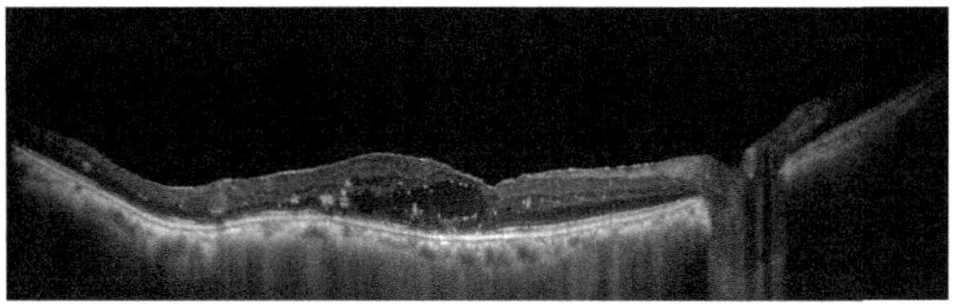

Fig. 3.6 OCT showing the 'pearl necklace sign'

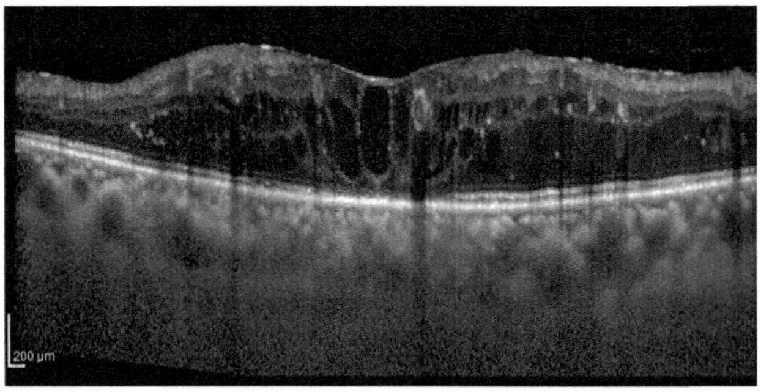

Fig. 3.7 OCT showing presence of bridging retinal processes between the cystic cavities

real aflibercept was seen in patients with SND compared to those without [35]. SND also responds significantly to dexamethasone implants as eyes without SND [36] (Fig. 3.8). However, there are studies which show that presence of SND is associated with poorer visual gains [34].

Disruption of the ELM is correlated with the presence and height of SND in eyes with DME, whereas ELM is intact in eyes without SND. This is because when ELM is intact, lipid extravasation due to breakdown of blood–retinal barrier collects anterior to the ELM causing outer retinal swelling. When ELM is disrupted, the fluid moves through the subretinal space causing SND [29]. Presence of SND is also associated with greater CMT and thicker choroid compared to eyes without SND.

3.3.8 Vitreomacular Interface

Vitreomacular traction which is described as a taut posterior hyaloid membrane is a sheet of posterior hyaloid along the posterior pole causing traction over the retina and macular distortion. This can be a cause of recalcitrant DME and requires surgical intervention in the form of pars plana vitrectomy and removal of the posterior hyaloid [37, 38] (Fig. 3.9).

3.3.9 Integrity of External Limiting Membrane and Ellipsoid Zone

Visual acuity directly correlates with the integrity of the ELM and EZ which indicates the health of the photoreceptors. Three grades of IS/OS junction, i.e., EZ involvement have been described—continuous, partly disrupted, completely disrupted. Eyes with intact EZ have better visual prognosis post treatment [36]. In DME, there can be loss of ELM and EZ focally or in a diffuse manner. Extensive ELM disruption was the strongest OCT biomarker to predict anti-VEGF resistance followed by tractional ERM. EZ disruption and DRIL had lower predictive value [39].

3.3.10 Photoreceptor Outer Segment

Another biomarker is the photoreceptor outer segment (PROS) which is the length between the photoreceptor inner and outer segment junction and the RPE. Length of PROS is

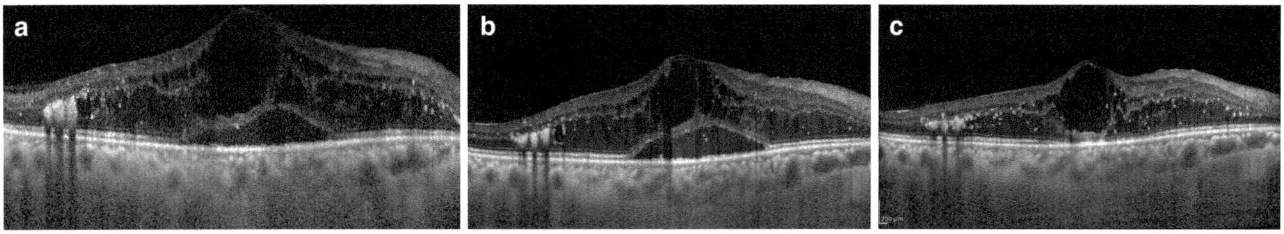

Fig. 3.8 OCT showing presence of CI-DME with neurosensory detachment (SND) (**a**) which did not respond to anti-VEGF injection (**b**) but showed resolution of SND to Ozurdex (Dexamethasone implant) (**c**)

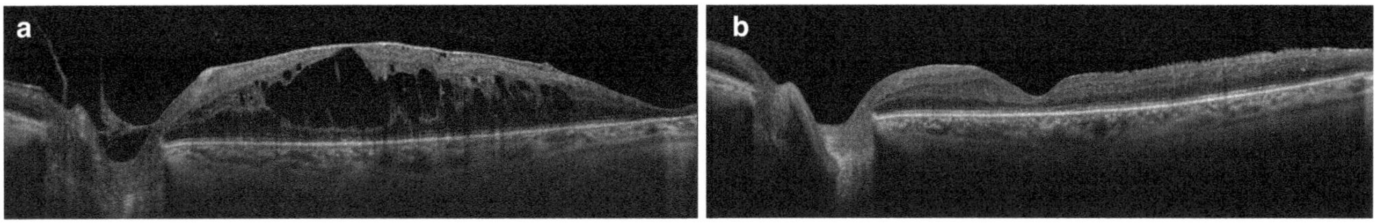

Fig. 3.9 Pre-operative OCT showing an epiretinal membrane with macular edema and increased retinal thickness (**a**) and post-operative OCT showing resolution of macular edema after vitrectomy and epiretinal membrane removal (**b**)

a better prognosticator of visual acuity than macular thickness in patients with DME, thus serving as a prognostic biomarker in eyes with DME [40].

3.3.11 Outer Retinal Layer Thickness [41]

It is the distance between the ELM and the RPE and is a sum of the length of the photoreceptors inner and outer segments. Decrease in outer retinal layer thickness [41] (ORL) can serve as a visual prognostic factor as even though DME can resolve, damage to photoreceptors can cause poor visual acuity. ORL thickness was found to correlate better with visual acuity than total foveal point thickness, i.e., the distance between the ILM and the RPE at the foveal centre.

3.3.12 Retinal Pigment Epithelium Thickness

Thickness of the RPE is an OCT biomarker for prediction of functioning of the outer blood–retinal barrier. Eyes with PDR and DME showed decreased RPE thickness in almost all quadrants, suggesting that degenerative changes may occur in a hypoxic environment [42]. This could be due to disruption of the RPE-photoreceptor complex caused by ischemia [43, 44]. In the same study, in the NPDR-DME group, there was a strong positive correlation between RPE thickness and CMT due to greater edema. This suggests that in NPDR, edema involves the entire retina and in PDR, edema is mainly due to ischemia. RPE thickness shows that staging of DR plays a role in DME.

3.3.13 Foveal Eversion

Foveal eversion is defined as a complete convex profile of the central fovea. It is associated with worse clinical and morphological outcomes in DME treated with both anti-VEGF and steroid, as well as higher retreatment in eyes treated with intravitreal steroid [45]. It is associated with higher frequency of persistent DME.

3.3.14 Parallelism

Parallelism [46] is a newer OCT feature reflecting the orientation of lines in the OCT image and represents the complexity of the photoreceptor-RPE complex alterations in DME. It is a potential OCT biomarker for visual prognosis in DME. It can reflect structural changes in photoreceptor layers, IS/OS junction and presence of HRF. Parallelism was found to be lower in eyes with DME as compared to normal eyes and positively correlated with visual acuity.

3.4 Choroidal Biomarkers

3.4.1 Subfoveal Choroidal Thickness

Subfoveal choroidal thickness (SFCT) is obtained using EDI-OCT scans. A greater baseline choroidal thickness is associated with greater decrease in CMT and better visual acuity gain to anti-VEGF therapy [47]. This is attributed to the fact that these eyes have intact choriocapillaris and a less ischemic outer retina, thus preserving the photoreceptors. SFCT decreased significantly after 3 monthly anti-VEGF injections, but it did not correlate with functional or anatomical outcomes or number of anti-VEGF injections.

3.4.2 Choroidal Vascularity Index

Choroidal vascularity index (CVI) is ratio of the choroidal luminal area to total choroidal area [48]. It has the advantage over choroidal thickness of being unaffected by ocular or systemic factors. It has been recently described as a novel OCT parameter to monitor progression of DR. PDR patients have been shown to have lower CVI than those with mild or moderate NPDR [49].

3.4.3 Hyperreflective Choroidal Foci

Hyperreflective choroidal foci (HCFs) [50] are hyperreflective foci seen in the choroidal layers in DME. They are probably secondary to migration from the retinal to the choroidal layers, with disruption of the external limiting membrane and ellipsoid zone, thus serving as a poor prognostic marker for visual acuity. They were found to be present significantly more in PDR than NPDR eyes.

3.5 OCT Angiography Biomarkers in Diabetic Macular Edema

3.5.1 Foveal Avascular Zone

Patients with diabetes are found to have a larger foveal avascular zone (FAZ) on the deep capillary plexus (DCP) slab on OCTA. Larger FAZ area has been shown to be associated with poor response to anti-VEGF therapy [51]. Increased FAZ and microaneurysms in the DCP but not superficial capillary plexus (SCP) have been predictive of response to anti-VEGF treatment in DME. FAZ dimension and vascular density can be used to evaluate the macular perfusion. Poor perfusion is associated with poor response to intravitreal therapy.

Larger FAZ is also seen in eyes with DRIL compared to eyes with no DRIL [52]. DME patients who show a poor response to anti-VEGF therapy demonstrate a larger FAZ in the DCP (Fig. 3.10).

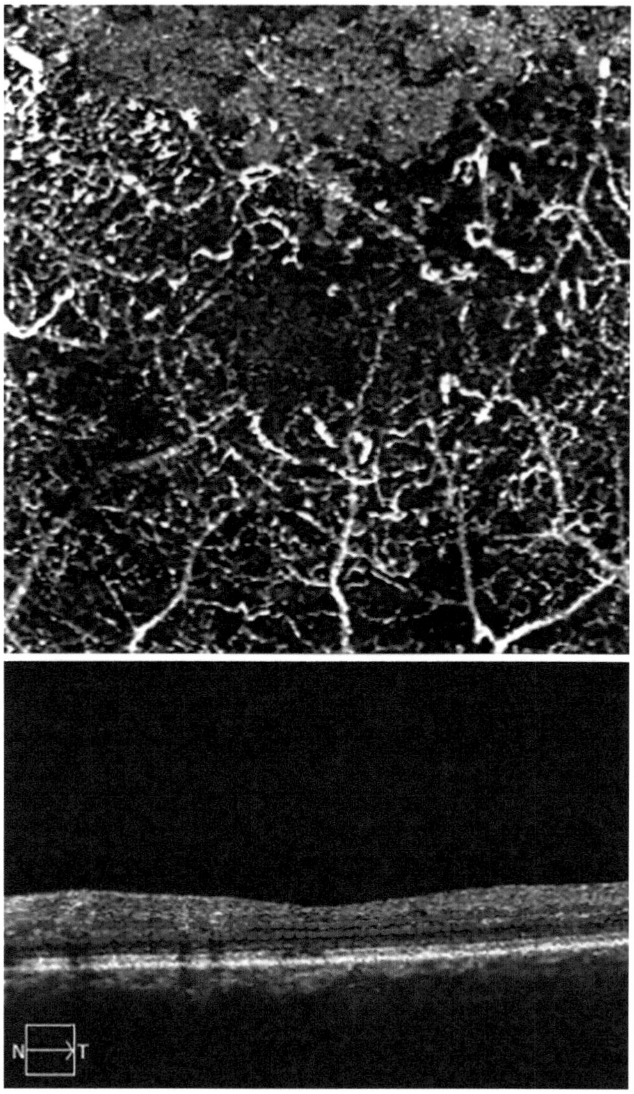

Fig. 3.10 OCTA showing enlargement of FAZ and lower vessel density at the DCP in a patient with poor visual outcomes due to macular ischemia after resolution of macular edema as seen in the structural OCT

3.5.1.1 Vessel Density in Superficial Capillary Plexus [53]

Lower parafoveal vessel density in the superficial layer correlates with poorer visual improvement after treatment with ranibizumab, i.e., poorer vascular perfusion itself results in poorer visual gain even after macular edema resolves. Eyes with DME have larger FAZ at the level of the SCP.

3.5.1.2 Loss of Deep Capillary Plexus

Deep capillary plexus (DCP) is the first affected in DME. Eyes with DME have significantly lower vessel densities at the DCP [54]. Extent of DCP loss and corresponding outer plexiform layer disruption in DME can be useful predictors of responsiveness to anti-VEGF treatment. Decreased vessel density (VD) in the DCP is associated with worse visual acuity, demonstrating that VD in DCP may reflect the capillary loss in patients with visual loss due to DME [55].

3.5.1.3 Middle Capillary Plexus

The middle capillary plexus (MCP) can provide further insights into the ischemic state of DR. MCP VD and flow index are found to decrease, and area of nonperfusion is found to increase with DR progression [56]. This is found to parallel changes in the DCP also.

3.6 Summary

The following is a summary of known OCT and OCTA biomarkers and their prognostic implications:

Prognostic marker	Indicator
Retinal biomarkers on OCT	
Retinal thickness	Not a reliable indicator Cross-sectional area of retinal tissue between plexiform layers is a better predictor
Disorganization of inner retinal layers (DRIL)	Increase in DRIL associated with worse visual acuity
Hyperreflective foci (HRF)	HRF responds well to both anti-VEGF and steroid therapy
Hard exudates	Subfoveal hard exudates respond better to intravitreal steroids
Cystoid spaces	Larger cysts in the ONL associated with macular ischemia and poorer visual prognosis
Pearl necklace sign	Subfoveal location has poor visual outcomes
Bridging retinal processes	Better visual acuity after anti-VEGF injection
Subfoveal neurosensory detachment (SND)	Responds well to both anti-VEGF and steroids Contrasting studies—some studies show better visual gains, some show poorer visual gains
Integrity of ellipsoid zone (EZ)	EZ integrity has better visual prognosis
Integrity of external limiting membrane (ELM)	Extensive ELM disruption predicts Anti VEGF-resistance
Length of Photoreceptor outer segment	Better visual acuity
Vitreomacular interface Taut posterior hyaloid membrane	Poorer prognosis—needs surgical intervention
RPE thickness	Correlates to severity of DR
Foveal eversion	Worse clinical and morphological outcomes in both anti-VEGF and steroid
Parallelism	Correlates with visual acuity, lower degree of parallelism in eyes with DME
Choroidal biomarkers on OCT	
Subfoveal choroidal thickness (SFCT)	Greater baseline SFCT better visual acuity gain to anti-VEGF therapy
Choroidal vascularity index	Increases with severity of DR
Hyperreflective choroidal foci	More significant in PDR eyes
OCTA biomarkers	
Foveal avascular zone (FAZ)	Larger FAZ is associated with poor perfusion and poor response to anti VEGF therapy
Superficial capillary plexus (SCP)	Lower vessel density in SCP is associated with poorer visual improvement after ranibizumab
Deep capillary plexus (DCP)	Greater DCP loss shows poorer response to anti-VEGF therapy and worse visual acuity
Middle capillary plexus (MCP)	MCP VD and flow index is found to decrease and area of non-perfusion is found to increase with DR progression

References

1. Eisma JH, Dulle JE, Fort PE. Current knowledge on diabetic retinopathy from human donor tissues. World J Diabetes. 2015;6(2):312–20.
2. Cheung N, Mitchell P, Wong TY. Diabetic retinopathy. Lancet. 2010;376:124–36.
3. Klaassen I, Van Noorden CJ, Schlingemann RO. Molecular basis of the inner blood–retinal barrier and its breakdown in diabetic macular edema and other pathological conditions. Prog Retin Eye Res. 2013;34:19–48.
4. Early Treatment Diabetic Retinopathy Study Research Group. Grading diabetic retinopathy from stereoscopic color fundus photographs—an extension of the modified Airlie House classification. ETDRS report number 10. Ophthalmology. 1991;98(5):786–806.
5. Bresnick GH. Diabetic macular edema. A review. Ophthalmology. 1986;93:989–97.
6. Schmitz-Valckenberg S, Holz FG, Bird AC, et al. Fundus autofluorescence imaging: review and perspectives. Retina. 2008;28:385–409.
7. Özmen S, Ağca S, Doğan E, et al. Evaluation of fundus autofluorescence imaging of diabetic patients without retinopathy. Arq Bras Oftalmol. 2019;82:412–6.
8. Trichonas G, Kaiser PK. Optical coherence tomography imaging of the macular oedema. Br J Ophthalmol. 2014;98(Suppl II):ii24–9. https://doi.org/10.1136/bjophthalmol-2014-305305.
9. Sikorski BL, Malukiewicz G, Stafiej J, Lesiewska-Junk H, Raczynska D. The diagnostic function of OCT in diabetic maculopathy. Mediat Inflamm. 2013;1:1–12.
10. Couturier A, Rey P-A, Erginay A, et al. Widefield OCT-angiography and fluorescein angiography assessments of nonperfusion in diabetic retinopathy and edema treated with anti-vascular endothelial growth factor. Ophthalmology. 2019;126:1685–94.
11. Borrelli E, Sacconi R, Querques L, et al. Quantification of diabetic macular ischemia using novel three-dimensional optical coherence tomography angiography metrics. J Biophotonics. 2020;11:e202000152.
12. Nguyen QD, Brown DM, Marcus DM, Boyer DS, Patel S, Feiner L, Gibson A, Sy J, Rundle AC, Hopkins JJ, Rubio RG. Ranibizumab for diabetic macular edema: results from 2 phase III randomized trials: RISE and RIDE. Ophthalmology. 2012;119(4):789–801.
13. Saxena S, Caprnda M, Ruia S, Prasad S, Fedotova J, Kruzliak P, Krasnik V. Spectral domain optical coherence tomography based imaging biomarkers for diabetic retinopathy. Endocrine. 2019;66(3):509–16.

14. Markan A, Agarwal A, Arora A, Bazgain K, Rana V, Gupta V. Novel imaging biomarkers in diabetic retinopathy and diabetic macular edema. Therap Adv Ophthalmol. 2020;12:2515841420950513.
15. Pelosini L, Hull CC, Boyce JF, et al. Optical coherence tomography may be used to predict visual acuity in patients with macular edema. Invest Ophthalmol Vis Sci. 2011;52:2741–8.
16. Sun JK, Lin MM, Lammer J, et al. Disorganization of the retinal inner layers as a predictor of visual acuity in eyes with center involved diabetic macular edema. JAMA Ophthalmol. 2014;132:1309–16.
17. Nadri G, Saxena S, Stefanickova J, Ziak P, Benacka J, Gilhotra JS, Kruzliak P. Disorganization of retinal inner layers correlates with ellipsoid zone disruption and retinal nerve fiber layer thinning in diabetic retinopathy. J Diabet Complications. 2019;33(8):550–3.
18. Vujosevic S, Bini S, Torresin T, Berton M, Midena G, Parrozzani R, Martini F, Pucci P, Daniele AR, Cavarzeran F, Midena E. Hyperreflective retinal spots in normal and diabetic eyes: B-scan and en face spectral domain optical coherence tomography evaluation. Retina. 2017;37(6):1092–103.
19. Bolz M, Schmidt-Erfurth U, Deak G, Mylonas G, Kriechbaum K, Scholda C, Diabetic Retinopathy Research Group Vienna. Optical coherence tomographic hyperreflective foci: a morphologic sign of lipid extravasation in diabetic macular edema. Ophthalmology. 2009;116(5):914–20.
20. Huang CH, Yang CH, Hsieh YT, Yang CM, Ho TC, Lai TT. Hyperreflective foci in predicting the treatment outcomes of diabetic macular oedema after anti-vascular endothelial growth factor therapy. Sci Rep. 2021;11(1):1–9.
21. Mao J, Zhang S, Zheng Z, et al. Prediction of anti-VEGF efficacy in diabetic macular oedema using intraocular cytokines and macular optical coherence tomography. Acta Ophthalmol. 2021;100(4):e891–8. https://doi.org/10.1111/aos.15008.
22. Kang JW, Lee H, Chung H, Kim HC. Correlation between optical coherence tomographic hyperreflective foci and visual outcomes after intravitreal bevacizumab for macular edema in branch retinal vein occlusion. Graefes Arch Clin Exp Ophthalmol. 2014;252(9):1413–21. https://doi.org/10.1007/s00417-014-2595-5.
23. Shin YU, Hong EH, Lim HW, et al. Quantitative evaluation of hard exudates in diabetic macular edema after short-term intravitreal triamcinolone, dexamethasone implant or bevacizumab injections. BMC Ophthalmol. 2017;17:182.
24. Wu J, Zhang C, Yang Q, Xie H, Zhang J, Qiu Q, Liu K, Luo D, Liu F, Zhang J. Imaging hyperreflective foci as an inflammatory biomarker after anti-VEGF treatment in neovascular age-related macular degeneration patients with optical coherence tomography angiography. Biomed Res Int. 2021;2021:6648191.
25. Yanoff M, Fine BS, Brucker AJ, et al. Pathology of human cystoid macular edema. Surv Ophthalmol. 1984;28:505–11.
26. Yalçın NG, Özdek Ş. The relationship between macular cyst formation and ischemia in diabetic macular edema. Turk J Ophthalmol. 2019;49:194–200.
27. Reznicek L, Cserhati S, Seidensticker F, et al. Functional and morphological changes in diabetic macular edema over the course of antivascular endothelial growth factor treatment. Acta Ophthalmol. 2013;91:e529–36.
28. Al Faran A, Mousa A, Al Shamsi H, et al. Spectral domain optical coherence tomography predictors of visual outcome in diabetic cystoid macular edema after bevacizumab injection. Retina. 2014;34:1208–15.
29. Vujosevic S, Torresin T, Berton M, Bini S, Convento E, Midena E. Diabetic macular edema with and without subfoveal neuroretinal detachment: two different morphologic and functional entities. Am J Ophthalmol. 2017;181:149–55. https://doi.org/10.1016/j.ajo.2017.06.026.
30. Gaucher D, Sebah C, Erginay A, Haouchine B, Tadayoni R, Gaudric A, Massin P. Optical coherence tomography features during the evolution of serous retinal detachment in patients with diabetic macular edema. Am J Ophthalmol. 2008;145(2):289–96.
31. Ozdemir H, Karacorlu M, Karacorlu S. Serous macular detachment in diabetic cystoid macular oedema. Acta Ophthalmol Scand. 2005;83(1):63–6.
32. Sonoda S, Sakamoto T, Yamashita T, Shirasawa M, Otsuka H, Sonoda Y. Retinal morphologic changes and concentrations of cytokines in eyes with diabetic macular edema. Retina. 2014;34(4):741–8.
33. Funatsu H, Yamashita H, Noma H, Mimura T, Yamashita T, Hori S. Increased levels of vascular endothelial growth factor and interleukin-6 in the aqueous humor of diabetics with macular edema. Am J Ophthalmol. 2002;133(1):70–7.
34. Sophie R, Lu N, Campochiaro PA. Predictors of functional and anatomic outcomes in patients with diabetic macular edema treated with ranibizumab. Ophthalmology. 2015;122:1395–401.
35. Korobelnik J-F, Lu C, Katz TA, et al. Effect of baseline subretinal fluid on treatment outcomes in VIVID-DME and VISTA-DME studies. Ophthalmol Retina. 2019;3:663–9.
36. Zur D, Iglicki M, Busch C, Invernizzi A, Mariussi M, Loewenstein A, Cebeci Z, Chhablani JK, Chaikitmongkol V, Couturier A, Fraser-Bell S. OCT biomarkers as functional outcome predictors in diabetic macular edema treated with dexamethasone implant. Ophthalmology. 2018;125(2):267–75.
37. Yamamoto T, Akabane N, Takeuchi S. Vitrectomy for diabetic macular edema: the role of posterior vitreous detachment and epimacular membrane. Am J Ophthalmol. 2001;132:369–77.
38. Ghassemi F, Bazvand F, Roohipoor R, et al. Outcomes of vitrectomy, membranectomy and internal limiting membrane peeling in patients with refractory diabetic macular edema and non-tractional epiretinal membrane. J Curr Ophthalmol. 2016;28:199–205.
39. Koc F, Güven YZ, Egrilmez D, Aydın E. Optical coherence tomography biomarkers in bilateral diabetic macular edema patients with asymmetric anti-VEGF response. In: Seminars in ophthalmology. Milton Park: Taylor & Francis; 2021. p. 1–8.
40. Forooghian F, Stetson PF, Meyer SA, et al. Relationship between photoreceptor outer segment length and visual acuity in diabetic macular edema. Retina. 2010;30:63–70.
41. Wong RLM, Lee JWY, Yau GSK, Wong IYH. Relationship between outer retinal layers thickness and visual acuity in diabetic macular edema. Biomed Res Int. 2015;2015:981471.
42. Damian I, Nicoara SD. Optical coherence tomography biomarkers of the outer blood—retina barrier in patients with diabetic macular oedema. J Diabetes Res. 2020;2020:8880586.
43. Reznicek L, Kernt M, Haritoglou C, Kampik A, Ulbig M, Neubauer AS. In vivo characterization of ischemic retina in diabetic retinopathy. Clin Ophthalmol. 2010;2011(5):31–5.
44. Boynton GE, Stem MS, Kwark L, Jackson GR, Farsiu S, Gardner TW. Multimodal characterization of proliferative diabetic retinopathy reveals alterations in outer retinal function and structure. Ophthalmology. 2015;122(5):957–67.
45. Arrigo A, Aragona E, Capone L, Lattanzio R, Zollet P, Bandello F. Foveal eversion: a possible biomarker of persistent diabetic macular edema. Ophthalmol Therapy. 2021;10(1):115–26.
46. Uji A, Murakami T, Unoki N, Ogino K, Horii T, Yoshitake S, Dodo Y, Yoshimura N. Parallelism for quantitative image analysis of photoreceptor–retinal pigment epithelium complex alterations in diabetic macular edema. Invest Ophthalmol Vis Sci. 2014;55(5):3361–7.
47. Rayess N, Rahimy E, Ying G-S, et al. Baseline choroidal thickness as a predictor for response to anti-vascular endothelial growth factor therapy in diabetic macular edema. Am J Ophthalmol. 2015;159:85–91.

48. Agrawal R, Gupta P, Tan K-A, et al. Choroidalvascularity index as a measure of vascular status of the choroid: measurements in healthy eyes from a population-based study. Sci Rep. 2016;6:21090.
49. Tan K-A, Laude A, Yip V, et al. Choroidal vascularity index—a novel optical coherence tomography parameter for disease monitoring in diabetes mellitus. Acta Ophthalmol. 2016;94:e612–6.
50. Roy R, Saurabh K, Shah D, et al. Choroidal hyperreflective foci: a novel spectral domain optical coherence tomography biomarker in eyes with diabetic macular edema. Asia Pac J Ophthalmol. 2019;8:314–8.
51. Salz DA, de Carlo TE, Adhi M, et al. Select features of diabetic retinopathy on swept-source optical coherence tomographic angiography compared with fluorescein angiography and normal eyes. JAMA Ophthalmol. 2016;134:644–50.
52. Moein H-R, Novais EA, Rebhun CB, et al. Optical coherence tomography angiography to detect macular capillary ischemia in patients with inner retinal changes after resolved diabetic macular edema. Retina. 2018;38:2277–84.
53. Hsieh YT, Alam MN, Le D, et al. OCT angiography biomarkers for predicting visual outcomes after ranibizumab treatment for diabetic macular edema. Ophthalmol Retina. 2019;3(10):826–34.
54. AttaAllah HR, Mohamed AA, Ali MA. Macular vessels density in diabetic retinopathy: quantitative assessment using optical coherence tomography angiography. Int Ophthalmol. 2019;39(8):1845–59.
55. Tang FY, Chan EO, Sun Z, Wong R, Lok J, Szeto S, Chan JC, Lam A, Tham CC, Ng DS, Cheung CY. Clinically relevant factors associated with quantitative optical coherence tomography angiography metrics in deep capillary plexus in patients with diabetes. Eye Vis. 2020;7(1):1–1.
56. Onishi AC, Nesper PL, Roberts PK, et al. Importance of considering the middle capillary plexus on OCT angiography in diabetic retinopathy. Invest Ophthalmol Vis Sci. 2018;59(5):2167–76.

4 Optical Coherence Tomography Angiography in Diabetic Macular Edema

Mariana Lafetá, Ricardo Luz Leitão Guerra, Josef Christian Huemer, and Eduardo A. Novais

4.1 Introduction

Diabetic retinopathy (DR) is one of the leading causes of blindness worldwide. It is the number one cause of blindness affecting the working-age population in developed countries. To prevent further sight loss from diabetes, it is essential to make an early diagnosis and predict prognosis to optimize treatment for each patient. The development of high-speed Fourier-domain detection, which forms the basis for both spectral domain (SD) and swept source (SS) optical coherence tomography (OCT) and OCT angiography (OCT-a) instruments, represented a decisive technological advance. Fourier-domain devices have substantially increased A-scan rates and signal-to-noise ratios compared to early time-domain devices. Thus, with such advanced imaging, it is possible to study potential biomarkers for disease activity and prognosis, allowing a better understanding of the underlying disease.

M. Lafetá
Department of Ophthalmology, H Olhos São Gonçalo, São Gonçalo, Brazil

R. L. L. Guerra
Retina Department, Leitão Guerra – Oftalmologia, Salvador, Brazil
e-mail: ricardo@leitaoguerra.com.br

J. C. Huemer
Medical Retina Service, Moorfields Eye Hospital NHS Foundation Trust, London, UK
e-mail: josef.huemer1@nhs.net

E. A. Novais (✉)
Department of Ophthalmology, The Federal University of São Paulo, School of Medicine, São Paulo, Brazil
e-mail: eduardo@novais.md

4.2 Diabetic Macular Edema Biomarkers in OCT

The use of OCT has become imperative in the follow-up of DR. The acquisition of high-definition cross-sectional scans allows for a better appreciation of retinal and choroidal anatomy in great detail. In diabetic macular edema (DME), many signs have been identified that may help physicians predict prognosis and define the best treatment.

4.2.1 Bridging Retinal Processes

Bridging retinal processes are vertical remnants of retinal tissue (Fig. 4.1), believed to be mainly constituted by Muller and bipolar cells stretched between cystic cavities and allow the connection between inner and outer retinal layers. Their presence is associated with better visual outcomes after treatment, and they represent a reliable biomarker for visual prognosis [1]. Eyes without bridging retinal processes tend to evolve to foveal atrophy and worse visual acuity, despite resolution of cystoid spaces [2].

4.2.2 Choroidal Vascular Index

The study of the choroid has shown new surprising results and has allowed the discovery of new parameters. Choroidal vascularity index (CVI) is described as the ratio of choroidal vascular area to total choroidal area (Fig. 4.2). Recent studies have found that diabetic patients may show decreased CVI, even in normal thickness choroids. These changes not only seem to correlate with the progression of DR, but they can appear before the onset of DR. Thus, CVI may be an essential biomarker allowing the detection of early ocular disease and also as a progression indicator [3–5].

S. Saxena et al. (eds.), *Diabetic Macular Edema*, https://doi.org/10.1007/978-981-19-7307-9_4

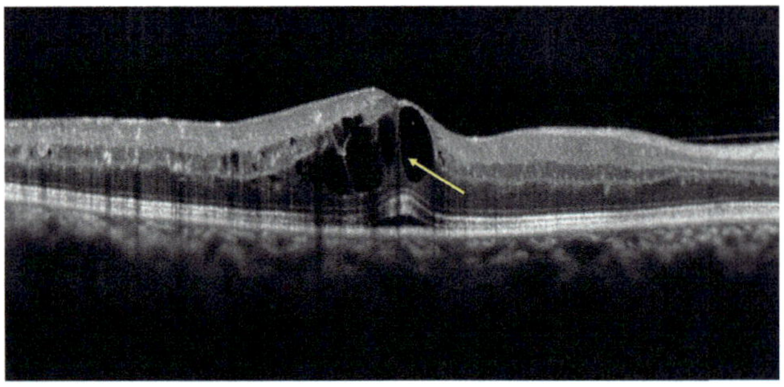

Fig. 4.1 Diabetic patient presenting intraretinal cystoid spaces separated by bridging retinal processes (yellow arrow). We can also observe the presence of a subfoveal neurosensory detachment and some hyperreflective retinal foci

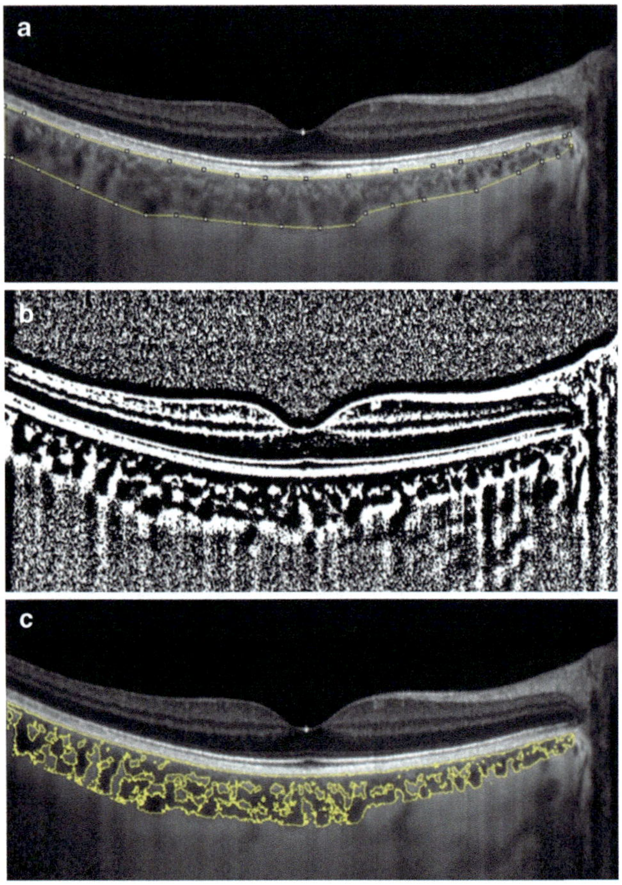

Fig. 4.2 (**a**) Boundaries are traced to calculate the total choroidal area (yellow lines); (**b**) the image is binarized (**b**), and a color threshold tool is used to select the dark pixels, representing the luminal area (yellow lines) (**c**). The CVI is calculated dividing luminal area by total choroidal area. OCT images, by Giuseppe Giannaccare. This image is available in the following link https://www.ncbi.nlm.nih.gov/core/lw/2.0/html/tileshop_pmc/tileshop_pmc_inline.html?title=Click%20on%20image%20to%20zoom&p=PMC3&id=7074450_jcm-09-00595-g001.jpg and is licensed under a Creative Commons Attribution-NonCommercial-NoDerivatives 4.0 International License—https://creativecommons.org/licenses/by-nc-nd/4.0/

4.2.3 Disorganization of Retinal Inner Layers

Disorganization of retinal inner layers (DRIL) can be defined as the inability to differentiate the retinal layers between the ganglion cell layer and the outer plexiform layer (Fig. 4.3). It is measured by its horizontal extent in the central retinal zone. It is believed that DRIL is a sign of damage in the structures located in the inner retinal layers, such as amacrine cells, bipolar cells, and axons [2]. When present, DRIL is usually associated with worse visual acuity and poor prognosis, especially if it is greater than 500 μm or >50% in the central 1000 μm zone. Presence of DRIL can be an important biomarker during DME treatment, allowing to predict visual prognosis. Indeed, an increase in DRIL is correlated to a decline in visual acuity, and a decrease in DRIL is correlated to better visual acuity [6]. In the context of macular capillary non-perfusion, DRIL has also been associated with the size of FAZ and with its presence in 84% of non-perfused areas [7–9]. If found in patients with no signs of DR, it can indicate early neural damage [4]. In conclusion, DRIL is an important biomarker for visual prognosis, disease severity, and vascular and other anatomic changes in DME.

4.2.4 Hyperreflective Retinal Foci and Hard Exudates

In the context of diabetes, hyperreflective retinal foci (HRF) reveal the presence of intraretinal lipoproteins that leak out from a break of the inner blood–retinal barrier, usually seen in inflammatory processes. Therefore, HRF may be important biomarkers for retinal inflammation. They are small, measuring less than 30 μm, their reflectivity is similar to the retinal nerve fiber layer (RNFL), and they do not cause backshadowing (Fig. 4.4). In OCT, their presence is usually noticed, at first, in the inner retinal layers (IRL), and then, they can move to the outer layers [10]. In patients presenting serous subfoveal detachment, subretinal HRF was described in association with subretinal hard exudates after detachment resolution [11]. Both anti-vascular endothelial growth factor (VEGF) therapy and corticosteroid implants have been shown to decrease HRF in number and size. However, corticosteroid implants showed better outcomes in patients with DME, probably due to its inflammatory etiology [10]. Recent studies suggest that patients with a higher number of HRF on OCT present with early recurrence of DME after steroid implants and should be followed closely.

Hard exudates are hyperreflective spots, similar to HRF but larger (>30 μm), and usually associated with back-

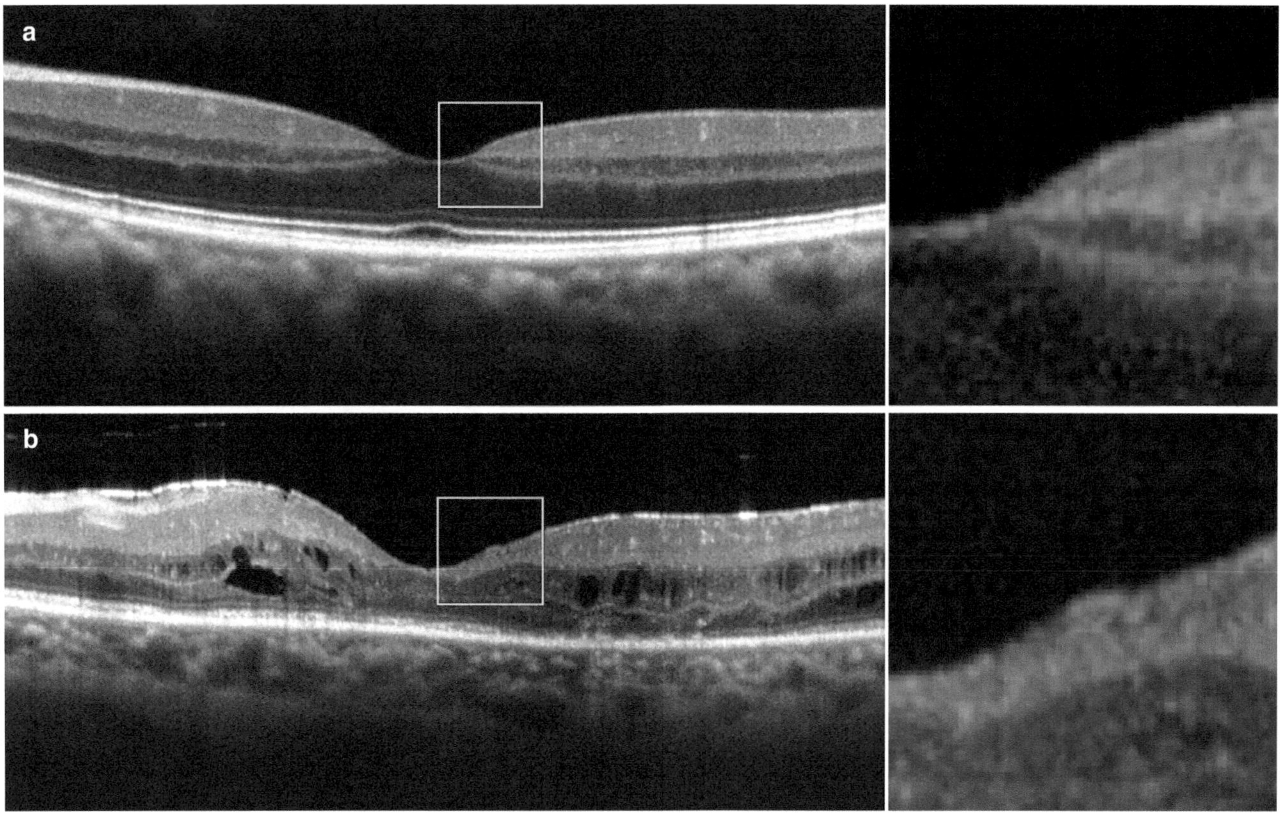

Fig. 4.3 Comparison between a (**a**) normal retina with organized inner retinal layers and (**b**) disorganized inner retinal layers (DRIL)

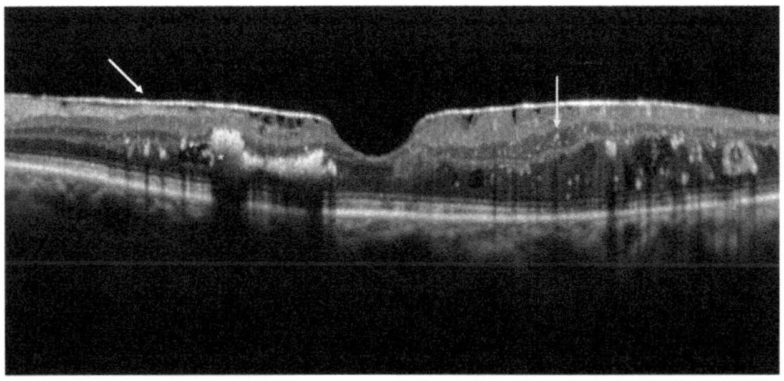

Fig. 4.4 Presence of confluent hard exudates (yellow asterisk), hyperreflective intraretinal foci (yellow arrow), and epiretinal membrane (white arrow)

shadowing (Fig. 4.4). They result from the breakdown of the inner blood–retinal barrier and are formed by accumulating lipid proteins. A high serum lipid level is associated with greater central macular involvement and hard exudates subfoveal accumulation [2]. DME with an expressive amount of hard exudates seems to respond better to intravitreal steroids than to anti-VEGF agents [12].

4.2.5 Hyperreflective Choroidal Foci

Hyperreflective choroidal foci (HCF) are similar to HRF but are located in the choroidal layers (Fig. 4.5) [13]. Similar dots were reported in Stargardt's disease, where choroidal dots were described as lipofuscin depositions. The pathophysiology of HCF is not quite elucidated yet, and a migration from the retina to the choroid after external limiting membrane (ELM) and ellipsoid zone (EZ) disruption is hypothesized. HCF have been associated with decreased visual acuity and are more prevalent in eyes with proliferative diabetic retinopathy (PDR) [2].

4.2.6 Intraretinal Cystoid Spaces

Intraretinal cystoid spaces (ICS) are hyporeflective oval-shaped findings localized between the inner and outer retina (Fig. 4.5). They represent extracellular fluid accumulation in the retina due to loss of inner blood–retinal barrier in patients with diabetes [14, 15]. The levels of VEGF play an important

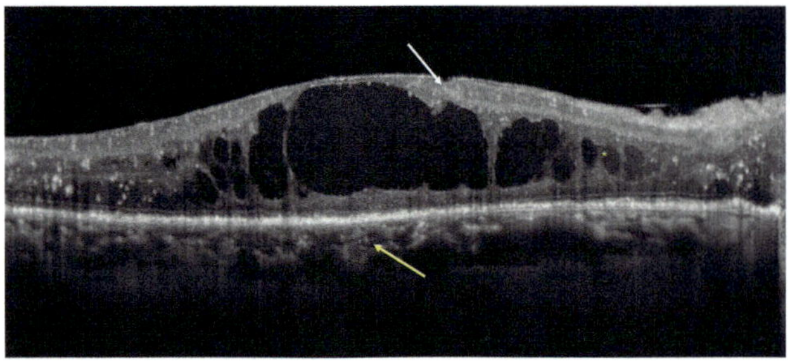

Fig. 4.5 Presence of discrete choroidal hyperreflective foci (yellow arrow), intraretinal cystoid spaces (yellow asterisk), hard exudates, and DRIL (white arrow)

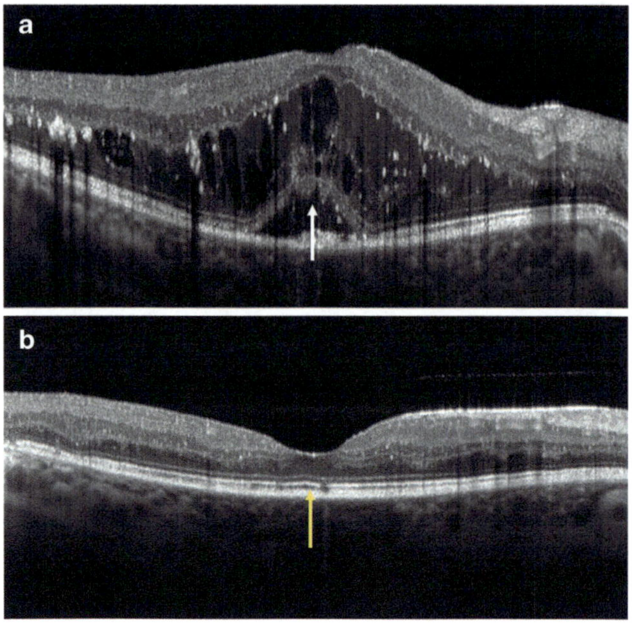

Fig. 4.6 (**a**) Diabetic macular edema with intraretinal cystoid spaces, hyperreflective intrarretinal foci, hard exudates, neurosensory subfoveal detachment with continuous external limiting membrane (ELM) and ellipsoid zone (EZ) (white arrow). (**b**) Same patient after anti-VEGF treatment with preserved ELM and EZ (yellow arrow)

role in ICS formation, and anti-VEGF therapy has shown to be an excellent treatment, with the reduction of vessel permeability and decrease of ICS in number and size [16]. In DME, the presence of cystoid spaces is related to worse visual outcomes [17]. In advanced stages, larger cysts (>200 μm) in the outer nuclear layer (ONL) can affect the integrity of photoreceptors, therefore being associated with worse outcomes when compared to smaller cysts in the inner retinal layers. The ICS can be completely hyporeflective or associated with hyperreflective signals within the cyst and can be categorized according to their size: small (<100 μm), large (101–200 μm), or giant (>200 μm). Cysts tend to increase in size, accordingly to the extent of macular ischemia, and hence present worse visual outcomes. Other characteristics may be associated with poorer prognosis, such as the location of the cysts and the degree of anatomical damage caused in inner and outer retinal layers by them [18].

4.2.7 Integrity of External Limiting Membrane and Ellipsoid Zone

The health of the outer retinal layers is directly related to visual outcomes. Retinal ELM and EZ are critical indicators of the integrity of the outer retina (Fig. 4.6). They can be classified as continuous, partly disrupted, or completely disrupted. Chronic DME may present more disrupted outer retinal layers and worse visual acuity results [11].

4.2.8 Retinal Thickness

In DME, the increased retinal thickness can be observed due to a breakdown of the blood–retinal barrier and extravasation of fluid into the retina. In SD-OCT, it is possible to measure the size of the edema and compare it with former scans as treatment is administrated (Fig. 4.7). Although central subfield thickness (CST) is an easy way to quantify the edema, it is not a good tool for evaluating DME's degree or prognosis studies. In fact, qualitative biomarkers seem to be more critical when predicting visual outcomes. In two patients with the same retinal thickness, resolution of DME can present different results, depending on the presence of bridging retinal processes, the extent of retinal involvement, presence or absence of DRIL, and other qualitative characteristics [19].

4.2.9 Photoreceptor Outer Segment

Photoreceptor outer segment (PROS) is defined by the distance between the retinal pigment epithelium (RPE) and the junction between the photoreceptor inner-outer segment. Their length appears to be lesser in patients with DR than in patients with no DR and showed a better correlation with visual acuity than other parameters such as macular thickness [20, 21].

4.2.10 Subfoveal Choroidal Thickness

Choroidal well-functioning is fundamental for retinal health, especially in the foveal area. Patients with greater choroidal thickness at baseline presented a better functional and anatomical response to treatment with anti-VEGF. Subfoveal choroidal thickness increases with the severity of DR, where the levels of VEGF may lead to vasodilation and increased choroidal thickness. These patients are thought to have less

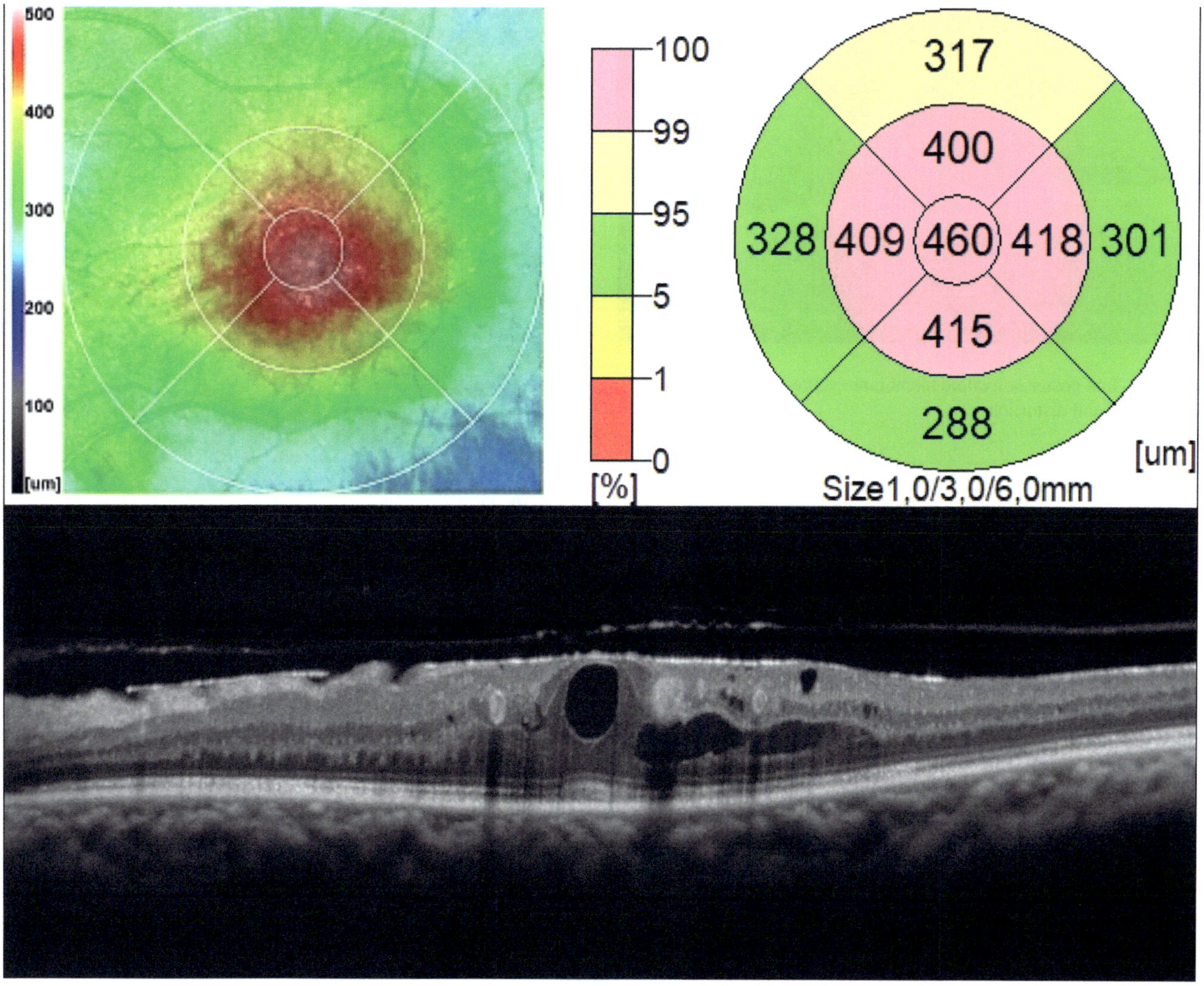

Fig. 4.7 Quantitative analysis showing the macular thickness maps and the corresponding B-scan

ischemic outer retina than those with the thinner choroid, presenting better visual outcomes after treatment [22].

4.2.11 Subfoveal Neurosensory Detachment

Subfoveal neurosensory detachment is present in 15–30% of patients with DME. In patients with hypoalbuminemia, changes in intravascular osmotic pressure and hydrostatic pressures can lead to fluid accumulation in the subretinal space (Fig. 4.8). Hence, subfoveal neurosensory detachment seems to directly relate to serum albumin levels, which can be a sensitive marker for detecting the presence of subretinal fluid (SRF) [23]. As for prognosis analysis, results regarding the presence of SRF are conflicting. While some studies show a protective role in final visual and anatomical outcomes, other studies demonstrate that SRF might be related to poor visual results [24, 25]. The RESTORE study and post-hoc analysis of the RISE/RIDE studies demonstrated that SRF at baseline was associated with better visual outcomes and better response to ranibizumab treatment. These eyes with SRF at baseline also seem to respond better to aflibercept treatment and dexamethasone implants [26, 27].

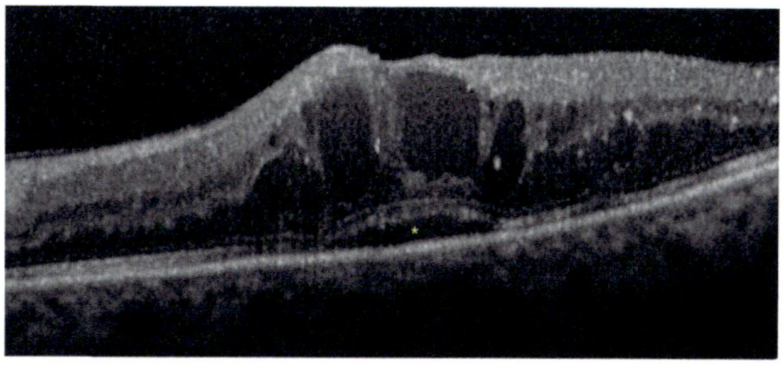

Fig. 4.8 Subfoveal neurosensory detachment (asterisk mark) associated with large intraretinal cystoid spaces

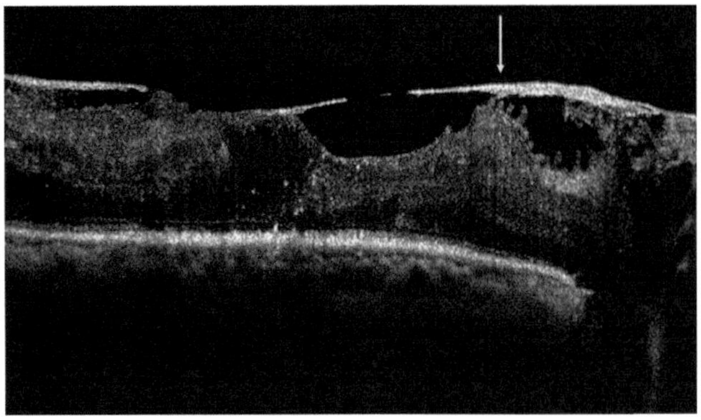

Fig. 4.9 Taut posterior hyaloid membrane (yellow arrow) causing retinal traction and distortion

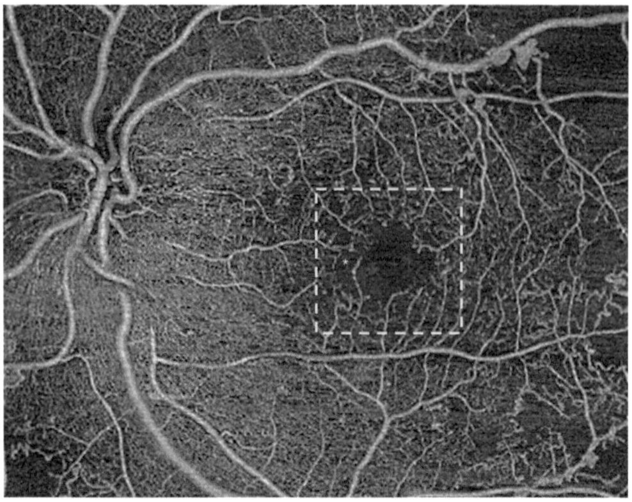

Fig. 4.10 OCT-a of a diabetic patient showing enlarged foveal avascular zone and increased intercapillary spacing (yellow asterisk)

Further studies are needed to affirm the exact effect of SRF in DME.

4.2.12 Taut Posterior Hyaloid Membrane

The vitreous body in diabetic patients can present different characteristics such as stronger adhesions, which may lead to an anomalous posterior vitreous detachment or retinal traction. Hyaloid can form a tight sheet in the posterior pole, resulting in retinal distortion and traction, defined as a taut posterior hyaloid membrane (Fig. 4.9). Patients presenting this feature may benefit from surgical treatment to remove the traction [2].

4.3 DME Biomarkers in OCT Angiography

OCT angiography allows a noninvasive study of retinal vascular plexuses in greater detail, allowing the study of each plexus separately, which helps better understand DR. New studies have described some particular findings present in patients with DME that could help treatment and follow-up.

4.3.1 Foveal Avascular Zone

OCT-a has allowed the study of the FAZ in greater detail (Fig. 4.10). Indeed, many parameters can be analyzed to assess changes in the FAZ, such as its axis ratio, area, or perimeter [28]. FAZ enlargement is a result of microvascular perifoveal occlusions [2].

A larger FAZ has been shown to be associated with more severe DR, thinner subfoveal choroidal thickness, shorter axial length, and lower body mass index (BMI) [29]. On deep plexus slabs, diabetic patients appear to have a larger FAZ than patients in the control group, FAZ enlargement, and loss of symmetry may appear even before the signs of DR. A larger FAZ is also associated with the presence of DRIL and with worse visual outcomes [30].

4.3.2 Intercapillary Spacing

Intercapillary spacing has shown to be a good indicator of early capillary dropouts and areas of ischemia (Fig. 4.10). Compared to VD and foveal avascular zone (FAZ), intercapillary spacing seems the most sensitive parameter for detecting vascular abnormalities. However, larger studies are necessary to confirm the importance of intercapillary spacing as a reliable biomarker [31].

4.3.3 Microaneurysms, Intraretinal Microvascular Abnormalities, Neovascularization, Nonperfusion Areas

OCT-a allows differentiating intraretinal microvascular abnormalities (IRMAs), that appear as localized areas of increased intraretinal blood flow from neovessels that grow above the ILM (Fig. 4.11). Studies have shown that OCT-a has higher detection rates of IRMAs than color fundus photography. Widefield OCT-a seems to be as sensitive as ultrawide field fluorescein angiography (FA) in detecting retinal and optic disc neovascularization (Fig. 4.11), also allowing to perception subtle changes of flow after treatment [32]. This modality also seems to have a higher sensitivity in detecting capillary non-perfusion since it is not affected by leakage (Fig. 4.12). Microaneurysms (MA) can also be stud-

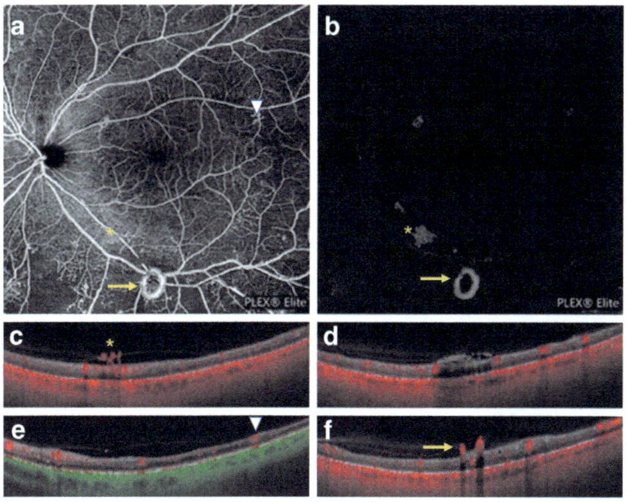

Fig. 4.11 Central 12×12 mm en face optical coherence tomography angiography (OCTA) segmented at the superficial (**a**) and vitreoretinal interface (**b**). OCTA B-scans at different levels illustrate various diabetic retinopathy signs: neovascularisation elsewhere (yellow star), seen as a preretinal hyperreflective material (PRHM) in the B-scan (**c**), with evident flow signals, which could be detected as a vascular network at the VRI level (**b**); intraretinal microvascular abnormalities (white arrowhead) seen on the en face OCTA at the superficial slab (**a**) as abnormally dilated blood vessels without any evident PRHM on the B-scan (**e**); preretinal hemorrhage characterized by PRHM with the absence of flow signals on OCTA B-scan along with backshadowing (**d**); vascular loops (yellow arrow) seen at the VRI level (**b**) and at the B-scan (**f**)

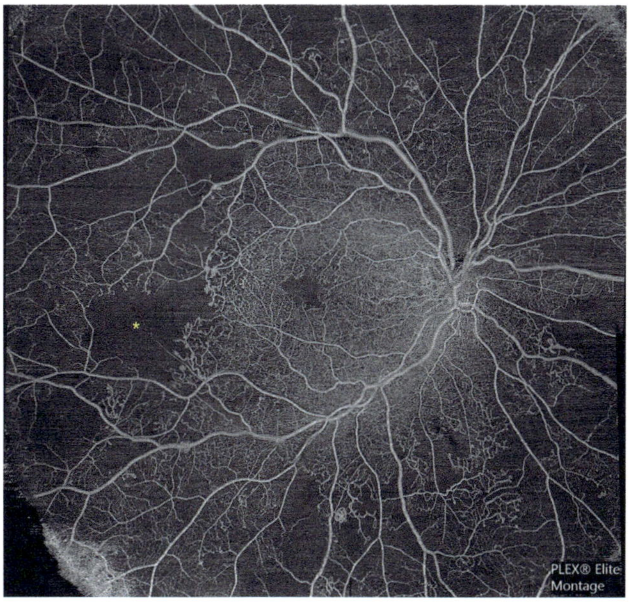

Fig. 4.12 Widefield OCT-a showing areas of nonperfusion (yellow asterisk), IRMAs, neovessels, reduced vascular density, and enlarged FAZ

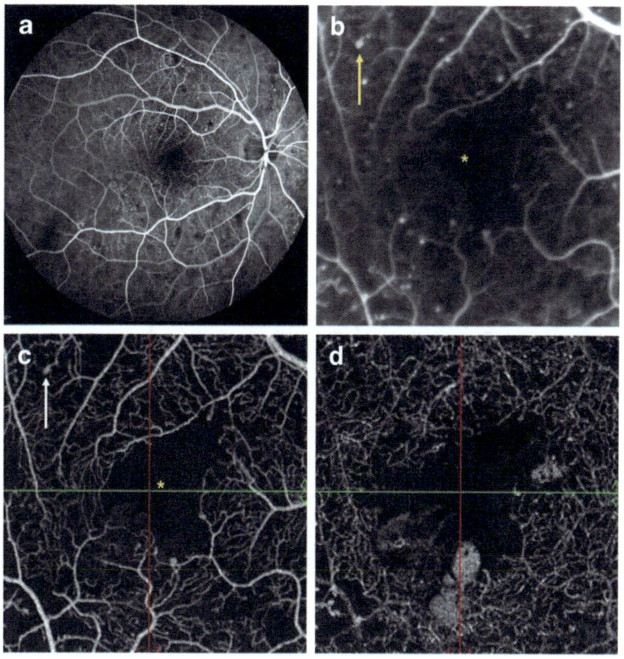

Fig. 4.13 Multimodal imaging of a 53-year-old patient with diabetic retinopathy. Foveal avascular zone (FAZ) and microaneurysms count comparison between fluorescein angiography (FA) and optical coherence tomography angiography (OCTA). (**a**) FA image. (**b**) 3 × 3 mm area of the FA showing the FAZ enlargement (yellow asterisk and microaneurysms (yellow arrow). (**c**) 3 × 3 mm OCTA of superficial capillary plexus showing the FAZ enlargement (yellow asterisk) and corresponding microaneurysm (white arrow). (**d**) OCTA of deep capillary plexus

ied in OCT-a (Fig. 4.13). There seems to be a relation between its location, visibility, and the development of extracellular fluid at 1 year. Deeper located MA, with the detectable flow, may be considered as biomarkers for the development of extracellular fluid accumulation in patients with NPDR [33].

4.3.4 Retinal Vascular Density

Vessel density (VD) can be measured by the ratio of vessel area to the total measured area [34]. The VD can decrease in diabetic patients, with or without DR, in both superficial (SCP) and deep capillary plexus (DCP) (Fig. 4.14) [35, 36]. Retinal VD does not seem to change after corticosteroids injections. Nevertheless, VD in the choriocapillaris seems to increase after the same treatment. Accordingly, VD in DCP seems to be significantly decreased in eyes with DME and is associated with worse visual outcomes. Indeed, the DCP supplies 10–15% of oxygen to the photoreceptors and changes in its morphology could indicate visual prognosis at early stages. In one study, lower VD in the DCP was the only indicator of non-proliferative diabetic retinopathy (NPDR) progression [37]. Studies suggest that VD is associated with the severity of DR, but some authors have pointed that, in eyes without predominantly peripheral lesions (PPL) that may be true, while in eyes presenting PPL, there was no association between VD and DR severity [38].

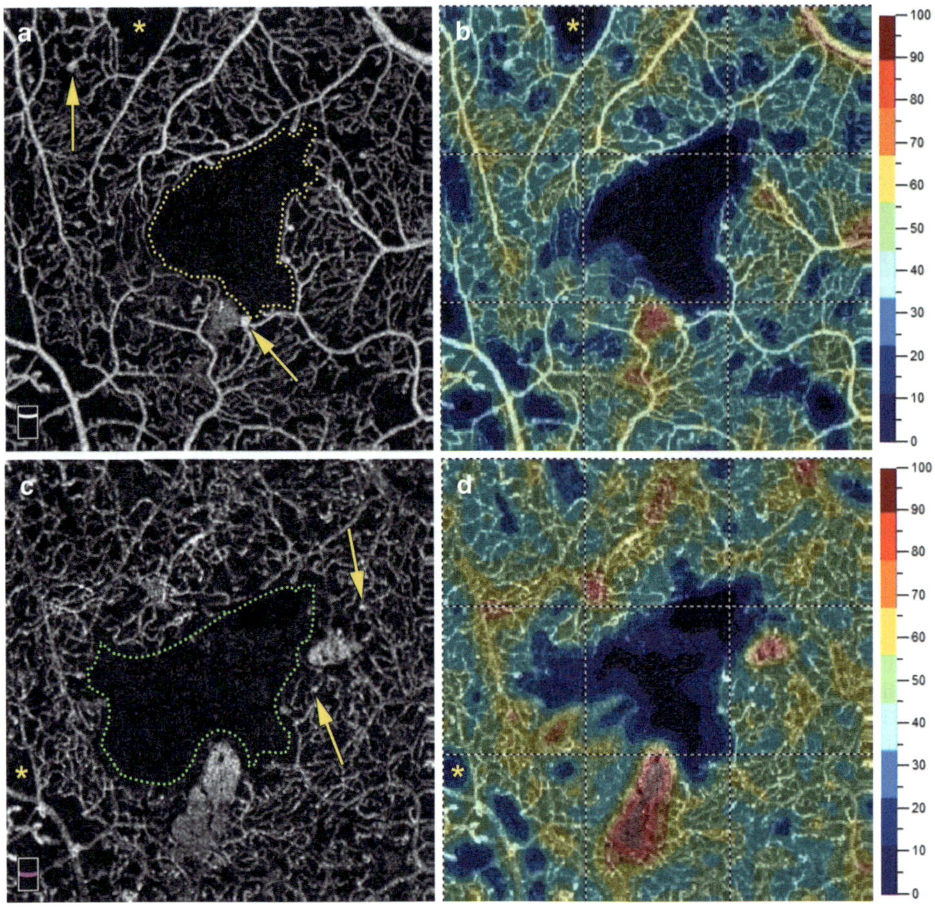

e

OCT Thickness ILM-RPE & Vessel Density

Density (%)	Section	Thickness (μm)
38.64	Whole Image	N/A
14.29	Fovea	271
41.04	ParaFovea	338
40.31	- Superior-Hemi	329
41.77	- Inferior-Hemi	346
41.40	- Tempo	322
40.06	- Superior	338
39.81	- Nasal	327
42.91	- Inferior	363

Grid-based Vessel Density (%)

40.98	41.94	40.01
40.30	15.16	45.02
37.73	47.11	39.48

OCT Thickness ILM-RPE & Vessel Density

Density (%)	Section	Thickness (μm)
45.78	Whole Image	N/A
19.02	Fovea	271
48.64	ParaFovea	338
46.79	- Superior-Hemi	329
50.48	- Inferior-Hemi	346
47.78	- Tempo	322
47.70	- Superior	338
46.32	- Nasal	327
52.75	- Inferior	363

Grid-based Vessel Density (%)

47.10	49.73	49.57
46.87	20.49	49.24
43.83	56.98	48.51

Fig. 4.14 Vascular density map of a diabetic patient. Superficial (**a**) and deep plexuses (**c**) show foveal avascular zone (FAZ) enlargement (dotted lines) and microaneurysms (yellow arrows). Yellow asterisks indicate areas of non-perfusion, which correlates to decreasedvascular density in both superficial (**b**) and deep plexuses (**d**). Quantitative vessel density analysis and its correlation with retinal OCT thickness (**e**)

4.3.5 Suspended Scattering Particles in Motion

Suspended scattering particles in motion (SSPiM) are extravascular signals that appear in OCT-a, inside retinal fluid pockets, near vascular–avascular junctions, more commonly in the Henle fiber layer (Fig. 4.15) [39]. SSPiM are not exclusively related to DME and can be found in other exudative maculopathies [40]. It is believed that extravasated lipids are involved in their formation, and in some patients, they decrease as hard exudates are formed [41].

In summary, recent developments in OCT and OCT-a have given us the basis for analyzing microstructural details of retina and choroid and have become obligatory in everyday practice in DR treatment. Biomarkers help detect subclinical disease and retinal vascular changes, even before clinically detectable changes, or development of visual symptoms, also giving us information about the prognosis after treatment and should be part of our practice in treating DR. The study of this noninvasive acquired imaging helps us understand the pathogenesis, assess the diagnosis, monitor disease progression, and respond to treatment.

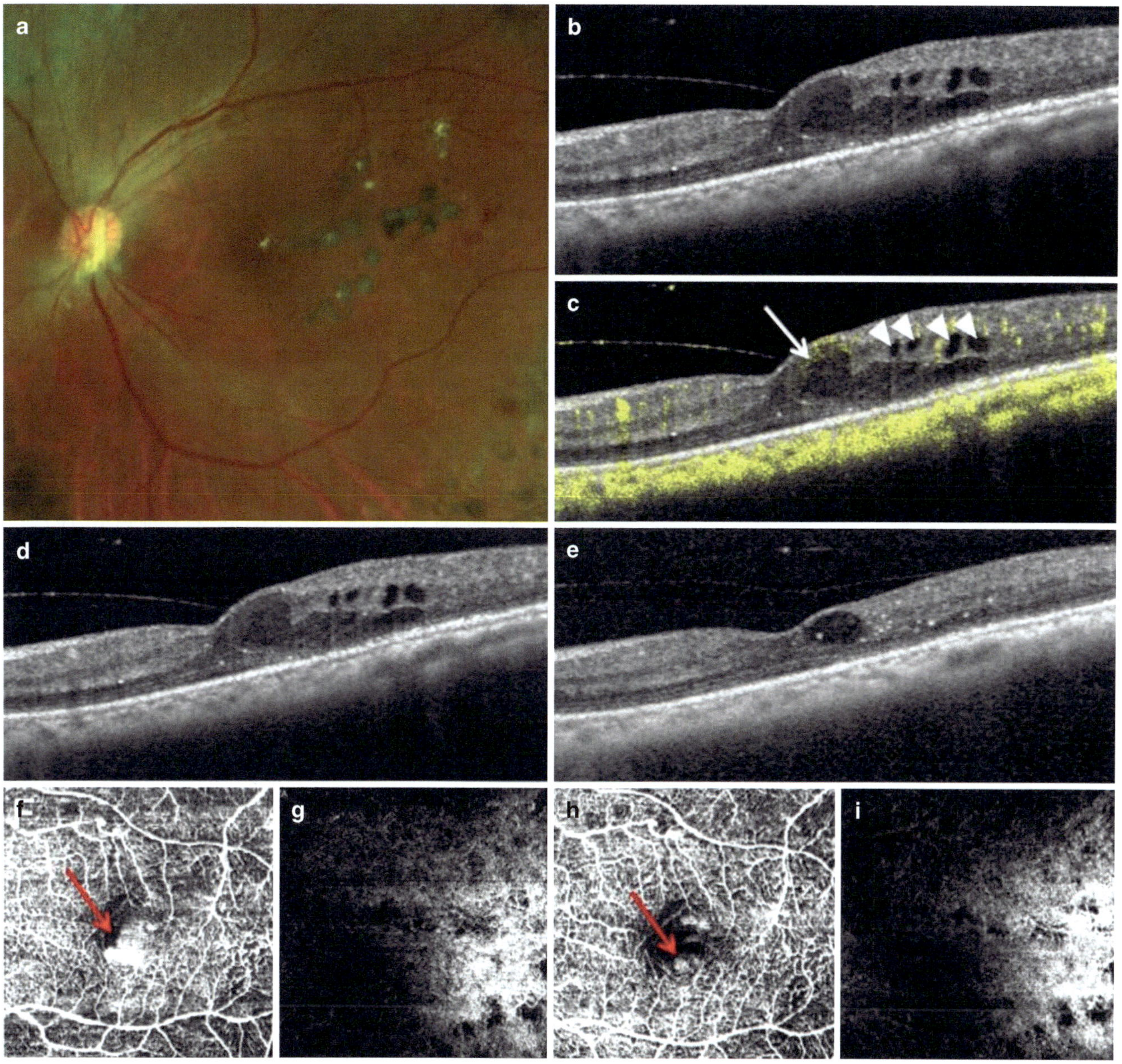

Fig. 4.15 Images of a patient with DME who underwent intravitreal triamcinolone injection, by Jaeryung Oh. (**a**) Fundus photograph. (**b**) Optical coherence tomography (OCT) image. There are several intraretinal cysts. (**c**) OCT image with optical coherence tomography angiography (OCTA) signal. The largest intraretinal cyst (arrow) has OCTA signal, while other intraretinal cysts do not have OCTA signal (arrowhead). (**d**) OCT image before treatment; the largest intraretinal cyst is 0.04 mm^2 in size. (**e**) OCT image 1 month after intravitreal triamcinolone injection; the largest intraretinal cyst size is 0.02 mm^2, a reduction of 48.14%. (**f**) OCTA image including inner nuclear layer (INL) with suspended scattering particles in motion (SSPiM) before treatment (arrow). (**g**) OCTA image including outer nuclear layer (ONL) without SSPiM before treatment. (**h**) OCTA image including INL with decreased SSPiM after treatment (arrow). (**i**) OCTA image including ONL without SSPiM after treatment. This image is available in the following link https://www.ncbi.nlm.nih.gov/core/lw/2.0/html/tileshop_pmc/tileshop_pmc_inline.html?title=Click%20on%20image%20to%20zoom&p=PMC3&id=6949280_41598_2019_55606_Fig3_HTML.jpg, and is licensed under a Creative Commons Attribution-NonCommercial-NoDerivatives 4.0 International License—https://creativecommons.org/licenses/by-nc-nd/4.0/

Financial Disclosure None.

Conflict of Interest None.

References

1. Al Faran A, Mousa A, Al Shamsi H, Al Gaeed A, Ghazi NG. Spectral domain optical coherence tomography predictors of visual outcome in diabetic cystoid macular edema after bevacizumab injection. Retina. 2014;34(6):1208–15.
2. Markan A, Agarwal A, Arora A, Bazgain K, Rana V, Gupta V. Novel imaging biomarkers in diabetic retinopathy and diabetic macular edema. Ther Adv Ophthalmol. 2020;12:2515841420950513.
3. Agrawal R, Gupta P, Tan KA, Cheung CM, Wong TY, Cheng CY. Choroidal vascularity index as a measure of vascular status of the choroid: measurements in healthy eyes from a population-based study. Sci Rep. 2016;6:21090.
4. Kim M, Ha MJ, Choi SY, Park YH. Choroidal vascularity index in type-2 diabetes analyzed by swept-source optical coherence tomography. Sci Rep. 2018;8(1):70.
5. Tan KA, Laude A, Yip V, Loo E, Wong EP, Agrawal R. Choroidal vascularity index - a novel optical coherence tomography parameter for disease monitoring in diabetes mellitus? Acta Ophthalmol. 2016;94(7):e612–e6.
6. Radwan SH, Soliman AZ, Tokarev J, Zhang L, van Kuijk FJ, Koozekanani DD. Association of disorganization of retinal inner layers with vision after resolution of center-involved diabetic macular edema. JAMA Ophthalmol. 2015;133(7):820–5.
7. Balaratnasingam C, Inoue M, Ahn S, McCann J, Dhrami-Gavazi E, Yannuzzi LA, et al. Visual acuity is correlated with the area of the foveal avascular zone in diabetic retinopathy and retinal vein occlusion. Ophthalmology. 2016;123(11):2352–67.
8. Das R, Spence G, Hogg RE, Stevenson M, Chakravarthy U. Disorganization of inner retina and outer retinal morphology in diabetic macular edema. JAMA Ophthalmol. 2018;136(2):202–8.
9. Nicholson L, Ramu J, Triantafyllopoulou I, Patrao NV, Comyn O, Hykin P, et al. Diagnostic accuracy of disorganization of the retinal inner layers in detecting macular capillary non-perfusion in diabetic retinopathy. Clin Exp Ophthalmol. 2015;43(8):735–41.
10. Hwang TS, Jia Y, Gao SS, Bailey ST, Lauer AK, Flaxel CJ, et al. Optical coherence tomography angiography features of diabetic retinopathy. Retina. 2015;35(11):2371–6.
11. Ota M, Nishijima K, Sakamoto A, Murakami T, Takayama K, Horii T, et al. Optical coherence tomographic evaluation of foveal hard exudates in patients with diabetic maculopathy accompanying macular detachment. Ophthalmology. 2010;117(10):1996–2002.
12. Shin YU, Hong EH, Lim HW, Kang MH, Seong M, Cho H. Quantitative evaluation of hard exudates in diabetic macular edema after short-term intravitreal triamcinolone, dexamethasone implant or bevacizumab injections. BMC Ophthalmol. 2017;17(1):182.
13. Roy R, Saurabh K, Shah D, Chowdhury M, Goel S. Choroidal hyperreflective foci: a novel spectral domain optical coherence tomography biomarker in eyes with diabetic macular edema. Asia Pac J Ophthalmol. 2019;8(4):314–8.
14. Fine BS, Brucker AJ. Macular edema and cystoid macular edema. Am J Ophthalmol. 1981;92(4):466–81.
15. Hee MR, Puliafito CA, Wong C, Duker JS, Reichel E, Rutledge B, et al. Quantitative assessment of macular edema with optical coherence tomography. Arch Ophthalmol. 1995;113(8):1019–29.
16. Reznicek L, Cserhati S, Seidensticker F, Liegl R, Kampik A, Ulbig M, et al. Functional and morphological changes in diabetic macular edema over the course of anti-vascular endothelial growth factor treatment. Acta Ophthalmol. 2013;91(7):e529–36.
17. Yanoff M, Fine BS, Brucker AJ, Eagle RC Jr. Pathology of human cystoid macular edema. Surv Ophthalmol. 1984;28(Suppl):505–11.
18. Deak GG, Bolz M, Ritter M, Prager S, Benesch T, Schmidt-Erfurth U, et al. A systematic correlation between morphology and functional alterations in diabetic macular edema. Invest Ophthalmol Vis Sci. 2010;51(12):6710–4.
19. Pelosini L, Hull CC, Boyce JF, McHugh D, Stanford MR, Marshall J. Optical coherence tomography may be used to predict visual acuity in patients with macular edema. Invest Ophthalmol Vis Sci. 2011;52(5):2741–8.
20. Forooghian F, Stetson PF, Meyer SA, Chew EY, Wong WT, Cukras C, et al. Relationship between photoreceptor outer segment length and visual acuity in diabetic macular edema. Retina. 2010;30(1):63–70.
21. Ozkaya A, Alkin Z, Karakucuk Y, Karatas G, Fazil K, Gurkan Erdogan M, et al. Thickness of the retinal photoreceptor outer segment layer in healthy volunteers and in patients with diabetes mellitus without retinopathy, diabetic retinopathy, or diabetic macular edema. Saudi J Ophthalmol. 2017;31(2):69–75.
22. Kim JT, Lee DH, Joe SG, Kim JG, Yoon YH. Changes in choroidal thickness in relation to the severity of retinopathy and macular edema in type 2 diabetic patients. Invest Ophthalmol Vis Sci. 2013;54(5):3378–84.
23. Tsai MJ, Hsieh YT, Shen EP, Peng YJ. Systemic associations with residual subretinal fluid after ranibizumab in diabetic macular edema. J Ophthalmol. 2017;2017:4834201.
24. Giocanti-Auregan A, Hrarat L, Qu LM, Sarda V, Boubaya M, Levy V, et al. Functional and anatomical outcomes in patients with serous retinal detachment in diabetic macular edema treated with ranibizumab. Invest Ophthalmol Vis Sci. 2017;58(2):797–800.
25. Seo KH, Yu SY, Kim M, Kwak HW. Visual and morphologic outcomes of intravitreal ranibizumab for diabetic macular edema based on optical coherence tomography patterns. Retina. 2016;36(3):588–95.
26. Antcliff RJ, Hussain AA, Marshall J. Hydraulic conductivity of fixed retinal tissue after sequential excimer laser ablation: barriers limiting fluid distribution and implications for cystoid macular edema. Arch Ophthalmol. 2001;119(4):539–44.
27. Korobelnik JF, Lu C, Katz TA, Dhoot DS, Loewenstein A, Arnold J, et al. Effect of baseline subretinal fluid on treatment outcomes in VIVID-DME and VISTA-DME studies. Ophthalmol Retina. 2019;3(8):663–9.
28. Johannesen SK, Viken JN, Vergmann AS, Grauslund J. Optical coherence tomography angiography and microvascular changes in diabetic retinopathy: a systematic review. Acta Ophthalmol. 2019;97(1):7–14.
29. Tang FY, Chan EO, Sun Z, Wong R, Lok J, Szeto S, et al. Clinically relevant factors associated with quantitative optical coherence tomography angiography metrics in deep capillary plexus in patients with diabetes. Eye Vis. 2020;7:7.
30. Salz DA, de Carlo TE, Adhi M, Moult E, Choi W, Baumal CR, et al. Select features of diabetic retinopathy on swept-source optical coherence tomographic angiography compared with fluorescein angiography and normal eyes. JAMA Ophthalmol. 2016;134(6):644–50.
31. Bhanushali D, Anegondi N, Gadde SG, Srinivasan P, Chidambara L, Yadav NK, et al. Linking retinal microvasculature features with severity of diabetic retinopathy using optical coherence tomography angiography. Invest Ophthalmol Vis Sci. 2016;57(9):519–25.
32. Cui Y, Zhu Y, Wang JC, Lu Y, Zeng R, Katz R, et al. Comparison of widefield swept-source optical coherence tomography angiography with ultra-widefield colour fundus photography and fluorescein angiography for detection of lesions in diabetic retinopathy. Br J Ophthalmol. 2021;105(4):577–81.

33. Parravano M, De Geronimo D, Scarinci F, Virgili G, Querques L, Varano M, et al. Progression of diabetic microaneurysms according to the internal reflectivity on structural optical coherence tomography and visibility on optical coherence tomography angiography. Am J Ophthalmol. 2019;198:8–16.
34. You Q, Freeman WR, Weinreb RN, Zangwill L, Manalastas PIC, Saunders LJ, et al. Reproducibility of vessel density measurement with optical coherence tomography angiography in eyes with and without retinopathy. Retina. 2017;37(8):1475–82.
35. Al-Sheikh M, Akil H, Pfau M, Sadda SR. Swept-Source OCT angiography imaging of the foveal avascular zone and macular capillary network density in diabetic retinopathy. Invest Ophthalmol Vis Sci. 2016;57(8):3907–13.
36. Carnevali A, Sacconi R, Corbelli E, Tomasso L, Querques L, Zerbini G, et al. Optical coherence tomography angiography analysis of retinal vascular plexuses and choriocapillaris in patients with type 1 diabetes without diabetic retinopathy. Acta Diabetol. 2017;54(7):695–702.
37. Veiby N, Simeunovic A, Heier M, Brunborg C, Saddique N, Moe MC, et al. Associations between macular OCT angiography and nonproliferative diabetic retinopathy in young patients with type 1 diabetes mellitus. J Diabetes Res. 2020;2020:8849116.
38. Ashraf M, Sampani K, Rageh A, Silva PS, Aiello LP, Sun JK. Interaction between the distribution of diabetic retinopathy lesions and the association of optical coherence tomography angiography scans with diabetic retinopathy severity. JAMA Ophthalmol. 2020;138(12):1291–7.
39. Kashani AH, Chen CL, Gahm JK, Zheng F, Richter GM, Rosenfeld PJ, et al. Optical coherence tomography angiography: a comprehensive review of current methods and clinical applications. Prog Retin Eye Res. 2017;60:66–100.
40. Liang MC, Vora RA, Duker JS, Reichel E. Solid-appearing retinal cysts in diabetic macular edema: a novel optical coherence tomography finding. Retin Cases Brief Rep. 2013;7(3):255–8.
41. Kashani AH, Green KM, Kwon J, Chu Z, Zhang Q, Wang RK, et al. Suspended scattering particles in motion: a novel feature of OCT angiography in exudative maculopathies. Ophthalmol Retina. 2018;2(7):694–702.

Targeted Screening of Macular Edema by Spectral Domain Optical Coherence Tomography for Progression of Diabetic Retinopathy: Translational Aspects

5

Sandeep Saxena, Carsten H. Meyer, Jagjit S. Gilhotra, and Levent Akduman

5.1 Introduction

Diabetic retinopathy (DR) is a major microvascular complication of diabetes mellitus. By the year 2025, population with diabetes is expected to increase to an estimated 300 million, with the most significant increase in the developing world [1]. Approximately 25% of people with diabetes have some form of DR. Diabetic retinopathy is the leading cause of visual impairment in the working-age individuals.

Diabetic macular edema (DME) usually results from the breakdown of the blood–retinal barrier. This leads to abnormal fluid accumulation in the retinal layers and resultant increased retinal thickness. Prevalence of DME is 5% within the first 5 years after diagnosis of diabetes mellitus and 15% at 15 years [2].

5.2 Spectral Domain Optical Coherence Tomography-Based Evaluation of Diabetic Macular Edema

Slit lamp biomicroscopic examination of the macula provides only a subjective evaluation of retinal thickness; however, it is not a reliable quantitative indicator of fluid accumulation. Spectral domain optical coherence tomography (SD-OCT) provides a highly reproducible and reliable quantitative measurement of macular thickness in DME [3].

SD-OCT-based macular thickness analysis, at the time of screening for DR, provides a reliable baseline evaluation for planning the management and follow-up. Central subfield thickness (CST) is defined as thickness of the central circle of diameter 1mm in the circular early treatment diabetic retinopathy study (ETDRS) grid map (Fig. 5.1). Cube average thickness (CAT) is defined as an overall average thickness for the internal limiting membrane–retinal pigment epithelium tissue layer over the entire 6 × 6 mm square scanned area.

The ETDRS definition of clinically significant macular edema (CSME) includes: center-involved and noncentral types. Center-involved DME accounts for retinal thickening within 500 μm of the center of the macula or, hard exudates within 500 μm from the center of the macula with thickening of the adjacent retina. The noncentral DME is defined as a zone of retinal thickening, 1 disc area or larger, any portion of which is located within 1 disc diameter from the center of the macula [4]. On SD-OCT, CST incorporates the central 1mm area as recognized on the ETDRS map, whereas cube average thickness (CAT) would also include noncentral type of DME.

Studies have documented OCT as a sensitive tool for detection of early retinal thickening [5]. Slit lamp examination correlates with findings on OCT except in few cases where OCT is instrumental in detecting thickening in the absence of hard exudates in the central macula. Further, OCT is also useful in cases with diffuse rather than focal macular thickening with minimal variation in retinal surface contour [6]. The ability of OCT in detection of the small variation in macular thickness among normal eyes as well as variation between right and left eye is suggestive of its high precision and sensitivity [7]. A sensitivity value of 0.81 (95% CI 0.74–0.86) and a specificity of 0.85 (95% CI 0.75–0.91) were observed in a meta-analysis study, which evaluated the presence of clinically significant macular edema with a central retinal thickness above a median cut-off range of 250 μm (230–300 μm) [8]. The probability of subclinical macular edema rises with progression to nonproliferative diabetic reti-

S. Saxena (✉)
Department of Ophthalmology, King George's Medical University, Lucknow, India

C. H. Meyer
Augenklinik, Davos, Switzerland

J. S. Gilhotra
Department of Ophthalmology, University of Adelaide, Adelaide, SA, Australia

L. Akduman
Department of Ophthalmology, Eye Institute, St Louis University, St. Louis, MO, USA

S. Saxena et al. (eds.), *Diabetic Macular Edema*, https://doi.org/10.1007/978-981-19-7307-9_5

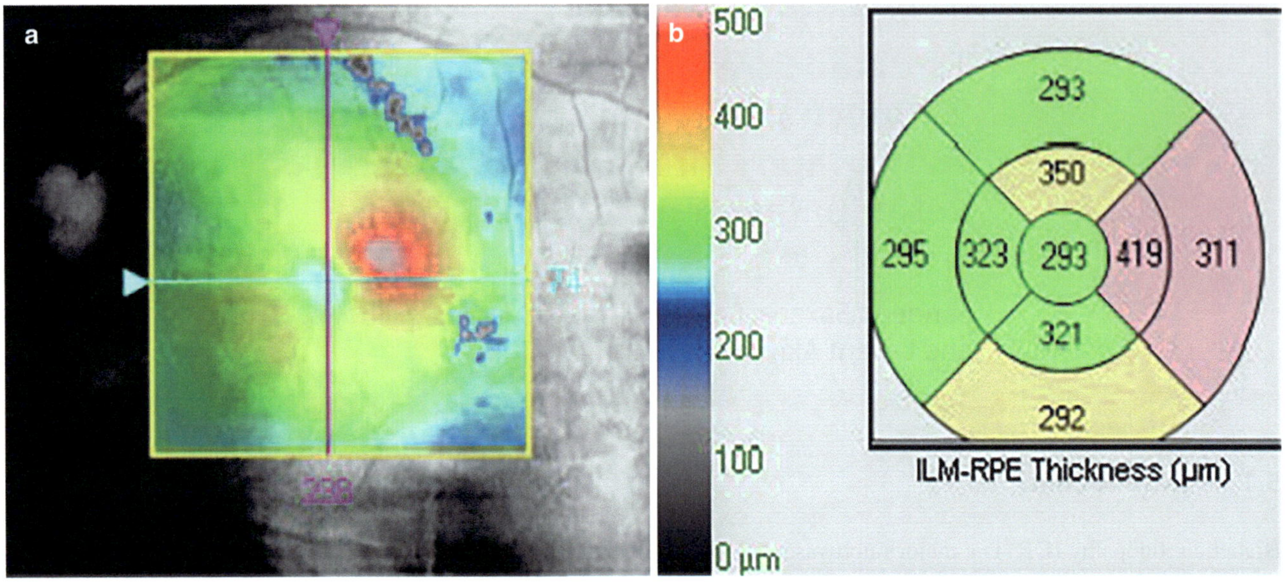

Fig. 5.1 (**a**) Color-coded internal limiting membrane–retinal pigment epithelium thickness overlap of 6 × 6 square mm macular cube. (**b**) ETDRS grid map shows numerical data for central subfield thickness within innermost circle

nopathy (NPDR) and proliferative diabetic retinopathy (PDR). Earlier studies have observed that besides individual baseline measurement, OCT is useful in detecting subclinical retinal thickening in advanced retinopathy without DME. Such cases of subclinical macular edema should be followed more closely as they are at increased risk of progression to DME [9]. Several studies have correlated OCT-based macular thickness with visual acuity in DME [10–12].

5.3 Vascular Endothelial Growth Factor and Diabetic Macular Edema

Vascular endothelial growth factor (VEGF) is a part of a subfamily of growth factors, functioning as signaling proteins, and involved in angiogenesis. Advanced glycation end products stimulate vascular endothelial growth factor (VEGF) expression [13–15]. VEGF serves as a biomolecule and is secreted from retinal pigment epithelial cells, pericytes, astrocytes, muller cells, glial cells, and endothelial cells. Multiple physiological and pathological effects, i.e., angiogenesis, vascular hyperpermeability, initiation of DR-like vascular changes, antithrombotic or prothrombotic responses, and neuroprotection can be attributed to VEGF [16].

Jain and associates observed that serum VEGF levels increased significantly as the severity of retinopathy increased from no diabetic retinopathy (no DR) to proliferative diabetic retinopathy (PDR) levels. Also, mean CST increased, whereas visual acuity decreased with severity of DR [17]. This has translational research significance (Figs. 5.2 and 5.3).

Ahuja and associates studied serum VEGF as a biomarker for severity of DR. They classified cases with DR according to ETDRS classification as mild NPDR, moderate NPDR, severe NPDR, early PDR, and advanced PDR. It was observed that serum VEGF levels served as simple, reliable, physician-friendly, and easy to comprehend biomolecular biomarker for severity of DR. Mean VEGF levels and CST were found to be significantly different among the study groups, highlighting that VEGF levels and CST increased with severity of DR. They also observed that significantly elevated levels of VEGF come into play even before the evidence of DR [18].

Ruia and Saxena observed a significant difference in CST and CAT in no DR, NPDR, and PDR study groups. An increase in CST and CAT was observed with increased severity of retinopathy. A positive correlation was also noted between CST and CAT. CST and CAT were observed to serve as surrogate markers for prognosticating the disease severity. This limited clinical data can be interpolated onto a population of diabetes mellitus with DR [19].

Increased serum VEGF levels have been observed to be associated with increased severity of DR and an increase in CST. Hence, an increase in CST indicates an increase in VEGF activity in the retina. An increase in CST and CAT, on SD-OCT, serves as a significant indicator of increased VEGF levels as well as increased severity of disease within the ETDRS grade of retinopathy, which may not be clinically evident. SD-OCT-based CST and CAT measurements provide reliable, objective, standard estimates for severity of retinopathy. Obtaining a precise baseline CST and CAT evaluation will be useful for detection of subtle variations in retinal thickening on follow-up for progression of disease.

With the advent of antivascular endothelial growth factor pharmacotherapy, the role of OCT for monitoring treatment in diabetic retinopathy has gained popularity as well as reli-

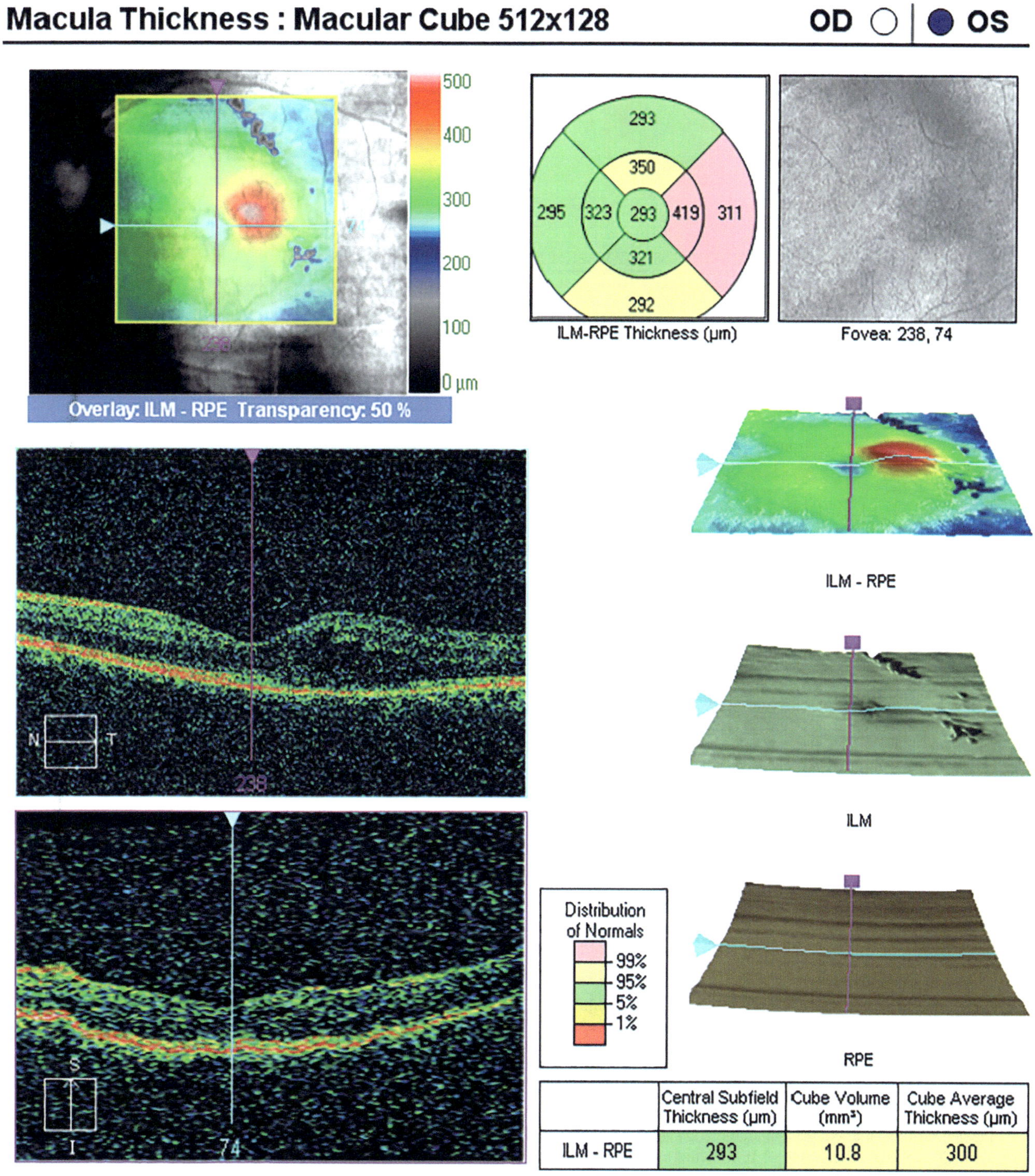

Fig. 5.2 Macular thickness: macular cube 512 × 128 scan obtained on SD-OCT showing diabetic macular edema approaching fovea on cross-sectional scan with central subfield thickness of 293 µm

ability. Screening with OCT will provide cost-effective timely intervention and better prognosis.

Targeted screening of DME, with OCT, would provide an effective tool for evaluating severity of disease. It would also be helpful in rationalizing decrease in visual acuity, on follow-up, with no change in clinically evident diabetic retinopathy. With the development of telemedicine, SD-OCT-based targeted screening of DME would serve as an appropriate tool for monitoring the progression of DR [20, 21].

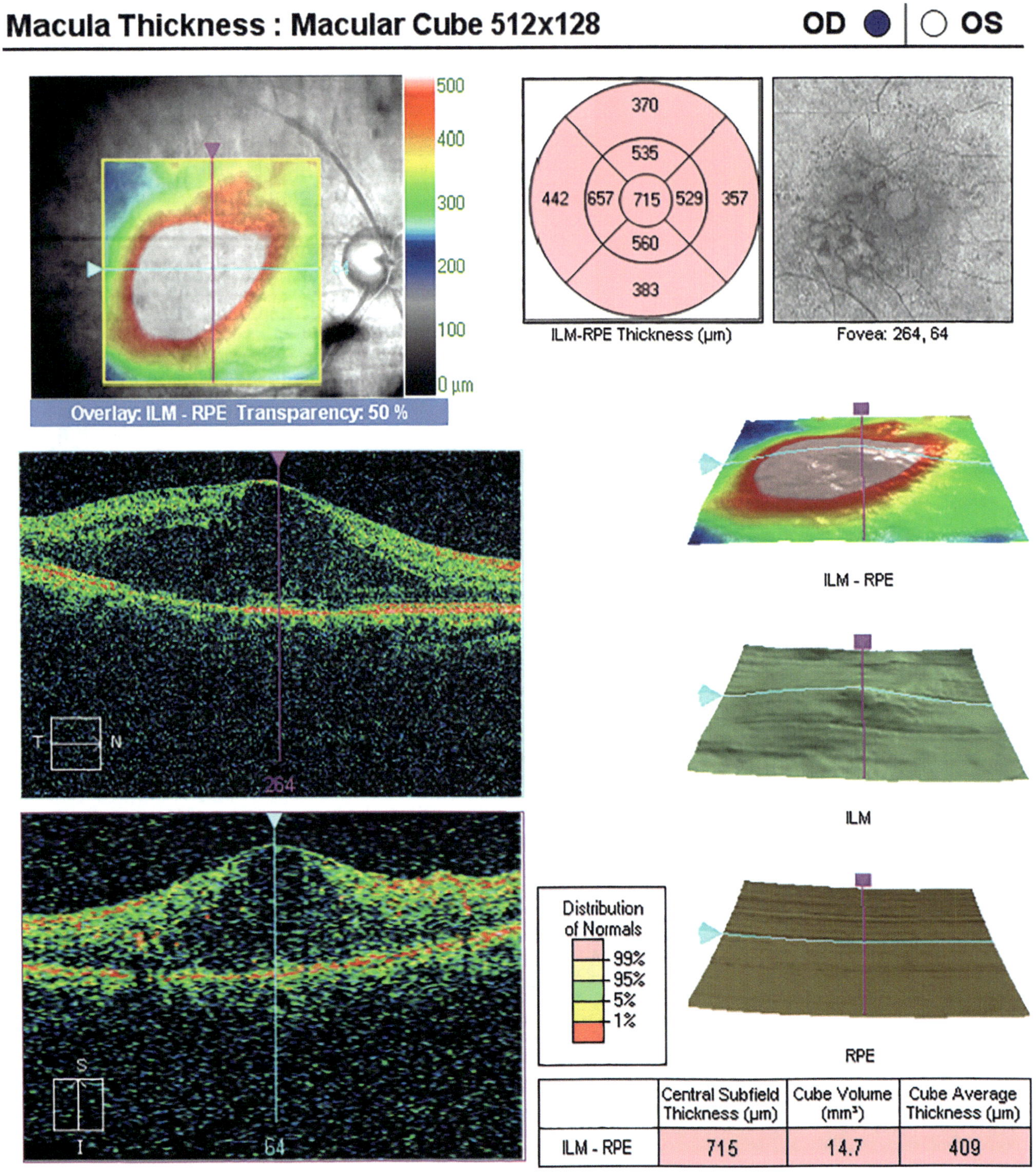

Fig. 5.3 Macular thickness: macular cube 512 × 128 scan obtained on SD-OCT showing severe diabetic macular edema involving fovea on cross-sectional scan with central subfield thickness of 715 µm

References

1. King H, Aubert RE, Herman WH. Global burden of diabetes, 1995-2025: prevalence, numerical estimates, and projections. Diabetes Care. 1998;21:1414–31.
2. Aiello LP, Gardner TW, King GL, Blankenship G, Cavallerano JD, et al. Diabetic retinopathy. Diabetes Care. 1998;21:143–56.
3. Goebel W, Kretzchmar-Gross T. Retinal thickness in diabetic retinopathy: a study using optical coherence tomography (OCT). Retina. 2002;22:759–67.
4. Early Treatment Diabetic Retinopathy Study Research Group. Photocoagulation treatment for diabetic macular edema. ETDRS report number 1. Arch Ophthalmol. 1985;103:1796–806.
5. Massin P, Erginay A, Haouchine B, Mehidi AB, Paques M, et al. Retinal thickness in healthy and diabetic subjects measured

using optical coherence tomography mapping software. Eur J Ophthalmol. 2001;12:102–8.
6. Hee MR, Puliafito CA, Duker JS, Reichel E, Coker JG, et al. Topography of diabetic macular edema with optical coherence tomography. Ophthalmology. 1998;105:360–70.
7. Krzystolik MG, Strauber SF, Aiello LP, Beck RW, Berger BB, Diabetic Retinopathy Clinical Research Network. Reproducibility of macular thickness and volume using Zeiss optical coherence tomography in patients with diabetic macular edema. Ophthalmology. 2007;114:1520–5.
8. Virgili G, Menchini F, Murro V, Peluso E, Rosa F, et al. Optical coherence tomography (OCT) for detection of macular oedema in patients with diabetic retinopathy. Cochrane Database Syst Rev. 2011;7:CD008081.
9. Browning DJ, Fraser CM, Clark S. The relationship of macular thickness to clinically graded diabetic retinopathy severity in eyes without clinically detected diabetic macular edema. Ophthalmology. 2008;115:533–9.
10. Browning DJ, Glassman AR, Aiello LP, Beck RW, Brown DM, Diabetic Retinopathy Clinical Research Network. Relationship between optical coherence tomography-measured central retinal thickness and visual acuity in diabetic macular edema. Ophthalmology. 2007;114:525–36.
11. Pelosini L, Hull C, Boyce JF, McHugh D, Stanford MR, et al. Optical coherence tomography may be used to predict visual acuity in patients with macular edema. Invest Ophthalmol Vis Sci. 2011;52:2741–8.
12. Alkuraya H, Kangave D, El-Asrar AMA. The correlation between optical coherence tomographic features and severity of retinopathy, macular thickness and visual acuity in diabetic macular edema. Int Ophthalmol. 2005;26:93–9.
13. Meleth AD, Agrón E, Chan CC, Reed GF, Arora K, Byrnes G, Csaky KG, Ferris FL, Chew EY. Serum inflammatory markers in diabetic retinopathy. Invest Ophthalmol Vis Sci. 2005;46:4295–301.
14. Mishra N, Saxena S, Shukla RK, Singh V, Meyer CH, Kruzliak P, Khanna VK. Association of serum N(ε)-Carboxy methyl lysine with severity of diabetic retinopathy. J Diabetes Complications. 2016;30(3):511–7. https://doi.org/10.1016/j.jdiacomp.2015.12.009. Epub 2015 Dec 11. PMID: 26782022.
15. Miyamoto K, Khosrof S, Bursell SE, Rohan R, Murata T, Clermont AC, Aiello LP, Ogura Y, Adamis AP. Prevention of leukostasis and vascular leakage in streptozotocin-induced diabetic retinopathy via intercellular adhesion molecule-1 inhibition. Proc Natl Acad Sci U S A. 1999;96(19):10836–41.
16. Joussen AM, Murata T, Tsujikawa A, Kirchhof B, Bursell SE, Adamis AP. Leukocyte-mediated endothelial cell injury and death in the diabetic retina. Am J Pathol. 2001;158:147–52.
17. Zhu Y, Zhang XL, Zhu BF, Ding YN. Effect of antioxidant N-acetylcysteine on diabetic retinopathy and expression of VEGF and ICAM-1 from retinal blood vessels of diabetic rats. Mol Biol Rep. 2012;39:3727–35.
18. Jain A, Saxena S, Khanna VK, Shukla RK, Meyer CH. Status of serum VEGF and ICAM-1 and its association with external limiting membrane and inner segment-outer segment junction disruption in type 2 diabetes mellitus. Mol Vis. 2013;19:1760.
19. Ahuja S, Saxena S, Akduman L, Meyer CH, Kruzliak P, Khanna VK. Serum vascular endothelial growth factor is a biomolecular biomarker of severity of diabetic retinopathy. Int J Retina Vitreous. 2019;5:1–6.
20. Ruia S, Saxena S. Targeted screening of macular edema by spectral domain optical coherence tomography for progression of diabetic retinopathy. Indian J Ocular Biol. 2016;1:102.
21. Olson J, Sharp P, Goatman K, Prescott G, Scotland G, et al. Improving the economic value of photographic screening for optical coherence tomography-detectable macular oedema: a prospective, multicentre, UK study. Health Technol Assess. 2013;17:1–142.

6 Anti-Vascular Endothelial Growth Factor Agents for Diabetic Macular Edema

Max Davidson and Aman Chandra

6.1 Treatment of Diabetic Macular Edema Before Anti-VEGF

Prior to the introduction of anti-VEGF agents in the twenty-first century, treatment of diabetic macular edema (DME) was limited to laser photocoagulation. The Early Treatment for Diabetic Retinopathy Study (EDTRS) was a randomized control trial (RCT) across 22 centers, involving 3711 patients with varying degrees of diabetic retinopathy (DR), and ran between 1979 and 1989 [1]. Its primary aim was to assess the efficacy of argon laser photocoagulation and aspirin therapy in preventing progression from early DR to more advanced DR. Each patient received one of four combinations of focal macular and scatter laser in one eye, initiated at various times during follow-up. The other eye was followed up closely and received scatter laser only if there was progression to high-risk pre-proliferative DR. One conclusion of the EDTRS was that scatter laser or pan-retinal photocoagulation may be delayed until the development of severe non-proliferative DR or early proliferative DR. Another outcome was to define "clinically significant macular edema" with criteria still used today, to determine which patients may benefit from laser treatment. Focal macular laser reduced the risk of moderate vision loss by 50% in this group of eyes. Chapter 10 explores the current use of laser for DME in more detail.

In the early 2000s, intravitreal steroids such as triamcinolone were trialed off-label in patients with DME, with better short-term visual improvement than laser. However, these came with a significant side effect profile such as raised intraocular pressure, glaucoma, and cataract. This chapter discusses how the introduction of anti-VEGF agents revolutionized the management of DME, causing not only reduced vision loss but significantly improved visual outcomes for patients with DME.

M. Davidson
Department of Ophthalmology, Southend University Hospital, Mid & South Essex NHS Foundation Trust, Southend-on-Sea, UK
e-mail: max.davidson@nhs.net

A. Chandra (✉)
Department of Ophthalmology, Southend University Hospital, Mid & South Essex NHS Foundation Trust, Southend-on-Sea, UK

Vision and Eye Research Unit, Anglia Ruskin University, Cambridge, UK
e-mail: a.chandra@nhs.net

6.2 History of VEGF Blockade Development [2]

> Pure retinal neovascularization is directly related to a tissue state of relative retinal anoxia. Under such circumstances, an unknown factor *x* develops in this tissue and stimulates new vessel formation, primarily from the capillaries and veins. (*George Wise, 1956*).

Initial attempts to identify this unknown "factor *x*" led to the isolation of acidic and basic fibroblast growth factors from the retina; however, further studies showed that these factors played only a small part in the angiogenic signaling cascade. It was not until 1994 when a landmark study in the *American Journal of Pathology* demonstrated that the hypoxic retina produces vascular endothelial growth factor (VEGF) [3]. In this study, retinas of nonhuman primates underwent laser photocoagulation to induce ischemia, resulting in neovascularization of the iris. Levels of VEGF messenger RNA and protein were elevated in a pattern that strongly suggested a role for VEGF in angiogenesis. Another report that year showed elevated levels of VEGF in ocular fluid isolated from eyes with new vessel growth compared to those without. A subsequent study demonstrated that injection of VEGF into a nonhuman primate eye is sufficient to cause new and porous vessels to grow in the retina as well as cause glaucoma, now a well-understood complication of neovascularization.

Angiogenesis was by this point recognized as an essential mechanism for tumor growth and survival. Bevacizumab, a humanized murine monoclonal antibody we will discuss at length in this chapter, entered phase I trials for the adjuvant treatment of colon cancer in 1997. Two years later marked

S. Saxena et al. (eds.), *Diabetic Macular Edema*, https://doi.org/10.1007/978-981-19-7307-9_6

the development of the pegylated anti-VEGF aptamer pegaptanib, which was then licensed to Eyetech pharmaceuticals (New York) under the trade name Macugen and entered into clinical trials for patients with neovascular ("wet") age-related macular degeneration (nAMD). Pegaptanib was the first aptamer approved for use in humans and was shown to bind specifically to the 165 isoform of VEGF ($VEGF_{165}$) and reduce vision loss associated with nAMD. It became the world's first licensed anti-angiogenic agent for ocular neovascularization in 2004 (see Table 6.1).

In diabetes, capillaries of the inner retinal layers are injured by hyperglycemia, inflammation, and oxidative stress, causing a breakdown of the inner blood–retinal barrier (BRB) and increased vascular permeability. Hard exudates seen in diabetic retinopathy are protein or lipid deposits that have leaked through damaged capillaries. When this process occurs at the macula, fluid can accumulate via these porous vessels causing DME. VEGF has been shown to promote vascular permeability in the retina via activation of the protein kinase C pathway, through phosphorylation of occludin, a protein localized to tight junctions between endothelial cells [7]. Other inflammatory cytokines which mediate vascular permeability, such as tumor necrosis factors alpha and beta, nitric oxide, and interleukin-1β are also raised in DME, which may explain why many patients do not respond to VEGF blockade [8].

Table 6.1 Structural, pharmacodynamic and pharmacokinetic parameters of antiangiogenic drugs

	Avastin (bevacizumab)	Lucentis (ranibizumab)	Eylea (aflibercept)
Structure	Humanized IgG1	Humanized Fab	r-fusion protein
Target	All VEGF-A isoforms	All VEGF-A isoforms	All VEGF-A/B, PlGF
Molecular weight (kDa)	149	48	115
Fc portion	Yes	No	Yes
Potency (IC_{50}) [4]	500–1476	88–1140	16–90
$t_{1/2}$ (human vitreous) [4]	6.7	7.2–9 days	–
$t_{1/2}$ (macaque vitreous) [5, 6]	2.8 days	2.3 days	2.2 days
$t_{1/2}$ (macaque vitrectomized) [5, 6]	1.5 days	1.4 days	1.5 days

Half-life figures for macaque monkeys are included due to inadequate human data comparing nonvitrectomized versus vitrectomized eyes. These figures illustrate higher drug clearance and possibly insufficient therapeutic level in vitrectomized eyes. Half-life data for Eylea in human vitreous is also missing in the literature

6.3 Anti-VEGF Agents for DME: The Present Day

Three intravitreal anti-VEGF agents dominate the global market for DME at the time of writing. We present each drug in turn including its structure, mechanism of action, and development history. We continue to discuss reported adverse effects and how these reflect in meta-analyses. At the end of this section, we comment briefly on the relative costs of the three agents and their cost-effectiveness in treating DME.

6.3.1 Avastin (Bevacizumab)

As previously mentioned, bevacizumab was developed originally for use as an anti-cancer agent. It is derived from a monoclonal antibody generated from mice immunized with 165-residue form of recombinant human VEGF. It was humanized by retaining the binding region and replacing the rest with a human full light chain and a human truncated IgG1 heavy chain, with some other substitutions. The resulting plasmid (93% human, 7% murine sequences) was transfected into Chinese hamster ovary cells which are now grown in industrial fermentation systems [9]. It has the molecular formula $C_{6638}H_{10160}N_{1720}O_{2108}S_{44}$ and molecular weight 149 kilodaltons (kDa).

Bevacizumab binds to the molecule VEGF, the key driver of angiogenesis, thus inhibiting the ability of VEGF to bind to its receptors VEGFR-1 and VEGFR-2 on the surface of endothelial cells. Reducing VEGF activity normalizes the existing tumor blood vessels and inhibits further neovascularization, thereby inhibiting tumor growth. It is manufactured under the trade name Avastin by Genentech, Inc. (California, USA) which operates as an independent subsidiary of Roche Products Limited. In 2004, Avastin received Food and Drug Administration (FDA) approval for systemic use in metastatic colon cancer, following which it has subsequently been approved for use in lung, breast, brain, kidney, ovarian, cervical, and liver cancers.

Avastin continues to be used "off-label" globally for DME. Preparation for intravitreal use involves manipulation of the authorized medicine to produce multiple aliquots, usually in plastic syringes (so-called compounding). The concentration of Avastin is 25 mg/mL for infusion; the standard dose for intravitreal injection is 1.25 mg, delivered in 0.05 mL of solution no more than once per month. It has a vitreous half-life of 6.7 days in humans. Potency is the amount of a drug required to produce a pharmacological effect and can be expressed by the half maximal inhibitory concentration (IC_{50}). Thus, a lower IC_{50} indicates a higher potency. As you can see from Table 6.1, estimated potency for Avastin varies but is the lowest of the three drugs.

6.3.2 Lucentis (Ranibizumab)

Initially bevacizumab was thought to be too large a molecule to diffuse into the choroid, so work began on developing a smaller anti-VEGF agent. Ranibizumab is an antigen-binding fragment (Fab) of the human A4.6.1 antibody. It lacks a fragment crystallizable region (Fc), allowing it to avoid Fc recycling and making it significantly smaller than the full-size antibody. Its smaller size is thought to assist penetration through the retina and faster systemic clearance, though it may also expedite clearance from the vitreous. It has the molecular formula $C_{2158}H_{3282}N_{562}O_{681}S_{12}$ and molecular weight 48 kDa.

Ranibizumab binds with high affinity to VEGF-A isoforms such as $VEGF_{110}$, $VEGF_{121}$, and $VEGF_{165}$, preventing these isoforms from binding to their receptors VEGFR-1 and VEGFR-2. It was licensed under the trade name Lucentis by Genentech, Inc. (California, USA) and now marketed under the same name in Europe by Novartis Pharmaceuticals UK Ltd. In 2006, it received FDA approval for the treatment of nAMD. It was subsequently approved for the treatment of macular edema following central and branch retinal vein occlusion (CRVO/BRVO) in 2010 and for DME in 2012. In 2015, Lucentis gained a further FDA license to treat DR in patients with DME, extended in 2017 to all patients with DR including those without DME. Since 2019 it has been licensed to treat retinopathy of prematurity.

Lucentis is supplied as a preservative-free, colorless to pale yellow, sterile solution placed in a single-use glass vial. There are two different concentrations: the 0.5 mg dose vial delivers 0.05 mL of 10 mg/mL ranibizumab; the 0.3 mg dose vial delivers 0.05 mL of 6 mg/mL ranibizumab. The recommended dose for DME is the latter 0.3 mg intravitreally no more than once per month. It has a vitreous half-life of 7.2–9 days in humans and greater potency than Avastin (see Table 6.1).

6.3.3 Eylea (Aflibercept)

Aflibercept was developed to try and improve the pharmacokinetics of VEGF binding. It is a recombinant protein consisting of sequences derived from two human VEGF receptors VEGFR-1 and VEGFR-2 which are fused to the Fc portion of human immunoglobulin G1 (IgG1). It is produced via transfection of Chinese hamster ovary cells in large industrial fermentation systems. It has the molecular formula $C_{4318}H_{6788}N_{1164}O_{1304}S_{32}$ and molecular weight 115 kDa.

Also known as "VEGF Trap," aflibercept acts as a soluble decoy receptor that binds VEGF-A, VEGF-B, and placental growth factor (PlGF) with higher affinity than their natural receptors, thus inhibiting the binding and activation of cell receptors. It is manufactured by Bayer plc under the trade name Eylea and initially gained FDA approval for nAMD in 2011. In 2012 it was granted a license for macular edema following CRVO. By the end of 2014 it was granted a license for the treatment of DME and macular edema following BRVO. In 2015 Eylea was licensed for DR in patients with DME and more recently extended to all DR patients with or without DME in 2019.

Eylea is supplied in vials with a concentration of 40 mg/mL containing at least 0.1 mL. This provides a usable amount to deliver the recommended single dose of 2 mg intravitreal aflibercept in 0.05 mL, to be given no more than once per month. No data on half-life in human eyes was available at the time of writing; however, its estimated potency is markedly higher than Avastin and Lucentis.

6.4 Adverse Effects of Anti-VEGF Agents

Systemically delivered anti-VEGF drugs, such as Avastin as an adjuvant to chemotherapy, are known to reduce vascular permeability, raise blood pressure, and increase the risk of thromboembolism [4]. In preclinical models, decoy VEGFR administration caused left ventricular dilatation and contractile dysfunction. This has been reflected clinically by an increased risk of heart failure in breast cancer patients treated with intravenous bevacizumab. In patients presenting with acute myocardial infarction, low serum VEGF measured after 7 days was associated with significantly increased risk of further cardiovascular or cerebrovascular event, compared to middle and higher levels. If anti-VEGF drugs can reach biologically active concentrations in the blood following intravitreal injection, patients receiving this treatment for DME and other retinal pathologies may be at risk of similar potential complications. Since these sequelae are rare in oncology patients and much rarer in ophthalmic patients, a study designed to detect meaningful difference would require a very large number of patients. Therefore, the best method we have of detecting true risk in this population is via meta-analysis of all available data.

Despite one DME RCT in detecting a higher rate of arterial thrombotic events with ranibizumab compared to bevacizumab and aflibercept [10], a meta-analysis of 21 systematic reviews on DME, nAMD, and RVO showed no detectable difference in the risk of systemic adverse events between anti-VEGF treatment and control nor between different anti-VEGF agents. There was, however, an association between ranibizumab and an increased risk of non-ocular hemorrhage in patients with nAMD, but not DME or RVO. This included epistaxis, hematuria, hematoma, ecchymosis, and gastrointestinal bleed [11].

Another recent meta-analysis of 74 RCTs supported this finding but found no overall association between intravitreal anti-VEGF and major cardiovascular events nor total mortality when compared to control agents. However, there was a significantly increased risk of mortality for the diabetic subgroup compared to nAMD and RVO subgroups [12]. An earlier meta-analysis considered fixed monthly treatment in DME only and found an increase in cerebrovascular events and death following 2 years of monthly aflibercept or 0.5 mg ranibizumab compared to sham or laser [13]. This suggests that total cumulative exposure to anti-VEGF may need to be considered when treating at-risk groups.

Patients with DME would fall into the at-risk vulnerable group. Alternatives such as intravitreal dexamethasone implant (explored in Chap. 8) may need to be considered early in these patients, particularly if there is limited response to anti-VEGF, or in vitrectomized eyes, where there is increased anti-VEGF clearance.

6.5 Treatment Regimens

6.5.1 When to Treat?

DME can be subclassified as center-involving (CIDME) and non-center-involving (non-CIDME). CIDME is defined by optical coherence tomography (OCT) as foveal involvement of abnormal intraretinal and/or subretinal fluid with concurrent thickening affecting the 1 mm diameter central subfield thickness. CIDME can be further subclassified according to the vision.

In the UK, the National Institute of Clinical Excellence recommends treatment of CIDME only if the eye has central retinal thickness (CRT) greater than or equal to 400 μm at the start of treatment.

In 2019, a multicenter DRCR.net trial showed that initial observation of patients with CIDME and visual acuity (VA) of 20/25 or better, resulted in no difference in long-term VA compared to initial laser or prompt aflibercept before visual loss. This suggests that in those with CIDME and good visual acuity, initial observation may be a reasonable approach.

6.5.2 PRN Regimen

In pro-re-nata (PRN) treatment regimes, the patient typically receives one intravitreal injection monthly until they have received three “loading” injections. After the first three visits, the patient is surveilled monthly with OCT, and the decision on further injections is based on vision and OCT evidence of intraretinal or subretinal fluid (IRF; SRF). The main challenge with this regimen is the burden on clinicians and patient of regular follow-up appointments.

6.5.3 Treat and Extend Regimen

An algorithm was developed by Freund et al. in 2015 which suggested that monthly injections should continue until a maximum response is achieved [14]. Maximum response was defined as:

1. Complete resolution of IRF and SRF without new retinal hemorrhage; or,
2. No further reduction of IRF or SRF on OCT for at least two consecutive visits in the absence of new retinal hemorrhage.
3. Some authors would also include in their definition:
4. No further flattening of serous or vascularized pigment epithelial detachments; and,
5. No further improvement in VA.

However, since visual changes fluctuate commonly in patients receiving multiple anti-VEGF injections, the consensus panel suggested VA should be used to guide treatment interval only in the context of clinical examination and OCT findings. While the disease remains stable, treatment intervals can be extended by up to 2 weeks at a time, with a standard maximum extension period of 12 weeks.

For minor signs of deterioration, the injection interval should be shortened by 1–2 weeks. Any major signs of deterioration should prompt immediate evaluation for the reason behind the change, followed by monthly injections until a maximum response is achieved for several consecutive patient visits (Table 6.2).

A recent meta-analysis on DME demonstrated superior visual outcomes in patients treated with aflibercept in a fixed dosing regimen than with a reactive regimen (PRN or treat and extend) [15]. This is explained by an increased number of injections and supports mounting evidence that frequency of injections influences final VA (Fig. 6.1) [16]. However, though fixed regimes are often employed during RCTs, they may often be impractical to continue in routine practice.

Table 6.2 Advantages of treat and extend versus PRN regimens

Advantages	Disadvantages
Better long-term visual outcomes Fewer recurrences	Risk of overtreating No identification of the patients that would remain stable without treatment
Fewer patient visits	
More guaranteed injections	
Potentially better adherence to follow-up	No stop criteria
Treatment tailored to patient	Higher cost from more injections

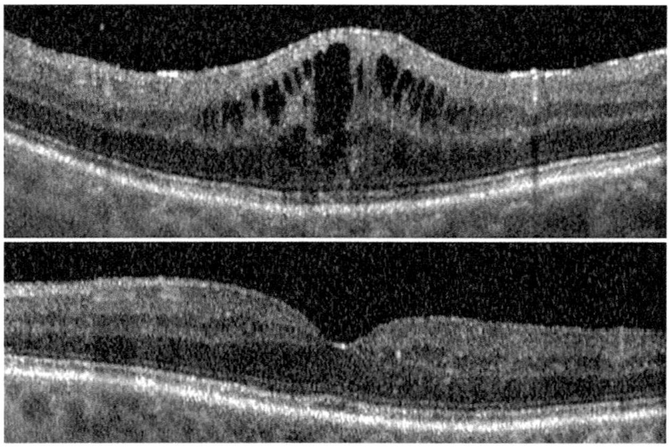

Fig. 6.1 Optical coherence tomography of an eye with DME. Top image shows significant intraretinal fluid (IRF) prior to initiation of anti-VEGF treatment. Bottom image shows complete resolution of IRF when reviewed 2 months after the fifth Eylea injection. Images obtained from the authors' ophthalmology department

6.6 Cost-Effectiveness

Ranibizumab and aflibercept are at least 20 times more expensive than bevacizumab in the western world [17]. Their estimated wholesale prices per dose are $60 for bevacizumab, $1170 for ranibizumab 0.3 mg, and $1850 for aflibercept. Considering the large number of injections required over the initial years of treatment, on average 17 over 5 years, this adds up to a substantial total cost. One RCT conducted by the Diabetic Retinopathy Clinical Research Network (DRCR.net) demonstrated a superior visual improvement at 1 year for patients with DME receiving aflibercept rather than ranibizumab or bevacizumab. This and other DRCR.net trials are discussed further in Chap. 5. Based on this RCT, the authors calculated quality-adjusted life-years (QALYs) according to visual acuities after 1 year of treatment for each agent. The incremental cost-effectiveness ratios of aflibercept and ranibizumab compared to bevacizumab were $1,110,000/QALY and $1,730,000/QALY, implying these agents would require a 90–95% reduction in price in order to become cost-effective ($100,000/QALY) relative to bevacizumab. The case for selecting aflibercept or ranibizumab over bevacizumab weakens further following data from a meta-analysis demonstrating that the advantage in visual recovery after 1 year of aflibercept observed in this DRCR.net trial is not upheld at 2 years [18].

6.7 Anti-VEGF Agents: Head-to-Head

According to a meta-analysis of 24 RCTs focusing on 6007 patients with DME and moderate vision loss, approximately 1 in 10 people improved vision by 3 or more lines with laser after 1 year, although on average there was no change in VA with laser after 1 year. Ranibizumab and bevacizumab both improved vision at 1 year in 3 out of 10 patients. Aflibercept achieved this gain in 4 out of 10 patients [19].

The RISE and RIDE trials compared ranibizumab with laser, and later the VISTA and VIVID trials compared aflibercept with laser. Neither these nor the following studies and meta-analyses demonstrated any additional benefit of macular laser when given alongside anti-VEGF therapy, thus laser is no longer routinely recommended in CIDME, but reserved for cases of non-CIDME.

A more recent meta-analysis looked at 1-year outcomes of 72 studies including RCTs and observational data of 45,032 eyes with DME. The authors detected a significantly superior visual result of +3.01 ETDRS letters for aflibercept when compared to bevacizumab [15].

Interestingly, subgroup analysis in several meta-analyses have identified that aflibercept gave better visual improvement than bevacizumab and ranibizumab *only for patients with low baseline VA* (those able to see fewer than 69 EDTRS letters). This effect was seen at 1 year but not at 2 years [8, 18].

Up to 30% of patients are resistant to current anti-VEGF therapy, likely due to the multifactorial pathophysiology of DME. Numerous cytokines are involved which may be the reason that targeting one particular factor such as VEGF can fail. However, there is evidence that switching treatment from ranibizumab or bevacizumab to aflibercept produces a significant improvement in VA gain and CRT in patients with persistent DME [20]. Intravitreal dexamethasone remains an alternative treatment option for unresponsive cases.

Adequate follow-up data is currently lacking to ascertain whether the superior effect at 1 year of aflibercept for patients with poor vision is maintained long-term. Importantly for less economically developed countries, all available data indicate non-inferiority in visual and anatomical outcomes with the cheapest agent, bevacizumab, versus ranibizumab.

6.8 Future of Anti-VEGF

Frequent intravitreal injections are expensive, may cause non-adherence and increase the risk of endophthalmitis, retinal detachment, elevated intraocular pressure and vitreous hemorrhage. Several novel anti-VEGF therapies are under development to address this problem.

6.8.1 Conbercept

Conbercept is a recombinant fusion protein containing Fc segments of human VEGFR-1, VEGFR-2, and IgG1. Its structure is similar to aflibercept but contains a VEGFR-2 kinase insert domain receptor Ig-like region 4 (KDRd4) which improves the 3D structure to increase its binding capacity for all VEGF isoforms and PlGF.

Conbercept was approved in China for DME in 2019 and showed excellent phase III 2-year results against sham treatment in the Sailing Study. Here, intravitreal conbercept or laser was given on a PRN regimen. A smaller retrospective study comparing conbercept and ranibizumab showed that on a PRN regimen, the number of conbercept injections required was significantly lower than for ranibizumab. Prospective results confirming this are awaited along with international approval of this medicine.

6.8.2 Beovu (Brolucizumab)

Brolucizumab is a humanized monoclonal single-chain Fv antibody fragment produced in *Escherichia coli* cells by recombinant DNA technology. The Fv portion of an IgG is the smallest fragment that maintains the full binding capacity of the intact antibody, thus the molecular weight of brolucizumab is only 26 kDa. Therefore, its main potential benefits are a higher concentration delivered per injection and less frequent dosing schedule.

Beovu was licensed for nAMD in 2019 and is currently in the phase III trials KESTREL and KITE to evaluate their potential use in DME. In August 2021, Novartis Pharmaceuticals announced 2-year results of 926 patients across 36 countries receiving either brolucizumab 6 mg or aflibercept 2 mg. In one treatment arm, Beovu was initially given every 6 weeks for a total of five doses and maintained with 12-weekly dosing unless patients demonstrated increased disease activity, in which case they were moved to 8-weekly dosing. At week 72, Beovu patients could be extended to 16-weekly dosing. Over 50% patients that completed an initial 12-week cycle were maintained on 12- or 16-weekly intervals until the end of the 2-year period. Brolucizumab was non-inferior to aflibercept in best-corrected VA at 2 years, with superior anatomical results and excellent safety profile.

6.8.3 Faricimab

Faricimab is a bispecific antibody, which simultaneously binds to both VEGF-A and angiopoietin-2 (Ang-2). It is composed of an anti-Ang-2 Fab fragment, an anti-VEGF-A Fab fragment, and a modified Fc region with molecular weight 150 kDa. Ang-2 is another upregulated factor in the ischemic retina causing vascular leakage and inflammation. In targeting both VEGF-A and Ang-2, faricimab aims to deliver improved results over longer treatment intervals.

In February 2021, Roche announced 1-year results of YOSEMITE and RHINE, two identical global phase III trials involving 1891 people and investigating the efficacy of faricimab in DME versus aflibercept. Treatment arms included 2-monthly faricimab vs personalized treatment intervals (PTI) of faricimab of up to 4-monthly injections, and faricimab demonstrated non-inferiority in vision gains compared to aflibercept at 1 year. Over 70% PTI patients achieved 3- or 4-monthly dosing at 1 year, and faricimab patients achieved better anatomical results.

6.9 Novel Therapies in Production [21]

6.9.1 Abicipar Pegol

Designed ankyrin repeat proteins are genetically engineered proteins that mimic antibodies with equal or better binding affinity and specificity. They are smaller, enabling better penetration with a longer half-life (>13 days) than ranibizumab (7.2 days). 8-weekly or 12-weekly abicipar pegol showed non-inferior results compared to ranibizumab delivered every 4 weeks in phase III SEQUOIA and CEDAR trials for patients with nAMD. To our knowledge, to date, no large trials have started in patients with DME.

6.9.2 Port Delivery System

Phase II trials in nAMD patients demonstrated safety and a 15-month refill time for port-delivered ranibizumab. Vitreous hemorrhage occurrence decreased toward the end of the trial as the surgical procedure was optimized. Phase III results for nAMD are awaited, along with studies on DME.

6.9.3 Thermosensitive Hydrogels

These hydrophilic polymers are liquid at room temperature and become solid at body temperature, allowing both intravitreal injection followed by sustained drug release. Each of bevacizumab, ranibizumab, and aflibercept has been tested in vitro, while the latter has shown sustained release over 6 months in nonhuman primates without toxic side effects.

6.9.4 Microparticles

Microparticles aggregate following exposure to vitreous and sink to form a depot at the base of the eye, leading to sustained release. Poly-lactic-co-glycolic acid (PLGA) is a biodegradable polymer of microparticles and forms the base for the FDA-approved dexamethasone intravitreal implant (Ozurdex, AbbVie-Allergan). The anti-VEGF agent sunitinib malate associated with PLGA is currently under phase IIb trial ALTISSIMO for DME.

6.9.5 Gene Therapy

In late 2017, voretigene neparvovec was the first FDA-approved retinal gene therapy for patients with RPE65-mediated inherited retinal dystrophies. Since DME pathogenesis has not been linked to single gene mutations, gene therapy for DME remains challenging and pre-clinical, but may 1 day offer long-term VEGF suppression.

6.10 Conclusion

Since the introduction of anti-VEGF agents two decades ago, there has been remarkable progress in patient outcomes for DME. However, this has been achieved at incredible cost and labor burden to healthcare systems, workforce, and patients. Newly approved therapies will increase costs further until longer-term strategies for VEGF suppression prove safe and efficacious. As discussed in Chap. 1, multiple other signaling pathways are involved in DME pathophysiology, which present alternative targets that need to be addressed alongside the advancement in anti-VEGF technology.

References

1. Early Treatment Diabetic Retinopathy Study Research Group. Treatment techniques and clinical guidelines for photocoagulation of diabetic macular edema. Early treatment diabetic retinopathy study report number 2. Ophthalmology. 1987;94:761–74. https://doi.org/10.1016/s0161-6420(87)33527-4.
2. Kim LA, D'Amore PA. A brief history of anti-VEGF for the treatment of ocular angiogenesis. Am J Pathol. 2012;181:376–9. https://doi.org/10.1016/j.ajpath.2012.06.006.
3. Miller JW, Adamis AP, Shima DT, et al. Vascular endothelial growth factor/vascular permeability factor is temporally and spatially correlated with ocular angiogenesis in a primate model. Am J Pathol. 1994;145:574–84.
4. Fogli S, Del Re M, Rofi E, et al. Clinical pharmacology of intravitreal anti-VEGF drugs. Eye (Lond). 2018;32:1010–20. https://doi.org/10.1038/s41433-018-0021-7.
5. Kakinoki M, Sawada O, Sawada T, et al. Effect of vitrectomy on aqueous VEGF concentration and pharmacokinetics of bevacizumab in macaque monkeys. Invest Ophthalmol Vis Sci. 2012;53:5877–80. https://doi.org/10.1167/iovs.12-10164.
6. Niwa Y, Kakinoki M, Sawada T, et al. Ranibizumab and Aflibercept: intraocular pharmacokinetics and their effects on aqueous VEGF level in vitrectomized and nonvitrectomized macaque eyes. Invest Ophthalmol Vis Sci. 2015;56:6501–5. https://doi.org/10.1167/iovs.15-17279.
7. Aiello LP, Bursell SE, Clermont A, et al. Vascular endothelial growth factor-induced retinal permeability is mediated by protein kinase C in vivo and suppressed by an orally effective beta-isoform-selective inhibitor. Diabetes. 1997;46:1473–80. https://doi.org/10.2337/diab.46.9.1473.
8. Furino C, Boscia F, Reibaldi M, et al. Intravitreal therapy for diabetic macular edema: an update. J Ophthalmol. 2021;2021:6654168. https://doi.org/10.1155/2021/6654168.
9. Lien S, Lowman HB. Therapeutic anti-VEGF antibodies. Handb Exp Pharmacol. 2008;181:131–50. https://doi.org/10.1007/978-3-540-73259-4_6.
10. Wells JA, Glassman AR, Ayala AR, et al. Aflibercept, Bevacizumab, or Ranibizumab for diabetic macular edema: two-year results from a comparative effectiveness randomized clinical trial. Ophthalmology. 2016;123:1351–9. https://doi.org/10.1016/j.ophtha.2016.02.022.
11. Thulliez M, Angoulvant D, Pisella P-J, et al. Overview of systematic reviews and meta-analyses on systemic adverse events associated with intravitreal anti-vascular endothelial growth factor medication use. JAMA Ophthalmol. 2018;136:557–66. https://doi.org/10.1001/jamaophthalmol.2018.0002.
12. Ngo Ntjam N, Thulliez M, Paintaud G, et al. Cardiovascular adverse events with intravitreal anti-vascular endothelial growth factor drugs: a systematic review and meta-analysis of randomized clinical trials. JAMA Ophthalmol. 2021;139:610. https://doi.org/10.1001/jamaophthalmol.2021.0640.
13. Avery RL, Gordon GM. Systemic safety of prolonged monthly anti-vascular endothelial growth factor therapy for diabetic macular edema: a systematic review and meta-analysis. JAMA Ophthalmol. 2016;134:21–9. https://doi.org/10.1001/jamaophthalmol.2015.4070.
14. Freund KB, Korobelnik J-F, Devenyi R, et al. Treat-and-extend regimens with anti-VEGF agents in retinal diseases: a literature review and consensus recommendations. Retina. 2015;35:1489–506. https://doi.org/10.1097/IAE.0000000000000627.
15. Veritti D, Sarao V, Soppelsa V, et al. Managing diabetic macular edema in clinical practice: systematic review and meta-analysis of current strategies and treatment options. Clin Ophthalmol. 2021;15:375–85. https://doi.org/10.2147/OPTH.S236423.
16. Falcão M. Impact of intravitreal Ranibizumab therapy on vision outcomes in diabetic macular edema patients: a meta-analysis. Ophthalmologica. 2020;243:243–54. https://doi.org/10.1159/000505070.
17. Ross EL, Hutton DW, Stein JD, et al. Cost-effectiveness of Aflibercept, Bevacizumab, and Ranibizumab for diabetic macular edema treatment: analysis from the diabetic retinopathy clinical research network comparative effectiveness trial. JAMA Ophthalmol. 2016;134:888–96. https://doi.org/10.1001/jamaophthalmol.2016.1669.
18. Pham B, Thomas SM, Lillie E, et al. Anti-vascular endothelial growth factor treatment for retinal conditions: a systematic review and meta-analysis. BMJ Open. 2019;9:e022031. https://doi.org/10.1136/bmjopen-2018-022031.
19. Virgili G, Parravano M, Evans JR, et al. Anti-vascular endothelial growth factor for diabetic macular oedema: a network meta-analysis. Cochrane Database Syst Rev. 2018;10:CD007419. https://doi.org/10.1002/14651858.CD007419.pub6.
20. Liu Y, Cheng J, Gao Y, et al. Efficacy of switching therapy to aflibercept for patients with persistent diabetic macular edema: a systematic review and meta-analysis. Ann Transl Med. 2020;8:382. https://doi.org/10.21037/atm.2020.02.04.
21. Chung SH, Frick SL, Yiu G. Targeting vascular endothelial growth factor using retinal gene therapy. Ann Transl Med. 2021;9:1277. https://doi.org/10.21037/atm-20-4417.

Agents Targeting Angiopoietin/Tie Pathway in Diabetic Macular Edema

7

Fanny L. T. Yip, Cherie Y. K. Wong, and Timothy Y. Y. Lai

7.1 Roles of Angiopoietin/Tie Pathway in Retinal Diseases and Diabetic Macular Edema

Neovascular age-related macular degeneration (nAMD), diabetic macular edema (DME), proliferative diabetic retinopathy (PDR), and retinal vascular occlusion (RVO) are among the leading causes of blindness worldwide [1]. One of the common features of these conditions is the destabilization of the mature vasculature, associated with increased vascular permeability, inflammation, and/or growth of new pathological abnormal vessels [2]. Vascular endothelial growth factor (VEGF) and the angiopoietin/tyrosine kinase with immunoglobulin-like and endothelial growth factor-like domains (Tie) pathway are the key players in this process.

The angiopoietin/Tie pathway regulates the development and maintenance of blood vessels (including angiogenesis and vascular permeability), homeostasis, and inflammation [3–5]. Angiopoietins are growth factors playing important roles in vascular development. Angiopoietin-1 (Ang-1) is expressed by mesenchymal cells, pericytes, and smooth muscle cells [3, 6], while angiopoietin-2 (Ang-2) is expressed at low levels by endothelial cells in the deep vascular plexus in mature vasculature [7]. The receptor component of the Ang/Tie pathway, Tie2, is a type I tyrosine kinase receptor expressed in the endothelium and on pericytes [8].

Under normal physiological conditions, Ang-1 is expressed at higher levels than Ang-2 [9, 10]. Ang-1 is a strong Tie2 receptor agonist [3, 5, 11]. It activates Tie2 by inducing its phosphorylation, leading to signaling through the pro-survival phosphatidylinositol 3-kinase-protein kinase B (PI3K-AKT) pathway, resulting in stabilization of the cortical actin cytoskeleton and vascular endothelial cadherins (VE-cadherins) at cellular junctions. In addition, Tie2 activation phosphorylates transcription factor forkhead box protein O1 (FOXO1), and thus suppresses the expression of its target genes including Ang-2. These stabilize newly formed vessels and cause their maturation by promoting endothelial cell survival, pericyte recruitment, and improved endothelial barrier function, therefore acting as a molecular brake to prevent vascular leakage and inflammation [12, 13].

In pathologic conditions such as hypoxia and hyperglycemia associated with nAMD or DME, Ang-2 is upregulated while Ang-1 continues to be expressed at a relatively consistent level. This leads to a higher Ang-2/Ang-1 ratio [14, 15]. The higher level of Ang-2 displaces Ang-1, thus inhibiting Ang-1/Tie2 activation [3, 5]. Ang-2/Tie2 signaling in the endothelial cells leads to pericyte detachment, which sensitizes the retinal vasculature to VEGF and other pro-inflammatory factors via activation of *FOXO1* target genes. One of these genes is *Ang-2*, so a positive feedback loop is created [3, 16]. Independently of Tie2, Ang-2 can also bind to integrins (e.g. $\alpha\nu\beta1$, $\alpha\nu\beta3$, $\alpha3\beta1$, and $\alpha5\beta1$) with a lower affinity to promote vascular destabilization [17, 18]. Another member of the angiopoietin/Tie pathway is the protein tyrosine phosphatase (VE-PTP), which is also upregulated under hypoxic conditions. The expression of VE-PTP is specific to endothelial cells, where it dephosphorylates and inactivates Tie2 [19].

Increased understanding of the role of angiopoietin/Tie pathway in the pathogenesis of retinal diseases including DME has contributed to the development of therapeutic agents targeting this key pathway. Studies have suggested that modulation of the angiopoietin/Tie pathway, along with VEGF-A inhibition, can restore vascular stability by enhancing pericyte coverage and blood–retinal barrier integrity. This reduces vascular leakage, pathological neovascularization, and tissue infiltration by inflammatory cells. In addition, Ang-2 inhibition reduces pro-inflammatory macrophage polarization and vascular responsiveness to VEGF and other pro-inflammatory cytokines, potentially contributing to prevention of sustained retinal inflammation [2, 10, 14, 19–23].

F. L. T. Yip · C. Y. K. Wong
Hong Kong Eye Hospital, Kowloon, Hong Kong

T. Y. Y. Lai (✉)
Department of Ophthalmology and Visual Sciences, Chinese University of Hong Kong, Kowloon, Hong Kong
e-mail: tyylai@cuhk.edu.hk

S. Saxena et al. (eds.), *Diabetic Macular Edema*, https://doi.org/10.1007/978-981-19-7307-9_7

Table 7.1 List of pharmacological agents targeting the angiopoietin/Tie pathway

Pharmacological agent	Mechanism of action	Route of administration	Current development status
Razuprotafib (AKB-9778)	Small molecule inhibitor of VE-PTP	Subcutaneous injection	Completed phase 2 for DME and DR
Nesvacumab	Fully human IgG1 monoclonal antibody inhibiting Ang-2	Intravitreal injection as a co-formulation with aflibercept	Completed phase 2 for DME Development currently discontinued
Faricimab (Vabysmo)	Bi-specific IgG1-based antibody inhibiting both Ang-2 and VEGF simultaneously	Intravitreal injection	Completed phase 2 and 3 for DME and nAMD. Approved by the US FDA for the treatment of DME and nAMD
AXT107	Type IV collagen-derived peptide that activates Tie-2 and inhibits VEGF-A and VEGF-C	Intravitreal injection	On-going phase 1/2a for DME and nAMD
BI 836880	Bi-specific single-domain antibody (nanobody) inhibiting both VEGF and Ang-2	Intravitreal injection	On-going phase 1 for nAMD

DME diabetic macular edema, *DR* diabetic retinopathy, *nAMD* neovascular age-related macular degeneration

In this chapter, we will explore the latest development in the pharmacological agents targeting the angiopoietin/Tie pathway for treating retinal diseases like DME (Table 7.1).

7.2 Razuprotafib (AKB-9778)

7.2.1 Razuprotafib Mechanism of Action

Razuprotafib (AKB-9778) is a small molecule inhibitor of VE-PTP which activates Tie2 independent of the presence of Ang-1 or Ang-2 [4, 13, 24]. It acts by binding and inhibiting the intracellular catalytic domain of VE-PTP, thereby stabilizing endothelial junctions [19, 25]. Administered as subcutaneous injections, razuprotafib has been investigated for treatment of various vascular complications associated with diabetes, including DME and diabetic nephropathy [26–30].

7.2.2 Phase 1 DME Study

A phase 1 trial in DME was conducted in 24 patients and revealed AKB-9778 with dosages of 15 mg or higher resulted in improvements in BCVA and reductions in OCT central subfield thickness (CST) in some eyes with no systemic safety issues identified [3].

7.2.3 Phase 2 TIME-2 Study

TIME-2 was a phase 2 study in which 144 patients with DME were randomized into three arms: (1) AKB-9778 monotherapy: subcutaneous AKB-9778 15 mg twice per day (BID) + monthly sham intraocular injections; (2) combination therapy: subcutaneous AKB-9778 15 mg BID + monthly 0.3 mg ranibizumab; or (3) ranibizumab monotherapy: subcutaneous placebo injections BID + monthly 0.3 mg ranibizumab [31].

At week 12, the mean CST reduction from baseline was significantly greater in the combination group (−164.4 ± 24.2 μm) compared with the ranibizumab monotherapy group (−110.4 ± 17.2 μm; $P = 0.008$). No significant difference in vision gains at week 12 was observed between the combined AKB-9778 and ranibizumab arm versus ranibizumab monotherapy (6.3 ± 1.3 vs. 5.7 ± 1.2 letters, respectively; $P = 0.74$). No notable mean changes from baseline at week 12 in CST or vision from baseline were observed with AKB-9778 monotherapy. AKB-9778 appeared to be well tolerated with no significant difference in serious adverse events between the three arms.

TIME-2a and TIME-2b studies were follow-up trials on the potential role of AKB-9778 for the treatment of diabetic retinopathy. In TIME-2a, comparable proportions of eyes manifested a ≥2-step improvement in diabetic retinopathy severity score (DRSS) in the ranibizumab, AKB-9778, and combination groups (8.8%, 10.0%, and 11.4%, respectively) [13, 32]. In TIME-2b, there was no significant difference between AKB-9778 and placebo groups in the proportions of eyes attaining a ≥2-step improvement in DRSS, showing that Tie2 activation likely requires concomitant VEGF suppression for optimal efficacy [13, 33]. No further studies of AKB-9778 has been announced since the completion of the TIME-2b study.

7.3 Nesvacumab + Aflibercept Coformulation (REGN910-3)

7.3.1 Nesvacumab Mechanism of Action

Nesvacumab is a fully human immunoglobulin G1 (IgG1) monoclonal antibody which selectively binds Ang-2 with high affinity and blocks its binding to Tie-2 receptors [34]. This in turn promotes more Ang1/Tie2 receptor binding and phosphorylation of the Tie2 pathway, leading to vascular stabilization. Nesvacumab was co-formulated with aflibercept for intravitreal injection.

7.3.2 Phase 1 Trial

In a phase 1 dose escalating study, 20 patients with nAMD or DME were allocated into the following arms (two patients with nAMD and two patients with DME per arm): (1) 0.5 mg nesvacumab +2 mg aflibercept; (2) 1 mg nesvacumab +2 mg aflibercept; (3) 3 mg nesvacumab +2 mg aflibercept; (4) 6 mg nesvacumab +2 mg aflibercept; and (5) 6 mg nesvacumab alone. Visual and anatomical improvements were noted in all doses, leading to further phase II studies in the ONYX study for nAMD and the RUBY study for DME [35, 36].

7.3.3 Phase 2 RUBY Study

RUBY was a double-masked, multicenter phase 2 study evaluating the use of nesvacumab and aflibercept coformulation in DME [37]. A total of 302 patients were randomized into three arms in a 1:2:3 ratio to receive low-dose combination (3 mg nesvacumab +2 mg aflibercept), high-dose combination (6 mg nesvacumab +2 mg aflibercept), or aflibercept monotherapy (2 mg) [38]. Patients received intravitreal injections every 4 weeks (Q4W) for a total of 12 weeks. After 12 weeks, patients were re-randomized to assess additional dosing regimens, including up to every 12 weeks (Q12W) administration of the high-dose combination and aflibercept monotherapy up to week 36. The primary endpoint was change from baseline in BCVA (Early Treatment Diabetic Retinopathy Study [EDTRS] letter score) at week 12 and week 36.

Results showed that combination of intravitreal nesvacumab and aflibercept did not provide additional visual acuity benefit over aflibercept monotherapy. Despite the similar visual outcome, patients treated with high-dose combination had significantly more reduction in mean central retinal thickness (CRT) compared to patients treated with aflibercept monotherapy at week 12 (least-square mean CRT change from baseline of −191.6 vs. −163.8 μm, respectively; $P = 0.0183$). In addition, significantly higher proportions of patients treated in the high-dose combination arm had complete resolution of fluid at the foveal center at week 12 compared with patients treated with aflibercept monotherapy (66.3% vs. 53.7%, respectively; $P = 0.0489$). The safety profiles of the nesvacumab/aflibercept coformulation were reported to be similar to aflibercept in patients with DME. However, since no additional visual benefit was shown in the nesvacumab/aflibercept coformulation group over aflibercept monotherapy, further clinical development of the nesvacumab and aflibercept coformulation has been discontinued.

7.4 Faricimab (RG7716)

7.4.1 Faricimab Mechanism of Action

Faricimab (RG7716) is a bispecific immunoglobulin G1–based antibody targeting both Ang-2 and VEGF-A, designed using Roche's proprietary CrossMAb technology for intraocular use [14]. It can bind Ang-2 and VEGF-A at the same time with high affinity and specificity [14, 15, 39]. The fragment crystallizable (Fc) portion was engineered to abolish binding interactions with neonatal Fc and Fc gamma receptors, therefore can reduce the risk of potential inflammation and can allow for a faster systemic clearance [14].

The dual inhibition of Ang-2 and VEGF with faricimab was shown to synergistically promote vascular stability and reduce vascular leakage compared with intravitreal anti-VEGF monotherapy in preclinical models [39]. The efficacy and safety of faricimab in patients with DME have been evaluated in the phase 2 BOULEVARD study and the phase 3 YOSEMITE and RHINE studies. Meanwhile, the ongoing RHONE-X study will further evaluate its long-term safety and tolerability.

7.4.2 Phase 2 BOULEVARD Study

BOULEVARD was a prospective, randomized, double-masked, multicenter phase 2 trial comparing the safety and efficacy of faricimab with ranibizumab in patients with DME [40]. It enrolled 229 patients (168 treatment-naive and 61 previously treated with anti-VEGF) who were 18 years of age or older with center-involving DME, best corrected visual acuity (BCVA) of 73 to 24 Early Treatment Diabetic Retinopathy Study (ETDRS) letters, and central subfield thickness (CST) of 325 μm or more. The treatment-naive patients were randomized in the ratio of 1:1:1 into receiving intravitreal faricimab 6 mg, faricimab 1.5 mg, or ranibizumab 0.3 mg. Patients previously treated with anti-VEGF were randomized 1:1 into receiving faricimab 6 mg or ranibizumab 0.3 mg. All patients were dosed monthly for 20 weeks, followed by an observation period up to week 36 to assess the durability. During the observation period, patients were evaluated every 4 weeks and received a single dose of ranibizumab 0.3 mg if they met the respecified re-treatment criteria based on BCVA and CST measurements.

The primary endpoint was the mean change in BCVA from baseline at week 24 in the treatment-naive patients. In the treatment-naive population, faricimab 6 mg–treated patients achieved statistically greater mean BCVA gains than those treated with ranibizumab 0.3 mg at week 24. The proportion of patients achieving ≥10-letter gains and the proportion of patients achieving CST ≤325 μm were both higher in the faricimab 6 mg group, compared with the faricimab 1.5 mg and ranibizumab 0.3 mg groups. The faricimab 6 mg and 1.5 mg groups demonstrated dose-related BCVA improvements and CST reductions. As for the effect on DR, there was a greater percentage of patients achieving one-step or more improvement in DRSS in the faricimab 6 mg group. For the durability, patients treated with faricimab 6 mg exhibited longer time to re-treatment during the observation period compared with the ranibizumab-treated patients. There were no new or unexpected safety signals with faricimab.

This study provided evidence that vascular stabilization mediated through the simultaneous inhibition of Ang-2 and VEGF-A can restore retinal anatomic features and function better than VEGF inhibition alone. It also demonstrated potential for the added benefit of Ang-2 inhibition in the management of DR.

7.4.3 Phase 3 RHINE and YOSEMITE Studies

RHINE and YOSEMITE are randomized, double-masked, non-inferiority phase 3 clinical trials to evaluate the efficacy and safety of faricimab in patients with DME [41]. The studies enrolled a total of 1891 patients across 353 sites in 31 countries with macular thickening secondary to DME involving the center of fovea with CST ≥325 μm and with BCVA of 73–25 letters. The patients were randomized into receiving faricimab 6 mg every 8 weeks (Q8W) after six initial Q4W doses, faricimab 6 mg with personalized treatment interval (PTI) after a minimum of four initial Q4W doses, and aflibercept 2 mg Q8W after five initial Q4W doses.

The six initial Q4W doses in the Q8W group was based on the phase 2 BOULEVARD trial [40], in which patients treated with faricimab showed continuous BCVA improvement with each Q4W dose up to week 24. The Q8W maintenance interval in this group was also supported by the BOULEVARD trial which demonstrated that 93% of patients had no disease reactivation 8 weeks after their last dose of faricimab 6 mg. In addition, assessments of the aqueous humor samples from a subset of patients treated with faricimab in the AVENUE phase 2 study showed suppression of ocular-free Ang-2 and VEGF-A for at least 8 weeks [42, 43]. Dosing intervals in the PTI group were determined by an automated algorithm based on the treat-and-extend concept, with dosing interval adjusted by 4-week intervals according to prespecified BCVA and CST criteria. The PTI protocol allowed for up to Q16W dosing intervals.

The primary endpoint was the mean BCVA change from baseline at 1 year, averaged over weeks 48, 52, and 65. The BCVA gains from baseline in the faricimab Q8W or faricimab PTI groups were non-inferior compared with the aflibercept group. The mean BCVA gains at 1 year for the faricimab Q8W, faricimab PTI, and aflibercept groups were 10.7, 11.6, and 10.9 ETDRS letters in the YOSEMITE study respectively, and 11.8, 10.8, and 10.3 ETDRS letters in the RHINE study, respectively. The studies also demonstrated superior anatomic outcomes in patients treated with faricimab, with more patients showing absence of DME and more patients showing absence of intraretinal fluid compared with the aflibercept groups. The change in mean CST also favored faricimab. In the faricimab PTI group, more than 70% of patients were on at least Q12W dosing intervals at week 52, showing the strong durability with faricimab. The median number of injections for the faricimab Q8W, faricimab PTI, and aflibercept Q8W groups were 10, 8, and 8, respectively. Faricimab was well tolerated in the study with no case of occlusive retinal vasculitis reported.

7.4.4 RHONE-X Study

RHONE-X study is an on-going multicentered long-term extension study designed to evaluate the long-term safety and tolerability of intravitreal faricimab injection using the PTI regime for DME patients who have completed the YOSEMITE or RHINE studies (ClinicalTrials.gov identifier NCT04432831). The first 16 weeks of this study is a masked period during which participants receive either faricimab or sham injection. Participants and physicians will be masked only to the faricimab treatment interval. After the week 16 treatment procedure, this study follows an open-label design. The primary outcome measures include the incidence and severity of ocular and systemic adverse events, number of participants with presence of anti-drug antibodies (ADAs) at baseline, and the incidence of ADAs during the study. It is expected to complete by 2023.

7.5 Other Potential Agents Targeting Angiopoietin/Tie Pathway for DME

7.5.1 AXT107

AXT107 is a synthetic 20-mer type IV collagen-derived self-forming gel peptide that activates Tie-2 pathway signaling and inhibits VEGF-A and VEGF-C [34]. Both the actions are mediated by AXT107's interaction with and disruption of integrin $\alpha_5\beta_1$ and integrin $\alpha_V\beta_3$ proteins [44, 45]. AXT107 disrupts integrin $\alpha_5\beta_1$ and allows Tie-2 receptors to cluster at endothelial cell junctions. These Tie-2 clusters are similar to Tie-2 superclusters that are formed naturally in response to Ang-1 exposure which are inactive without a bound ligand. The junctional clustering of Tie-2 induced by AXT107 allows both Ang-1 and even Ang-2, which normally acts as an antagonist of Tie-2 and an inducer of vascular leakage, to function as a strong agonist of Tie-2 and promoter of vascular integrity. Tie-2 phosphorylation and activation promotes vascular stability and health.

With the same mechanism of converting the pro-inflammatory Ang-2 into a strong agonist of Tie-2 pathway by promoting junctional clustering of Tie-2, AXT107 suppresses TNF-α-induced vascular inflammation in endothelial cells and prevents IκBα degradation. The recovery of IκBα prevents NF-κB nuclear localization and blocks NF-κB-induced inflammatory responses. AXT107 also disrupts integrin $\alpha_V\beta_3$ and prevents their binding to VEGFR2, thereby reducing VEGF-bound VEGFR2 phosphorylation and downstream signaling.

In animal models, AXT107 has been shown to suppress neovascularization, decreases vascular permeability, and reduces inflammation [34]. AXT107 is delivered by intravitreal injection as a self-assembling gel depot formation which might have the potential to be dosed once per year. A phase 1/2a study (CONGO) is currently ongoing to assess the safety, tolerability, bioactivity, and duration of action of a single intravitreal injection of 0.1 mg, 0.25 mg, or 0.5 mg AXT107 in approximately 18 subjects (up to 6 subjects per dose) with DME. The study is expected to be completed in May 2022 [46].

7.5.2 BI 836880

Developed by Boehringer Ingelheim, BI 836880 is a humanized bi-specific single-domain antibody (nanobody) which binds both VEGF and Ang-2 in a similar manner to faricimab, along with a albumin-binding domain for better durability with half-life extension. It is administered via intravitreal injection [35]. A phase I study is ongoing to evaluate the safety and tolerability of BI 836880 in 45 nAMD patients, while no study in DME has been performed so far (ClincalTrial.gov identifier NCT03861234). The phase I study contains a single rising dose segment, which is followed by a multiple rising dose segment. The study is expected to be completed by August 2022.

7.6 Summary

Over the past two decades, intravitreal anti-VEGF monotherapy has been the standard of care treatment for patients with DME. Although, anti-VEGF therapy can result in substantial visual gain in the majority of patients, many patients will require multiple repeated injections causing significant treatment burden. Therefore, it is desirable to have other treatment options which have the potential improve the durability of existing treatment while keeping the visual improvement efficacy [47].

As highlighted in this chapter, the angiopoietin/Tie2 pathway is another therapeutic target for the treatment of DME. Pathologic conditions including DME and nAMD will result in angiogenic switch, causing increase in Ang-2/Ang-1 ratio. This will lead to inhibition of Tie2 activation, making the blood vessels more sensitivity to the effects of VEGF-A, thereby causing vascular permeability, angiogenesis, and increase in susceptivity to inflammation. It has been demonstrated that the levels of Ang-2 is upregulated in the vitreous samples of patients with retinal diseases such as nAMD, DME, PDR, and RVO [14]. Preclinical data in a murine CNV model also demonstrated that dual inhibition of VEGF and Ang-2 can result in greater reduction in CNV leakage with increased durability compared with inhibiting VEGF alone [48]. Based on the positive results in the use of faricimab in the phase 3 RHINE and YOSMITE studies for DME and in the phase 3 TENAYA and LUCERNE studies for nAMD [41, 49], faricimab has been approved by the US Food and Drug Administration (FDA) in January 2022 for the treatment of both DME and nAMD. It is being marketed under the trade name Vabysmo by Genentech/Roche. With further research and on-going clinical trials, more pharmaceutical agents targeting the angiopoietin/Tie pathway might become available in the future for the treatment of DME and other macular diseases.

References

1. Flaxman SR, Bourne RRA, Resnikoff S, et al. Global causes of blindness and distance vision impairment 1990–2020: a systematic review and meta-analysis. Lancet Glob Health. 2017;5:e1221–34.
2. Joussen AM, Ricci F, Paris LP, Korn C, Quezada-Ruiz C, Zarbin M. Angiopoietin/Tie2 signalling and its role in retinal and choroidal vascular diseases: a review of preclinical data. Eye (Lond). 2021 May;35(5):1305–16.
3. Saharinen P, Eklund L, Alitalo K. Therapeutic targeting of the angiopoietin-TIE pathway. Nat Rev Drug Discov. 2017;16:635–61.
4. Campochiaro PA, Peters KG. Targeting Tie2 for treatment of diabetic retinopathy and diabetic macular edema. Curr Diab Rep. 2016;16:126.
5. Huang H, Bhat A, Woodnutt G, et al. Targeting the ANGPT-TIE2 pathway in malignancy. Nat Rev Cancer. 2010;10:575–85.
6. Augustin HG, Koh GY, Thurston G, Alitalo K. Control of vascular morphogenesis and homeostasis through the angiopoietin-Tie system. Nat Rev Mol Cell Biol. 2009;10:165–77.
7. Oshima Y, Deering T, Oshima S, et al. Angiopoietin-2 enhances retinal vessel sensitivity to vascular endothelial growth factor. J Cell Physiol. 2004;199:412–7.
8. Teichert M, Milde L, Holm A, Stanicek L, Gengenbacher N, Savant S, et al. Pericyte-expressed Tie2 controls angiogenesis and vessel maturation. Nat Commun. 2017;8:16106.
9. Imhof BA, Aurrand-Lions M. Angiogenesis and inflammation face off. Nat Med. 2006;12:171–2.
10. Fiedler U, Reiss Y, Scharpfenecker M, Grunow V, Koidl S, Thurston G, et al. Angiopoietin-2 sensitizes endothelial cells to TNF-a and has a crucial role in the induction of inflammation. Nat Med. 2006;12:235–9.
11. Makinde T, Agrawal DK. Intra and extravascular transmembrane signalling of angiopoietin-1-Tie2 receptor in health and disease. J Cell Mol Med. 2008;12:810–28.
12. Parikh SM. Angiopoietins and Tie2 in vascular inflammation. Curr Opin Hematol. 2017;24:432–8.
13. Heier JS, Singh RP, Wykoff CC, Csaky KG, Lai TYY, Loewenstein A, Schlottmann PG, Paris LP, Westenskow PD, Quezada-Ruiz

C. The angiopoietin/tie pathway in retinal vascular diseases: a review. Retina. 2021;41(1):1–19.
14. Regula JT, Lundh von Leithner P, Foxton R, et al. Targeting key angiogenic pathways with a bispecific CrossMAb optimized for neovascular eye diseases. EMBO Mol Med. 2016;8:1265–88.
15. Regula JT, Lundh von Leithner P, Foxton R, et al. Targeting key angiogenic pathways with a bispecific CrossMAb optimized for neovascular eye diseases. EMBO Mol Med. 2019;11:e10666.
16. Hammes HP, Lin J, Wagner P, Feng Y, Vom Hagen F, Krzizok T, et al. Angiopoietin-2 causes pericyte dropout in the normal retina: evidence for involvement in diabetic retinopathy. Diabetes. 2004;53:1104–10.
17. Felcht M, Luck R, Schering A, Seidel P, Srivastava K, Hu J, et al. Angiopoietin-2 differentially regulates angiogenesis through TIE2 and integrin signaling. J Clin Invest. 2012;122:1991–2005.
18. Hakanpaa L, Sipila T, Leppanen V-M, Gautam P, Nurmi H, Jacquemet G, et al. Endothelial destabilization by angiopoietin-2 via integrin β1 activation. Nat Commun. 2015;6:5962.
19. Shen J, Frye M, Lee BL, Reinardy JL, McClung JM, Ding K, et al. Targeting VE-PTP activates TIE2 and stabilizes the ocular vasculature. J Clin Invest. 2014;124:4564–76.
20. Scholz A, Lang V, Henschler R, Czabanka M, Vajkoczy P, Chavakis E, et al. Angiopoietin-2 promotes myeloid cell infiltration in a β2-integrin–dependent manner. Blood. 2011;118:5050–9.
21. Srivastava K, Hu J, Korn C, Savant S, Teichert M, Kapel SS, et al. Postsurgical adjuvant tumor therapy by combining anti- angiopoietin-2 and metronomic chemotherapy limits metastatic growth. Cancer Cell. 2014;26:880–95.
22. Benest AV, Kruse K, Savant S, Thomas M, Laib AM, Loos EK, et al. Angiopoietin-2 is critical for cytokine-induced vascular leakage. PLoS One. 2013;8:e70459.
23. Lee S-J, Lee C-K, Kang S, Park I, Kim YH, Kim SK, et al. Angiopoietin-2 exacerbates cardiac hypoxia and inflammation after myocardial infarction. J Clin Invest. 2018;128:5018–24.
24. Campochiaro PA, Sophie R, Tolentino M, et al. Treatment of diabetic macular edema with an inhibitor of vascular endothelial-protein tyrosine phosphatase that activates Tie2. Ophthalmology. 2015;122:545–54.
25. Frye M, Dierkes M, Küppers V, et al. Interfering with VE-PTP stabilizes endothelial junctions in vivo via Tie-2 in the absence of VE-cadherin. J Exp Med. 2015;212(13):2267–87.
26. Yabkowitz R, Meyer S, Yanagihara D, et al. Regulation of tie receptor expression on human endothelial cells by protein kinase C-mediated release of soluble tie. Blood. 1997;90(2):706–15.
27. Akwii RG, Mikelis CM. Targeting the Angiopoietin/Tie pathway: prospects for treatment of retinal and respiratory disorders. Drugs. 2021;81(15):1731–49.
28. Pournaras CJ, et al. Regulation of retinal blood flow in health and disease. Prog Retin Eye Res. 2008;27(3):284–330.
29. Saint-Geniez M, D'Amore PA. Development and pathology of the hyaloid, choroidal and retinal vasculature. Int J Dev Biol. 2004;48(8–9):1045–58.
30. Dreher Z, Robinson SR, Distler C. Muller cells in vascular and avascular retinae: a survey of seven mammals. J Comp Neurol. 1992;323(1):59–80.
31. Campochiaro PA, Khanani A, Singer M, et al. Enhanced benefit in diabetic macular edema from AKB-9778 Tie2 activation combined with vascular endothelial growth factor suppression. Ophthalmology. 2016;123(8):1722–30.
32. Aerpio Press Release. Aerpio therapeutics announces presentation of positive results of Akb-9778 in patients with diabetic retinopathy from time-2 phase 2a study. 2016. https://www.businesswire.com/news/home/20160210006109/en/Aerpio-Therapeutics-Announces-Presentation-Positive-Results-AKB-9778. Accessed 5 Jan 2022.
33. Aerpio Corporate Presentation. 2019. https://ir.aerpio.com/static-files/7ec12cbe-9bfd-41e4-98fb-569070cd1bf1. Accessed 5 Jan 2022.
34. Nguyen QD, Heier JS, Do DV, et al. The Tie2 signaling pathway in retinal vascular diseases: a novel therapeutic target in the eye. Int J Retina Vitreous. 2020;6:48.
35. Khanani AM, Russell MW, Aziz AA, et al. Angiopoietins as potential targets in management of retinal disease. Clin Ophthalmol. 2021;15:3747–55.
36. Regeneron Pharmaceuticals. An open-label, dose-escalation study of the safety and tolerability of intravitreal (IVT) REGN910–3 and IVT REGN910 in patients with either neovascular AMD or DME [Internet]. clinicaltrials.gov; 2016. https://clinicaltrials.gov/ct2/show/NCT01997164. Accessed 5 Jan 2022.
37. ClinicalTrials.gov. Anti-vasculaR Endothelial Growth Factor plUs anti-angiopoietin 2 in Fixed comBination therapY: evaluation for the Treatment of Diabetic Macular Edema (RUBY). Tarrytown, NY: Regeneron Pharmaceuticals. https://clinicaltrials.gov/ct2/show/NCT02712008. Accessed 5 Jan 2022.
38. Boyer DS. Intravitreal Nesvacumab+Aflibercept in diabetic macular edema: the phase 2 RUBY Trial. Invest Ophthalmol Vis Sci. 2018;59(9):3620.
39. Schaefer W, Regula JT, Bähner M, et al. Immunoglobulin domain crossover as a generic approach for the production of bispecific IgG antibodies. Proc Natl Acad Sci U S A. 2011;108:11187–92.
40. Sahni J, Patel SS, Dugel PU, et al. Simultaneous inhibition of angiopoietin-2 and vascular endothelial growth factor-A with faricimab in diabetic macular edema: BOULEVARD phase 2 randomized trial. Ophthalmology. 2019;126:1155–70.
41. Wykoff CC, Abreu F, Adamis AP, et al. Efficacy, durability, and safety of intravitreal faricimab with extended dosing up to every 16 weeks in patients with diabetic macular oedema (YOSEMITE and RHINE): two randomised, double-masked, phase 3 trials. Lancet. 2022;399(10326):741–55.
42. Sahni J, Dugel PU, Patel SS, et al. Safety and efficacy of different doses and regimens of faricimab vs ranibizumab in neovascular age-related macular degeneration: the AVENUE phase 2 randomized clinical trial. JAMA Ophthalmol. 2020;138:955–63.
43. Csaky K, Cheik D, Foxton R, et al. Data supporting the sustained efficacy of Faricimab, a bispecific antibody neutralizing both Angiopoietin-2 and VEGF-A. In: Presented at American Academy of Ophthalmology Subspecialty Day; October 11-12, 2019; San Francisco, CA, USA.
44. Mirando AC, Shen J, Silva RLE, et al. A collagen Iv-derived peptide disrupts alpha5beta1 integrin and potentiates Ang2/Tie2 signaling. JCI Insight. 2019;4:e122043.
45. Silva RLE, Kanan Y, Mirando AC, et al. Tyrosine kinase blocking collagen iv-derived peptide suppresses ocular neovascularization and vascular leakage. Sci Transl Med. 2017;9:eaai8030.
46. ClinicalTrials.gov. Safety and bioactivity of AXT107 in subjects with diabetic macular edema (CONGO). https://clinicaltrials.gov/ct2/show/NCT04697758. Accessed 5 Jan 2022.
47. Chia MA, Keane PA. Beyond anti-VEGF: can faricimab reduce treatment burden for retinal disease? Lancet. 2022;399(10326):697–9.
48. Foxton RH, Uhles S, Grüner S, Revelant F, Ullmer C. Efficacy of simultaneous VEGF-A/ANG-2 neutralization in suppressing spontaneous choroidal neovascularization. EMBO Mol Med. 2019;11(5):e10204.
49. Heier JS, Khanani AM, Quezada Ruiz C, et al. Efficacy, durability, and safety of intravitreal faricimab up to every 16 weeks for neovascular age-related macular degeneration (TENAYA and LUCERNE): two randomised, double-masked, phase 3, non-inferiority trials. Lancet. 2022;399(10326):729–40.

8 DRCR.net Trials for Diabetic Macular Edema

Mariacristina Parravano, Eliana Costanzo, Riccardo Sacconi, and Giuseppe Querques

8.1 Introduction

The Diabetic Retinopathy Clinical Research Network (DRCR.net) was formed in 2002 through a National Eye Institute and National Institute of Diabetes and Digestive and Kidney Diseases-sponsored cooperative agreement, to create a network enable to facilitate collaborations and multicenter clinical research on Diabetic Retinopathy (DR), Diabetic Macular Edema (DME), and associated conditions [1].

In the last two decades (2003–2021), the DRCR.net conducted 35 multicenter studies, in 131 active clinical sites by 420 investigators, publishing 113 scientific papers (available online at https://public.jaeb.org).

The most relevant results of the studies conducted since here promoted the use of anti-vascular endothelial growth factor (VEGF) therapy as effective alternative to panretinal photocoagulation (PRP) in patients affected by proliferative diabetic retinopathy (PDR) and as first-line therapy in case of visual impairment due to DME, established treatment algorithms for intravitreal agents and also helped to better understand the use of different imaging modalities, as optical coherence tomography (OCT), OCT-angiography (OCTA), fluorescein angiography (FA), and wide-field devices, in the DR/DME management [1].

Since 2017 the network was extended to all retinal disease, creating the DRCR Retina Network.

Table 8.1 summarized all DRCR.net protocols, reporting the major findings on DME and DR management and treatment. Specific DME protocols will be focused on in the following sections.

M. Parravano · E. Costanzo
IRCCS-Fondazione Bietti, Rome, Italy

R. Sacconi · G. Querques (✉)
Department of Ophthalmology, IRCCS Ospedale San Raffaele, University Vita-Salute, Milan, Italy

S. Saxena et al. (eds.), *Diabetic Macular Edema*, https://doi.org/10.1007/978-981-19-7307-9_8

Table 8.1 DRCR.net trials for diabetic macular edema

Protocol	Title/description	Study period	Major findings for DME/DR
A	A Pilot Study of Laser Photocoagulation for Diabetic Macular Edema	2003–2008	Focal/grid laser in non-CI CSME eyes was associated with relative stable VA and retinal thickness measurements and decreased FA leakage area at 1 year
B	A Randomized Trial Comparing Intravitreal Triamcinolone Acetonide and Laser Photocoagulation for Diabetic Macular Edema	2004–2008	Over 2 and 3 years, focal/grid laser was more effective and has fewer side effects than intravitreal triamcinolone
D	Evaluation of Vitrectomy for Diabetic Macular Edema Study	2004–2009	Following vitrectomy performed for DME and vitreomacular traction, retinal thickening was reduced in most eyes. It might consider vitrectomy for DME in eyes with at least moderate vision loss and vitreomacular traction
E	A Pilot Study of Peribulbar Triamcinolone Acetonide for Diabetic Macular Edema	2004–2007	In cases of DME with good visual acuity, peribulbar triamcinolone, with or without focal photocoagulation, was unlikely to be of substantial benefit
C	Temporal Variation in Optical Coherence Tomography Measurements of Retinal Thickening in Diabetic Macular Edema	2004–2005	Although on average there are slight decreases in retinal thickening during the day, most eyes with DME have little meaningful change in OCT central subfield thickening between 8 a.m. and 4 p.m.
H	A Phase 2 Evaluation of Anti-VEGF Therapy for Diabetic Macular Edema: Bevacizumab (Avastin)	2005–2008	First multicenter RCT demonstrating anti-VEGF (bevacizumab) can reduce DME in some eyes
F	An Observational Study of the Development of Diabetic Macular Edema Following Scatter Laser Photocoagulation	2005–2008	Among eyes with PDR treated with PRP, clinically meaningful differences are unlikely in visual acuity or macular edema following application of PRP in 1 sitting compared with 4 sittings
G	Subclinical Diabetic Macular Edema Study	2005–2009	Although subclinical DME may be uncommon, approximately one-quarter and one-half of eyes with subclinical DME will progress to more definite thickening or be judged to need treatment for DME within 2 years after its identification
K	The Course of Response to Focal Photocoagulation for Diabetic Macular Edema	2006–2008	After focal/grid laser for DME, in eyes with a definite reduction, but not resolution, of central edema, 23%–63% will continue to improve without additional treatment
I	Intravitreal Ranibizumab or Triamcinolone Acetonide in Combination with Laser Photocoagulation for Diabetic Macular Edema	2007–2013	Intravitreal ranibizumab with prompt or deferred laser is more effective than laser alone at increasing visual acuity in eyes with center-involved DME
J	Intravitreal Ranibizumab or Triamcinolone Acetonide as Adjunctive Treatment to Panretinal Photocoagulation for Proliferative Diabetic Retinopathy	2007–2010	The addition of 1 intravitreal triamcinolone or 2 ranibizumab injections in eyes receiving focal/grid laser for DME and PRP was associated with better visual acuity and decreased macular edema (by 14 weeks)
L	Evaluation of Visual Acuity Measurements in Eyes with Diabetic Macular Edema	2007–2010	Autorefraction is not an acceptable substitute for manual refraction for most clinical trials with primary outcomes dependent on best-corrected VA
O	Comparison of Time Domain OCT and Spectral Domain OCT Retinal Thickness Measurement in Diabetic Macular Edema	2009–2013	Thickness reproducibility appeared similar between different devices (RTVue and Stratus). Conversion equations to transform RTVue measurements to Stratus-equivalent values within 10% of the observed Stratus RT are feasible. CRT measurement changed greater than 10% when using the same machine or 20% when switching from Stratus to RTVue, after conversion to Stratus equivalents
P	A Pilot Study in Individuals with Center-Involved DME Undergoing Cataract Surgery	2009–2010	No definitive conclusions for the heterogeneity of pre and post-surgical macular edema management
Q	An Observational Study in Individuals with Diabetic Retinopathy without Center-Involved DME Undergoing Cataract Surgery	2009–2011	In eyes with DR without concurrent central-involved DME, presence of non-central DME immediately prior to cataract surgery, or history of DME treatment, may increase risk of developing central-involved macular edema 16 weeks after cataract extraction

N	An Evaluation of Intravitreal Ranibizumab for Vitreous Hemorrhage Due to Proliferative Diabetic Retinopathy	2010–2012	The clinically important difference between ranibizumab and saline at the rate of vitrectomy by 16 weeks (short term) and 52 weeks (long term) in eyes with VH from PDR was lower than expected Short term secondary outcomes including visual acuity improvement, increased PRP completion rates, and reduced recurrent VH rates suggest biologic activity of ranibizumab
M	Effect of Diabetes Education during Retinal Ophthalmology Visits on Diabetes Control	2011–2014	Addition of personalized education and risk assessment during retinal ophthalmology visits, as assessed in the study, did not result in HbA1c improvement compared with usual care over 1 year
R	A Phase II Evaluation of Topical NSAIDs in Eyes with Non Central Involved DME	2011–2013	In eyes with non-central DME and good visual acuity, topical NSAIDs for 1 year likely did not have a meaningful effect on OCT-measured retinal thickness
S	Prompt Panretinal Photocoagulation versus Intravitreal Ranibizumab with Deferred Panretinal Photocoagulation for Proliferative Diabetic Retinopathy	2012–2018	2015: Visual acuity at 2 years with ranibizumab is non-inferior to (not worse than) PRP for PDR 2018: • Mean change in VA with ranibizumab similar to PRP at 5 years • Substantial VA loss rare (6% in each group) • Visual field loss progressed in both groups in years 2–5; difference between groups • Diminished • Vitreous hemorrhage in almost 50% of both groups
GEN	Genes in Diabetic Retinopathy Project	2012–recruiting	
T	A Comparative Effectiveness Study of Intravitreal Aflibercept, Bevacizumab and Ranibizumab for Diabetic Macular Edema	2012–2018	• For eyes with DME and moderate or worse visual acuity loss (20/50 or worse) at baseline, on average, aflibercept results in superior visual acuity results compared with bevacizumab and ranibizumab 0.3-mg at 1 year and continues to be superior to bevacizumab at 2 years • For eyes with DME and initial visual acuity 20/32–20/40, on average, visual acuity results using bevacizumab, ranibizumab 0.3-mg, and aflibercept are similar at 1 year and 2 years
V	Treatment for Central-Involved Diabetic Macular Edema in Eyes with Very Good Visual Acuity	2013–2018	• Among eyes with center-involved DME and GOOD visual acuity (20/25 or better), VA loss after 2 years was similar regardless of whether initial management was aflibercept, laser, or observation • Each treatment strategy resulted in a 20/20 mean vision
U	Short-term Evaluation of Combination Corticosteroid + Anti-VEGF Treatment for Persistent Central-Involved Diabetic Macular Edema Following Anti-VEGF Therapy	2014–2017	Although its use is more likely to reduce retinal thickness and increase intraocular pressure, the combination of dexamethasone and ranibizumab does not improve visual acuity at 24 weeks more than ranibizumab alone among eyes with persistent DME following anti-VEGF therapy
AA	Peripheral Diabetic Retinopathy (DR) Lesions on Ultrawide-field Fundus Images and Risk of DR Worsening Over Time	2015	Imaging by the ETDRS 7-field and UWF imaging systems have moderate to substantial agreement when determining the severity of DR within the 7 standard fields
W	Intravitreous Anti-VEGF Treatment for Prevention of Vision Threatening Diabetic Retinopathy in Eyes at High Risk	2016–2022	• 2-year results: among eyes with moderate to severe NPDR, the proportion of eyes that developed PDR or vision-reducing CI-DME was lower with periodic aflibercept compared with sham treatment. However, through 2 years, preventive treatment did not confer visual acuity benefit compared with observation plus treatment with aflibercept only after development of PDR or vision-reducing CI-DME • The 4-year results will be important to assess longer-term visual acuity outcomes

(continued)

Table 8.1 (continued)

Protocol	Title/description	Study period	Major findings for DME/DR
AB	Intravitreous Anti-VEGF vs. Prompt Vitrectomy for Vitreous Hemorrhage from Proliferative Diabetic Retinopathy	2016–2020	• In eyes with vitreous hemorrhage from PDR, there was no significant difference in mean VA letter score over 24 weeks following initial treatment of aflibercept versus vitrectomy with PRP • Vision improved more quickly with vitrectomy, but long-term vision was similar • Considering the range of the confidence interval, a clinically important benefit in favor of initial vitrectomy with photocoagulation over 24 weeks cannot be excluded
TX	A Comparative Effectiveness Study of Intravitreal Aflibercept, Bevacizumab and Ranibizumab for Diabetic Macular Edema—Follow-up Extension Study	2017–2019	In the protocol extension, the mean VA improved from baseline to 5 years without protocol-defined treatment after follow-up ended at 2 years Although mean retinal thickness was similar at 2 and 5 years, mean VA worsened during this period
AC	Randomized Trial of Intravitreous Aflibercept versus Intravitreous Bevacizumab + Deferred Aflibercept for Treatment of Central-Involved Diabetic Macular Edema	2017–follow-up	
AD	PROMINENT-Eye Ancillary Study: Diabetic Retinopathy Outcomes in a Randomized Trial of Pemafibrate versus Placebo	2017–2018	
AH	Single-Arm Study Assessing the Effects of Pneumatic Vitreolysis on Macular Hole	2018–2020	In most eyes with VMT, PVL induced hyaloid release. In eyes with FTMH, PVL resulted in hole closure in approximately one third of eyes. These studies were terminated early because of safety concerns related to retinal detachments and retinal tears
AG	Randomized Clinical Trial Assessing the Effects of Pneumatic Vitreolysis on Vitreomacular Traction	2018–2020	
AE	A Pilot Study Evaluating Photobiomodulation Therapy for Diabetic Macular Edema	2019	Photobiomodulation, as given in this study, while safe and well tolerated, was not found to be effective for the treatment of CI-DME in eyes with good vision
AJ	Vitreous Proteomics in Eyes with a Macular Hole	2020–recruiting	Biobanking of vitreous samples
AF	A Randomized Trial Evaluating Fenofibrate for Prevention of Diabetic Retinopathy Worsening	2021–recruiting	
AK	Home OCT Monitoring System: Feasibility Study	2021–recruiting	

8.2 Protocol A: A Pilot Study of Laser Photocoagulation for Diabetic Macular Edema

Protocol A was conducted between 2003 and 2008 to report visual acuity (VA) and anatomic changes (imaged by OCT, FA, and fundus photography) from baseline to 12 months after focal/grid photocoagulation in eyes with non-center involved (non-CI) clinically significant macular edema (CSME).

In this protocol, 22 diabetic eyes were enrolled. Laser was associated with relative stable VA and retinal thickness measurements and decreased FA leakage area at 1-year, confirming the recommendation of Early Treatment Diabetic Retinopathy Study (ETDRS) of using focal/grid laser in non-CI CSME eyes [2, 3].

However, another factor has been recognized to have a key role in the abnormal vascular permeability of diabetic eyes: the vascular endothelial growth factor (VEGF) leading to investigate the use of anti-VEGF to treat DME [1].

8.3 Protocol B: A Randomized Trial Comparing Intravitreal Triamcinolone Acetonide and Laser Photocoagulation for Diabetic Macular Edema

The protocol B included 306 DME patients with VA between 20/40 and 20/320, comparing focal/grid laser with triamcinolone acetonide (1 mg and 4 mg).

In the laser arm an improvement in BCVA was seen at 2- and 3-year follow-up (FU) visits (+5 ETDRS letters) versus no changes in VA in both triamcinolone groups. Furthermore, patients who have received triamcinolone showed a cumulative risk of cataract surgery by 3 years of 46% and 83%, respectively, in 1 mg and 4 mg group compared to 31% of laser group.

Results from Protocol B did not show long-term benefits of intravitreal triamcinolone [4, 5].

8.4 Protocol H: A Phase 2 Evaluation of Anti-VEGF Therapy for Diabetic Macular Edema: Bevacizumab (Avastin)

The protocol H was the first phase 2 randomized clinical trial (RCT) using bevacizumab to treat DME [6]. It was conducted between 2005 and 2008 enrolling 121 patients randomized to receive bevacizumab (1.25 mg or 2.5 mg) every 6 weeks or focal photocoagulation alone or combined with intravitreal injections (five arms). The objectives were to assess the dose, the dose interval, the effect, and the safety of this promising drug.

This important DRCR.net pilot study demonstrated a short-term effect (at 12 weeks) in terms of reduction of CRT and improvement of VA after intravitreal injections of bevacizumab [1, 6]. The dose of 1.25 mg appeared to have the same effect of 2.5 mg, and the interval injection of 4 weeks seemed to be more appropriate compared to 6 weeks.

8.5 Protocol I: Intravitreal Ranibizumab or Triamcinolone Acetonide in Combination with Laser Photocoagulation for Diabetic Macular Edema

Protocol I was a phase 3 study conducted between 2007 and 2013 to assess the efficacy of anti-VEGF in the treatment of DME. Protocol B has already demonstrated the efficacy of anti-VEGF treatment of DME, showing that focal/grid photocoagulation in eyes with center-involved DME produced gradual visual acuity improvement of ≥2 lines in about 30% of eyes after 2 years, although approximately 20% of laser treated eyes worsen by ≥2 lines. Concerning intravitreal triamcinolone, protocol B suggested that triamcinolone treatment without laser was not superior to macular photocoagulation [5].

Protocol I was a definitive study on the efficacy and safety of anti-VEGF therapy for DME. The study consisted of 854 eyes from 691 diabetic patients, randomized in four treatment arms: ranibizumab (0.5 mg) plus prompt focal/grid laser (within 1 week), ranibizumab (0.5 mg) plus deferred laser for persistent macular edema (>6 months), triamcinolone (4 mg) plus prompt macular laser (within 1 week), and macular laser plus sham injections [7].

At baseline all patients in all groups had a VA of 20/50 and CRT between 371 and 401 μm.

At 1 and 2 years intravitreal ranibizumab with immediate or deferred laser was more effective in comparison with laser. In the first year, both ranibizumab groups showed an improvement in VA of +9 ETDRS letters versus +4 letters of triamcinolone group and +3 letters of macular laser plus sham injections. The mean number of injections was between 8 and 9 in ranibizumab groups. In the second year, the efficacy was maintained in both ranibizumab groups with a decline of VA in triamcinolone and sham groups, with a mean number of injections that was of 2 and 3 in ranibizumab plus prompt and deferred laser, respectively [8].

The 3-year FU results concluded that, for ranibizumab regimen, prompt laser was no better and possibly worse than deferred laser, with a visual gain that was similar to that observed in the first two previous years [9].

Interesting results emerged from the 5-year analysis, in fact the VA gain at 1 year, was maintained to 5 years (+7.2 letters for ranibizumab plus prompt laser and + 9.8 letters for ranibizumab plus deferred laser), concomitant with diminishing need for treatment over time (one and two injections in the third years, reaching no injections at 5 years). On the other hand, the long-term results from protocol I also showed that, despite treatments, almost 6% of patients lost ≥15 letters at 5 years with no differences between prompt and deferred laser groups. Interestingly, in the ranibizumab plus deferred laser groups, 56% of eyes did not receive laser treatments prior to the 5-year visit [10].

8.6 Protocol T: A Comparative Effectiveness Study of Intravitreal Aflibercept, Bevacizumab, and Ranibizumab for Diabetic Macular Edema

Aflibercept was an anti-VEGF molecule introduced in 2011 to treat macular edema, in addition to bevacizumab and ranibizumab.

The DRCR.net Protocol T was a randomized multicenter study conducted between 2012 and 2018 in 89 sites, comparing the efficacy and the safety of these three medications for DME [11]. Aflibercept and ranibizumab have been approved by FDA for DME treatment, while bevacizumab was not approved for intraocular use, and it is used as "off-label."

Protocol T study enrolled patients affected by type 1 and type 2 diabetes, with a visual acuity between 20/32 or worse and 20/320 or better, with a center-involved DME, without history of anti-VEGF treatment in the last 12 months or any other DME treatment in the last 4 months. The patients enrolled were 224 in aflibercept group, and 218 in both bevacizumab and ranibizumab group, respectively.

The primary outcome was the change in visual acuity at 1-year adjusted for baseline VA. The treatment algorithm was the same for all anti-VEGF drug: repeat injections every 4 weeks (q4) if eye improved or worsened. The improvement/worsening was defined as ≥5 letter change from last injection or ≥10% CRT change on OCT from last injection. The injections could be deferred if VA was 20/20 or better and CRT was normal or, at or after 24 weeks, VA and OCT were stable after two consecutive injections. Furthermore, the injections could be resumed if VA or OCT worsened during FU. The laser treatment might be started at or after 24 weeks in case of persistent DME not improving after at least two injections.

In the full cohort, at 1 year, all drugs improved VA with a statistically significant difference in favor of aflibercept versus bevacizumab (+13 letters and +10 letters, respectively, $p < 0.001$) and no differences between aflibercept and ranibizumab.

The subgroup analysis revealed no differences between drugs in patients with a baseline VA from 20/32 to 20/40, with a mean change of +8 letters for all treatment arms and half of patients that gained >10 letters in all groups. Interesting results emerged from the subgroup analysis for patients with baseline VA of 20/50 or worse; in these patients, mean VA letter score was +18.9 in the aflibercept group, +14.2 in the ranibizumab group, and +11.8 in the bevacizumab group with a statistically significant difference in aflibercept group ($p < 0.001$ aflibercept vs. bevacizumab and $p = 0.0031$ aflibercept vs. ranibizumab, respectively).

At 1 year, all three anti-VEGF produced similar VA improvement with an advantage of aflibercept over the other agents in patients with worse initial VA.

In terms of CRT reduction, all agents significantly reduced the OCT CRT most evident in the aflibercept group. The subgroup analysis revealed that both in patient with better and worse initial VA, aflibercept and ranibizumab showed a similar effect on CRT and both significantly reduced the CRT in comparison with bevacizumab. In patients with initial thicker OCT CRT, aflibercept was more effective than others [12].

The interaction with baseline VA seen at 1 year was also evident at 2 years: at worse levels of initial VA, aflibercept was more effective at improving VA [13].

At 1 and 2 years, laser treatments were indicated per protocol less frequently in the aflibercept group [13].

Protocol T showed no differences in terms of safety between drugs at 1 and 2 years [13].

Results from Protocol I and Protocol T showed that, despite treatments, 40% of DME eyes experienced persistent macular edema after at least 6 monthly injections, and 32% of them had a concomitant visual loss; similar results were found for aflibercept and ranibizumab with a higher percentage of unresolved DME for bevacizumab-treated eyes [14, 15].

8.7 Protocol TX: A Comparative Effectiveness Study of Intravitreal Aflibercept, Bevacizumab, and Ranibizumab for Diabetic Macular Edema: Follow-Up Extension Study

The 5-year extension of Protocol T was the Protocol TX that recruited 317 patients (68% of protocol T participants), with the objective to provide information about treatment course, and VA and DME for 3 years after Protocol T were stopped. Of note, the treatments from 2 to 5 years were at investigator discretion.

About 95% of patients received at least one retinal examination since Protocol T with a mean number of 14 visits between 2 and 5 years, and 70% of patients received at least one treatment in this period (38% aflibercept, 32% bevacizumab, 19% ranibizumab, 10% corticosteroid, 8% focal/grid laser, 10% panretinal photocoagulation) [16].

Concerning the anti-VEGF treatments since Protocol T, globally 32% of patients did not receive anti-VEGF injections between 2 and 5 years [16].

The mean change in VA at 5 years was +7.4 letters, with a decline of −4.7 letters between 2 and 5 years (+8 letters aflibercept, +7.6 letters ranibizumab, +6.6 letters bevacizumab), on average all patients demonstrated visual gain from baseline, but mean VA worsened [16].

The mean change in OCT CRT at 5 years was −154 μm, with similar results for all anti-VEGF molecules, interestingly no changes in retinal thickness were detected between 2 and 5 years [16].

The results from Protocol TX highlighted the importance to create strategies for a long-term DME management.

8.8 Protocol U: Short-Term Evaluation of Combination Corticosteroid + Anti-VEGF Treatment for Persistent Central-Involved Diabetic Macular Edema Following Anti-VEGF Therapy

Protocol U was a phase 2 trial conducted between 2014 and 2017 enrolling 236 eyes with the objective to evaluate the role of steroids as adjuvant therapy in eyes that showed persistent macular edema (see the conclusion paragraph on Protocol T).

Eligibility criteria were VA 20/32 to 20/320, CI-DME despite at least three anti-VEGF injections (in 20 weeks) prior to enrollment. The study protocol consisted of a run-in phase in which three additional ranibizumab injections were given every 4 weeks, at this point 129 out of 236 patients were randomized to receive monthly ranibizumab plus dexamethasone implant (given at baseline and again at 3 months as needed) (65 eyes) versus monthly ranibizumab alone (64 eyes) for 6 months. The mean VA change was similar in both the groups (+3 letters for ranibizumab and + 2.7 in the combination group), independently from initial VA.

An interesting result was that 11% of eyes in the combination group had >15 letters improvement vs. 2% of ranibizumab group ($p = 0.03$). The lens status did not influence the final VA, but the study was not sufficiently sized to determine whether treatment response might differ by lens status.

The retinal thickness reduction was prominent in the combination group (−62 μm vs. −110 μm for ranibizumab and combination group, respectively; $P < 0.001$).

In the combination group, an important percentage of patients received ocular anti-hypertensives (20% of eyes).

The conclusion of this trial was that the use of dexamethasone reduced the retinal thickness more effectively than ranibizumab alone but did not improve the final VA in eyes with persistent macular edema, with a significant risk of intraocular pressure increase [15].

References

1. Sun JK, Jampol LM. The diabetic retinopathy clinical research network (DRCR.net) and its contributions to the treatment of diabetic retinopathy. Ophthalmic Res. 2019;62:225–30.
2. Scott IU, Danis RP, Bressler SB, et al. Effect of focal/grid photocoagulation on visual acuity and retinal thickening in eyes with non-center-involved diabetic macular edema. Retina. 2009;29:613–7.
3. Danis RP, Scott IU, Qin H, et al. Association of fluorescein angiographic features with visual acuity and with optical coherence tomographic and stereoscopic color fundus photographic features of diabetic macular edema in a randomized clinical trial. Retina. 2010;30:1627–37.
4. Diabetic Retinopathy Clinical Research N, Beck RW, Edwards AR, et al. Three-year follow-up of a randomized trial comparing focal/grid photocoagulation and intravitreal triamcinolone for diabetic macular edema. Arch Ophthalmol. 2009;127:245–51.
5. Bressler NM, Edwards AR, Beck RW, et al. Exploratory analysis of diabetic retinopathy progression through 3 years in a randomized clinical trial that compares intravitreal triamcinolone acetonide with focal/grid photocoagulation. Arch Ophthalmol. 2009;127:1566–71.
6. Diabetic Retinopathy Clinical Research N, Scott IU, Edwards AR, et al. A phase II randomized clinical trial of intravitreal bevacizumab for diabetic macular edema. Ophthalmology. 2007;114:1860–7.
7. Diabetic Retinopathy Clinical Research N, Elman MJ, Aiello LP, et al. Randomized trial evaluating ranibizumab plus prompt or deferred laser or triamcinolone plus prompt laser for diabetic macular edema. Ophthalmology. 2010;117:1064–1077e1035.
8. Elman MJ, Bressler NM, Qin H, et al. Expanded 2-year follow-up of ranibizumab plus prompt or deferred laser or triamcinolone plus prompt laser for diabetic macular edema. Ophthalmology. 2011;118:609–14.
9. Diabetic Retinopathy Clinical Research N, Elman MJ, Qin H, et al. Intravitreal ranibizumab for diabetic macular edema with prompt versus deferred laser treatment: three-year randomized trial results. Ophthalmology. 2012;119:2312–8.
10. Elman MJ, Ayala A, Bressler NM, et al. Intravitreal Ranibizumab for diabetic macular edema with prompt versus deferred laser treatment: 5-year randomized trial results. Ophthalmology. 2015;122:375–81.
11. Diabetic Retinopathy Clinical Research N, Wells JA, Glassman AR, et al. Aflibercept, bevacizumab, or ranibizumab for diabetic macular edema. N Engl J Med. 2015;372:1193–203.
12. Wells JA, Glassman AR, Jampol LM, et al. Association of baseline visual acuity and retinal thickness with 1-year efficacy of Aflibercept, Bevacizumab, and Ranibizumab for diabetic macular edema. JAMA Ophthalmol. 2016;134:127–34.
13. Wells JA, Glassman AR, Ayala AR, et al. Aflibercept, Bevacizumab, or Ranibizumab for diabetic macular edema: two-year results from a comparative effectiveness randomized clinical trial. Ophthalmology. 2016;123:1351–9.
14. Parravano M, Costanzo E, Querques G. Profile of non-responder and late responder patients treated for diabetic macular edema: systemic and ocular factors. Acta Diabetol. 2020;57:911–21.
15. Maturi RK, Glassman AR, Liu D, et al. Effect of adding dexamethasone to continued Ranibizumab treatment in patients with persistent diabetic macular edema: a DRCR network phase 2 randomized clinical trial. JAMA Ophthalmol. 2018;136:29–38.
16. Glassman AR, Wells JA 3rd, Josic K, et al. Five-year outcomes after initial Aflibercept, Bevacizumab, or Ranibizumab treatment for diabetic macular edema (protocol T extension study). Ophthalmology. 2020;127:1201–10.

Effect of Anti-VEGF Therapy on Inner and Outer Retinal Layers on Spectral-Domain Optical Coherence Tomography in Diabetic Macular Edema

9

Nibha Mishra and Sandeep Saxena

9.1 Introduction

Diabetic macular edema (DME) is the commonest cause of vision loss in diabetic retinopathy (DR) [1]. Diabetic macular edema occurs at any stage of DR, affecting about 20% of patients with type 1 diabetes mellitus (DM) and 14–25% with type 2 DM during a 10-year follow-up [2]. Chronic hyperglycaemia leads to several molecular changes which results in blood–retinal barrier breakdown resulting in DME. Vascular endothelial growth factor (VEGF) plays a critical role in the pathogenesis of DME. Thus, anti-VEGF agents are considered to be the gold standard in the treatment of DME. Spectral-domain optical coherence tomography (SD-OCT) provides detailed visualization and delineation of retinal layers. Several OCT biomarkers have been used to predict treatment response in patients with DME treated with intravitreal anti-VEGF agents.

9.2 Pathogenesis of Diabetic Macular Oedema: Role of Vascular Endothelial Growth Factor

Diabetic macular edema is mediated by multiple complex mechanisms in its pathogenesis [3–5]. Hyperglycaemia in DM results in the formation of advanced glycation end products (AGEs) [6]. AGEs act on retinal pigment epithelium (RPE) and endothelial pericytes to stimulate VEGF expression [7–9]. VEGF, also known as vascular permeability factor (VPF), is a potent angiogenic factor and was first described as an essential growth factor for vascular endothelial cells and an endothelial cell-specific mitogen [10]. VEGF is a sub-family of growth factors, the platelet-derived growth factor family of cystine-knot growth factors and act as an important signalling protein involved in angiogenesis [11].

The balance between angiogenic (VEGF) and antiangiogenic factors pigment epithelium-derived factor (PEDF) secreted by RPE is crucial for progression of disease. This balance is important to maintain the structural integrity of the outer retina and choriocapillaries [12]. RPE dysregulation due to oxidative stress and inflammatory reactions may lead to abnormal angiogenesis and tissue hypoxia as a result of activation of VEGF [13, 14]. Downregulation of PEDF expression by elevated glucose concentration in cultured human RPE cells has been documented [15]. This increased expression of VEGF leads to breakdown of outer blood–retinal barrier. The breakdown of outer BRB leads to DME. Inflammation, characterized by leukostasis, accumulation of macrophages, intercellular adhesion molecule-1 activation (ICAM-1), inflammatory mediators (IL-6, MCP-1), and prostacyclin upregulation, is associated with capillary nonperfusion and breakdown of the blood–retina barrier leading to DME [13, 16]. In vitro studies have also documented a dual role of VEGF in regulating the permeability of endothelial blood–retinal barrier and retinal–RPE barrier. Cultured vascular endothelial cells have been observed to express increased vascular permeability in the presence of VEGF. In contrast, transepithelial resistance of cultured RPE cells, measure of RPE barrier function, has been observed to increase on exposure to VEGF [17]. Experimental studies have also documented that interaction of RPE and endothelial cells results in loss of barrier function of RPE. This was observed to be mediated by VEGF [15, 18].

N. Mishra (✉) · S. Saxena
Department of Ophthalmology, King George's Medical University, Lucknow, Uttar Pradesh, India

S. Saxena et al. (eds.), *Diabetic Macular Edema*, https://doi.org/10.1007/978-981-19-7307-9_9

9.3 Pathomorphology of Different Layers of Retina in Diabetic Macular Edema

Clinically thickening of the sensory retina and vascular lesions are noted in DME. Histologic studies show cystoid spaces mainly in the inner nuclear layer (INL) and the outer plexiform layer (OPL) and contribute partly to macular thickening [19–21]. Electron microscopy revealed accumulation of the extracellular fluid and intracytoplasmic swelling of the Müller also contribute to DME.OCT shows different foveal morphologies in DME—cystoid macular edema (CME), serous retinal detachment (SRD), and sponge-like diffuse retinal swelling [22]. Individual lesions have been delineated in the individual retinal layers. OCT showed cystoid spaces mainly in the INL and OPL [23, 24]. Extracellular fluids pool between the outer segments, and RPE is present in SRD. Sponge-like retinal swelling at the fovea occurs in the OPL. Vitreomacular traction also contributes to macular thickening in DME [25–27]. Sponge-like retinal swelling especially is often accompanied by pathological findings in the vitreomacular interface, and vitreomacular interface abnormalities contribute to thickening of the retinal parenchyma in the OPL at the fovea, as in the case of idiopathic epiretinal membrane (ERM) [28]. It was also reported that vitreomacular interface abnormalities might also induce SRD in DME, and OCT sometimes shows cystoid spaces with vitreoretinal abnormalities as with idiopathic macular holes [29, 30].

Hemodynamic circulation was found to play a causative role in the pathogenesis of DME [31]. Resistive index (RI) has been characterized as a marker of vascular resistance. Resistive index increases with increasing resistance, with vascular compliance taken into account [32]. Orbital RI was observed to be a useful marker for early diagnosis and follow-up of DR [33]. In a study on ocular hemodynamic, Mendivil et al. found a significant differences in flow velocities in ophthalmic artery (OA), central retinal artery (CRA), and short posterior ciliary arteries between healthy and diabetic patients [34]. Ocular blood flow velocity was found to be lower in advanced diabetic retinopathy patients as compared to normal. Several ocular blood flow studies have been done in patients with DR. Basement membrane thickening, pericyte loss, rise in the levels of ICAM-1, oxidative stress, rheological fluctuations, and decreased capillary perfusion led to damage of the retinal capillary endothelium. This results in fluid leakage out of the capillaries resulting in DME, capillary closure, and decreased capillary blood flow. These changes lead to decreased blood supply to retina which results in retinal ischemia and increased VEGF release [35–37]. Total retinal blood flow was found to be reduced in conjunction with raised levels of aqueous angiogenic cytokines in patients with diabetic retinopathy [38]. Increase in RI of CRA is correlated with severity of DR. Central retinal artery supplies the inner six layers of retina. Increase in RI of CRA, related to the vascular endothelium damage, was found to correlate significantly with severity of retinopathy. It has been demonstrated that deep capillary plexus (DCP) provides around 10–15% of oxygen to photoreceptor inner segment, particularly during dark adaptation [39]. Deep capillary plexus is located on outer side of inner nuclear layer. It receives its branches from CRA. In systemic hypoxia, blood supply to outer retina through inner retinal vessels becomes even more important, as choroidal vasculature has no autoregulatory mechanism [40]. Hence, it fails to autoregulate in such a setting [41]. Central retinal artery, through DCP, contributes to vascular supply of outer retina. On optical coherence tomography angiography (OCTA), DCP ischemia has been found to be associated with disruption of the outer retina, including thinning of the outer nuclear layer and photoreceptor disruption [42].

RPE cells are dependent on choroid for its metabolic needs. Resistive index of OA increases with severity of DR leading to choroidal blood supply being hampered due to lack of autoregulation. Thus, an increase in RI of OA also impairs blood supply of RPE resulting in structural changes expressed as topographical alterations in RPE on SD-OCT. RPE is essential for maintenance of retinal photoreceptors integrity and function. Alterations in RPE also correlated with EZ disruption. Studies have shown negative correlation between grades of EZ disruption and visual acuity [43]. Recent studies have shown RI of OA as a sensitive bioimaging biomarker for the severity of DR [44]. It can be concluded that with increased severity of DR, an increase in RI of OA results in decrease in blood flow to RPE. This leads to RPE topographic alterations and resultant decrease in visual acuity (VA). RI of OA is one of the important factors causing RPE topographical alterations [45].

9.4 SD-OCT-Based Changes in Inner Retinal Layers in Diabetic Macular Edema

Disorganization of inner retinal layers is defined as the inability to delineate the inner retinal layer boundaries, any of the boundaries of the ganglion cell layer–inner plexiform (GCL-IPL) complex, inner nuclear layer, and outer plexiform layer. If intraretinal cysts are observed in the outer nuclear layer, resulting in overall retinal thickening, but the inner retinal layers could be still demarcated, then DRIL was not considered to be present. Loss of the normal foveal contour does not constitute DRIL by itself unless there is concurrent loss of retinal layer boundaries.

Disorganization of the retinal inner layers affecting 50% or more of the central 1-mm-wide zone centred on the fovea (foveal DRIL) is associated with worse VA. This holds true even in eyes with reduced vision despite edema resolution or, conversely, in eyes with good vision despite concurrent edema [46].

The mechanisms by which DRIL affects VA is not clear and requires further histological studies. The inability to segment retinal layer boundaries due to disruption likely represents an anatomic interruption in the visual transmission pathway. Disruption has been hypothesized to result when bipolar axons snap after their elasticity limit has been exceeded due to edema [47]. Disorganization of the retinal inner layers could represent disorganization or destruction of cells within inner retinal layers, including bipolar, amacrine, or horizontal cells, and indicates a disruption of pathways that transmit visual information from the photoreceptors to the ganglion cells.

9.5 SD-OCT-Based Changes in Outer Retinal Layers in Diabetic Macular Edema

Pathogenesis of DR is complex involving multiple molecular pathways occurring due to deranged metabolism in DM. The long-standing hyperglycaemia leads to protein glycosylation resulting in the formation of AGE. Advanced glycation end products have an effect through their effect on retinal microvasculature, VEGF, ICAM-1, nitrosative and oxidative stress, and vitamin D and calcium metabolism.

AGEs and their receptor activation lead to endothelial dysfunction and release of proangiogenic factors resulting in pericyte apoptosis, vascular inflammation, and angiogenesis damaging the vascular components of the retina [48, 49]. This leads to leakage and fluid accumulation resulting in macular edema. AGE increases the expression of VEGF in retinal pericytes and RPE cells [50]. Healthy retina requires interaction between its photoreceptors and the RPE. An intact ELM has been highlighted as a prerequisite for an intact EZ [51]. DME is known to be associated with ELM and EZ disruption [52, 53]. Jain et al. classified ELM and EZ disruption: grade 0—no disruption of ELM and photoreceptor ellipsoid zone; grade 1—ELM disrupted and ellipsoid zone intact; grade 2—both ELM and ellipsoid zone disrupted [51] (Fig. 9.1).

ELM comprises of attachment of outer process of glial muller cells to one another and also to inner photoreceptor segments which has been demonstrated in animal model [54]. They revealed that tight junctions existed in the ELM between glial muller cells and photoreceptors. Occludin is the key component of tight junctions. In ELM, occludin was found to be organized between the glial muller cells and the photoreceptors, thus the ELM should be considered as part of a retinal barrier. In DME glial Muller cells at the level of ELM are swollen and lose their occludin content. ELM junctions thus could be considered as unique regulatory targets in treatment. VEGF alters tight junctions and promotes vascular permeability in many retinal diseases. Murukami et al. noted the role of occludin in the regulation of endothelial barrier properties [55].

The EZ serves as a clinical indicator of photoreceptor integrity. Biologically EZ consists of mitochondria mainly enabling higher levels of energy consumption within the photoreceptors [56]. Mitochondrial dysfunction occurs in the photoreceptors at fovea in DME. Absence of the subfoveal EZ on SD-OCT corresponds to the reduced reflectivity or anatomic absence of the EZ. Sharma et al. classified EZ disruption. Disruption of EZ was graded as Grade-0: intact EZ, Grade-1: focal subfoveal disruption of EZ, Grade-2: global disruption of EZ within macular cube (Fig. 9.2).

Studies demonstrating early retinal damage in experimental diabetes have observed morphological changes in RPE [57]. Oxidative stress has been found to result in lipid peroxidation and oxidation of glycated proteins in the diabetic retina [58]. An association of nitrosative and oxidative stress with retinal photoreceptor ellipsoid zone and topographical changes in RPE has been demonstrated [59]. Experimental studies have shown interaction of RPE and endothelial cells results in loss of barrier function of RPE which was mediated by VEGF. The balance between VEGF and antiangiogenic factor PEDF secreted by RPE is crucial for progression

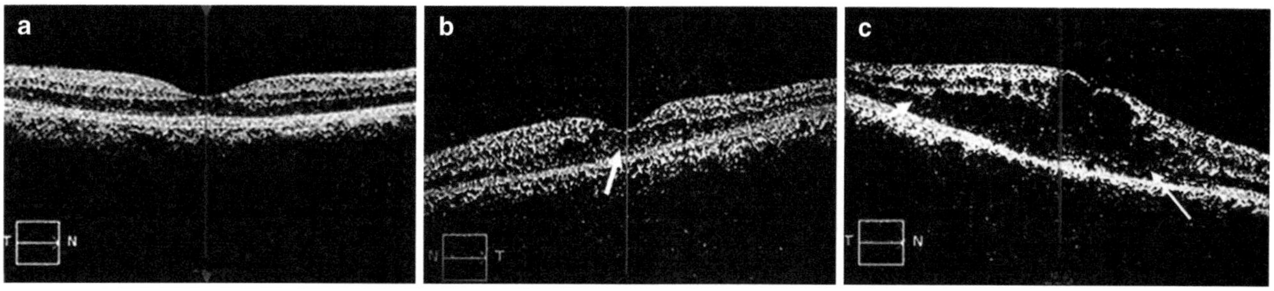

Fig. 9.1 Disruption of external limiting membrane (ELM) and ellipsoid zone (EZ) was graded as Grade-0: ELM and E intact (**a**); Grade-1: Focal subfoveal disruption of ELM and EZ intact (**b**); Grade-2: Disruption of ELM and EZ within macular cube (**c**)

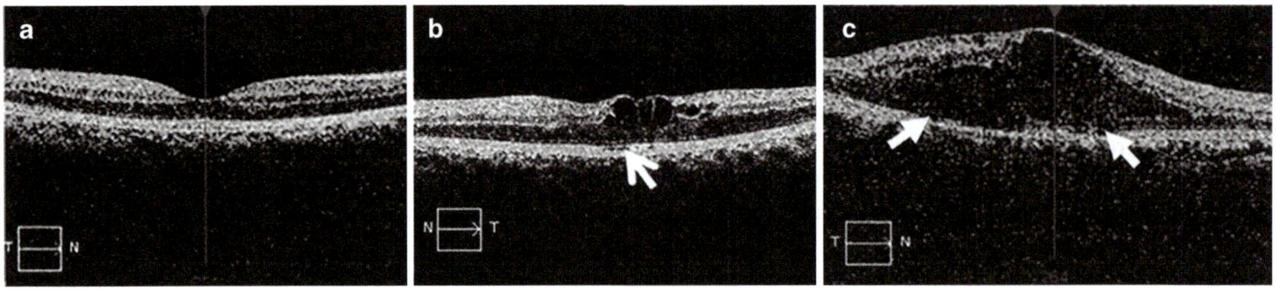

Fig. 9.2 Grades of ellipsoid zone (EZ) disruption as Grade-0: intact EZ (**a**); Grade-1: focal subfoveal disruption of EZ (**b**); Grade-2: global disruption of EZ within macular cube (**c**)

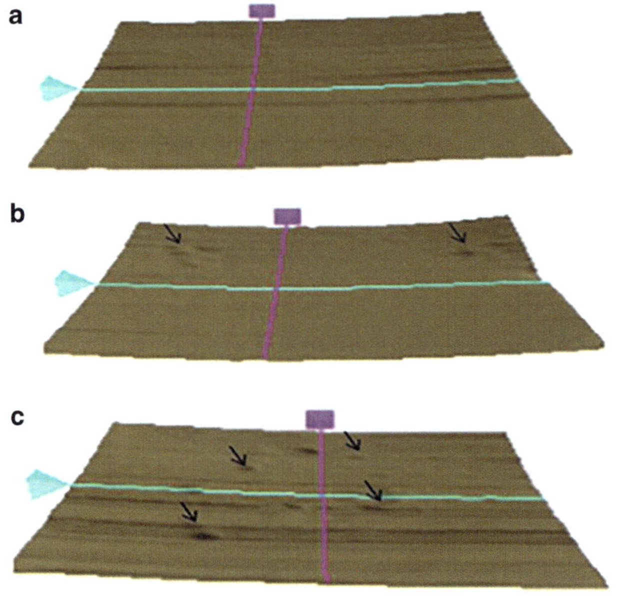

Fig. 9.3 Retinal pigment epithelium (RPE). RPE alterations were graded as: grade 0, no RPE alterations (**a**); grade 1, RPE alterations in up to two quadrants (**b**); and grade 2, RPE alterations in more than two quadrants (**c**)

of DR [60]. The VEGF secreted by RPE is essential for maintaining the structural integrity of the outer retina and choriocapillaris. RPE topography was studied on the SD-OCT segmentation map and RPE alterations were graded as: grade 0, No RPE alterations; grade 1, RPE alterations in up to two quadrants; and grade 2, RPE alterations in more than two quadrants [59] (Fig. 9.3).

Retinal VEGF induces ICAM-1 expression leading to leukostasis and breakdown of blood–retinal barrier [61]. Jain et al. demonstrated the correlation of VEGF and ICAM-1 on ELM and EZ disruption [51]. Advanced glycation end products trigger oxidative stress generation resulting in inflammatory and thrombogenic reactions. Mitochondrial superoxide generation plays an important role in the formation and accumulation of AGEs under diabetic conditions [62]. Sharma et al. showed nitric oxide and oxidative stress in DR is associated with disruption of ELM and EZ [59]. Increased serum anti-myeloperoxidase antibody levels have been found to be associated with ELM and EZ disruption in DR [63]. Deranged metabolism in DM leads to compromised nutritional status. Vitamin D deficiency has been found to be associated with disruption ELM and EZ [64]. Vitamin D also plays an important role in regulating calcium homeostasis. Increased serum ionized calcium induces retinal photoreceptor apoptosis resulting in ELM and EZ disruption in DR [65].

9.6 Role of Anti-VEGF Therapy in DME

Anti-VEGF agents have become the mainstay of treatment for DME. Anti-VEGF drugs ranges from aptamers (pegaptanib), antibodies to VEGF (bevacizumab), antibody fragments to VEGF (ranibizumab), and fusion proteins combining a receptor for VEGF with the Fc fragment of an immunoglobulin (aflibercept and conbercept). The antibodies and fusion proteins bind all isoforms of VEGF-A; fusion proteins additionally bind VEGF-B and placental growth factor. Fusion proteins have higher affinity for VEGF and thus have potential for less frequent injection frequency in the treatment of DME [66, 67].

Bevacizumab is Food and Drug Administration (FDA)-approved for the treatment of advanced solid cancers, but is widely used off-label in the treatment of DME. It is less expensive than the FDA-approved ocular anti-VEGF drugs [68]. Ziv-aflibercept is systemically formulated aflibercept in a buffered solution with a higher osmolarity than aflibercept [69].

The first anti-VEGF drug used to treat DME was pegaptanib which selectively blocks the 165-isoform of VEGF [70]. But superior results were obtained with anti-VEGF drugs that blocked all isoforms of VEGF. The efficacy of bevacizumab and ranibizumab was established in randomized controlled clinical trials in 2010 and that of aflibercept in 2014 [71, 72]. A prospective, randomized, comparative effectiveness trial of these three drugs showed no difference in efficacy of the three drugs in eyes with centre-involved

DME and visual acuity of 20/40 or better at 1 or 2 years of follow-up [73]. However, in eyes with visual acuity of 20/50 or worse, aflibercept was better than ranibizumab and bevacizumab at 1 year, whereas at 2 years, aflibercept and ranibizumab showed similar results, but it remained superior to bevacizumab [74].

9.7 Changes in Inner and Outer Layers of Retina Post Anti-VEGF Therapy Based on SD-OCT

Comyn et al. and Wells et al. found that there is significant reduction of Central Subfield Thickness (CST) and Cube Average Thickness (CAT) in patients of DME after anti-VEGF treatment [75, 76]. It was also found that the magnitude of CST reduction in several treatment regimens was associated with a better visual acuity outcome [47, 77, 78].

Improvement in SD-OCT parameters used as biomarkers of DME comprising of DRIL, ELM, and EZ were evident following intervention. DRIL has been suggested to be a strong predictor of VA in eyes with DME [46]. Therefore, DRIL can be used as a biomarker for predicting future VA. It was observed that improvement in VA was more evident in patients associated with improvement of DRIL. This suggests that restoration of DRIL is directly related to improvement in VA. DRIL has been shown to correlate with EZ disruption. DRIL is thought to correlate to regions where bipolar, horizontal, and amacrine cell synaptic connections have been disrupted, thus resulting in interruption of the transmission pathway between the ganglion cells and photoreceptors, leading to decrease in VA [79]. Anti-VEGF therapy improves DRIL, leading to restoration of synaptic connections and transmission of impulses from photoreceptors which results in improvement of VA. Similar findings were observed with regard to ELM and EZ disruption in DME. Percentage disruption of EZ has been found to correlate with decrease in VA in DME. Integrity of ELM and EZ has been reported to be a positive predictor for visual outcome [80–82]. Kang et al. demonstrated that the strongest predictor of final VA was the status of EZ integrity followed by status of ELM [83]. Decrease in logMAR VA was more pronounced in patients which was associated with restoration of ELM and EZ.

Hareedy et al. reported improvement in photoreceptor integrity took place after second and third dose of ranibizumab with improvement in VA and colour vision [84]. A statistically significant relation was found between colour vision and EZ after the first injection, but the correlation after the second and third injections was much more significant. Improvement in VA significantly correlated with EZ after the second and third injection [84]. The restoration of foveal photoreceptor microstructure following anti-VEGF therapy was associated with improvement in VA. A larger foveal photoreceptor microstructure defect was associated with lower VA. Patients with larger foveal photoreceptor microstructure defects at baseline had lesser VA improvements. The improvement in foveal photoreceptor microstructure integrity was associated with VA improvement [85]. Chatzerelli et al. reported noteworthy restoration of EZ photoreceptors in patients of DME following intravitreal ranibizumab after 12 months follow-up. The improvement in EZ defect size was dependent on the pattern of DME on SD-OCT [86].

Omri et al. demonstrated in animal model that ELM comprised of attachment of outer process of glial Muller cells to one another and also to inner photoreceptor segments [54]. It was reported that tight junctions (TJ) exist in the ELM. Ultrastructural analysis showed that TJ exist between glial Muller cells and photoreceptors. Occludin, a protein, is a main component of TJ. Occludin is organized between the glial Muller cells and the photoreceptors at the ELM. They proposed that the ELM should be considered as part of a retinal barrier that may be disrupted in various pathological conditions. In diabetic retinopathy, the glial Muller cells are swollen, and they also lose their occludin content at the ELM level. Hence, ELM junctions could be unique regulatory targets in treatment. Murukami et al. highlighted in animal model studies that retinal endothelial cells on treatment with VEGF resulted in occludin phosphorylation, ubiquitination, and fragmentation of TJ [55]. They demonstrated that occludin had an important role in the regulation of barrier properties and might serve as a possible therapeutic target. In SD-OCT based study, it was noted that an increase in VEGF was associated with increased severity of DR and sequential ELM and EZ disruption, highlighting that an intact ELM was a prerequisite for an intact EZ in DME.

De et al. provided insight into the mechanism of ELM and EZ restoration after anti-VEGF therapy. Anti-VEGF therapy led to restoration of barrier effect of ELM. The ELM was found to restore first followed by EZ restoration in DME [87] (Fig. 9.4).

Intravitreal anti-VEGF therapy was found to be associated with improvement in the grade of RPE alterations and in turn improvement of VA (Fig. 9.5). Healthy RPE has functional intact tight junctions which are required for the effective and controlled removal of fluid from the subretinal space [88]. Various growth factors secreted by RPE maintain the structural integrity of choriocapillaris, endothelium, and photoreceptors. These growth factors are important for both endothelial cell differentiation and photoreceptor differentiation [89–91]. RPE is vital for the preservation of photoreceptor excitability. This is achieved by various mechanisms: stabilizing the ion composition of the subretinal space [92, 93]. It sheds photoreceptor outer segments by phagocytosis, and rebuilding light-sensitive outer segments from the base

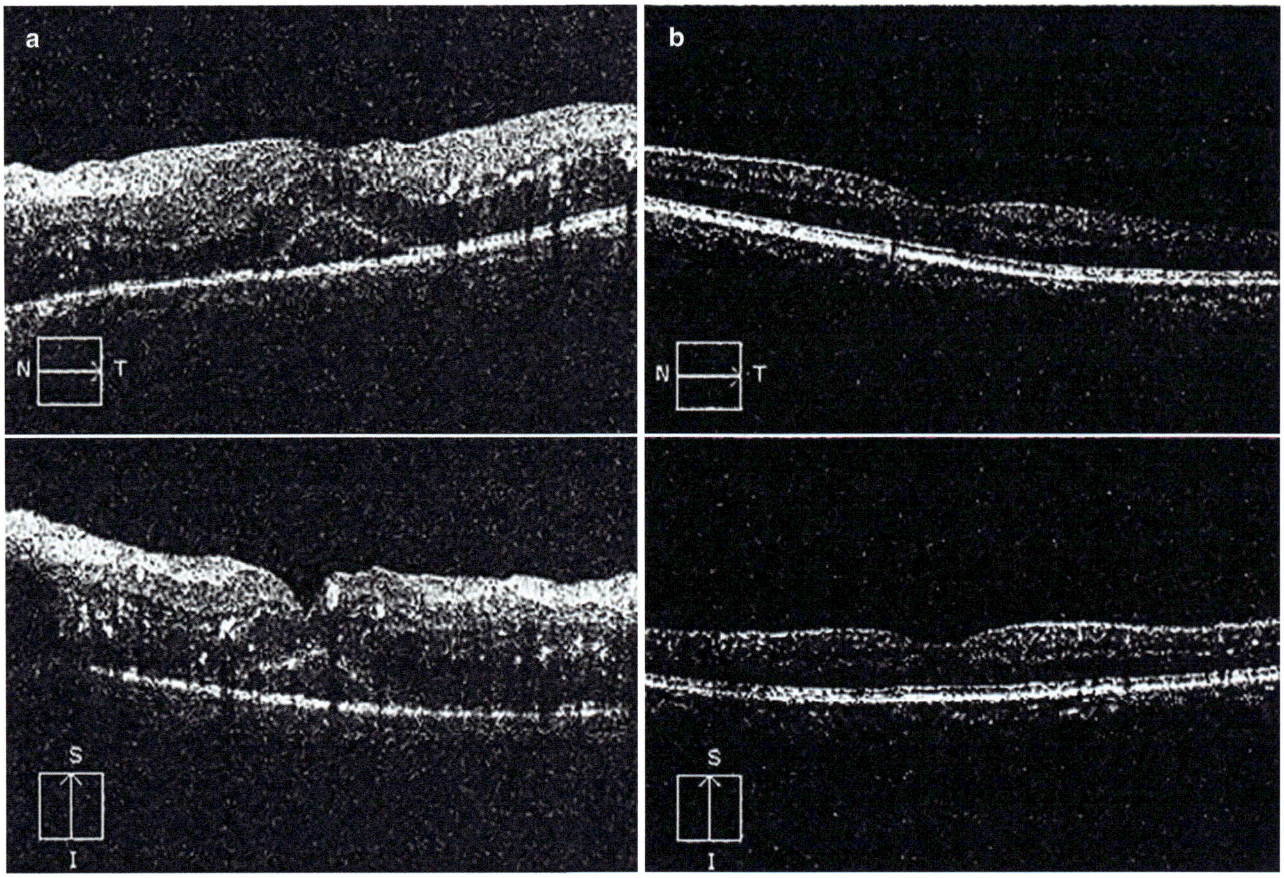

Fig. 9.4 (**a**) Disorganisation of retinal inner layers (DRIL), ellipsoid zone (EZ), and external limiting membrane (ELM) disruption. Figure (**b**) shows restoration of DRIL, ELM, and EZ

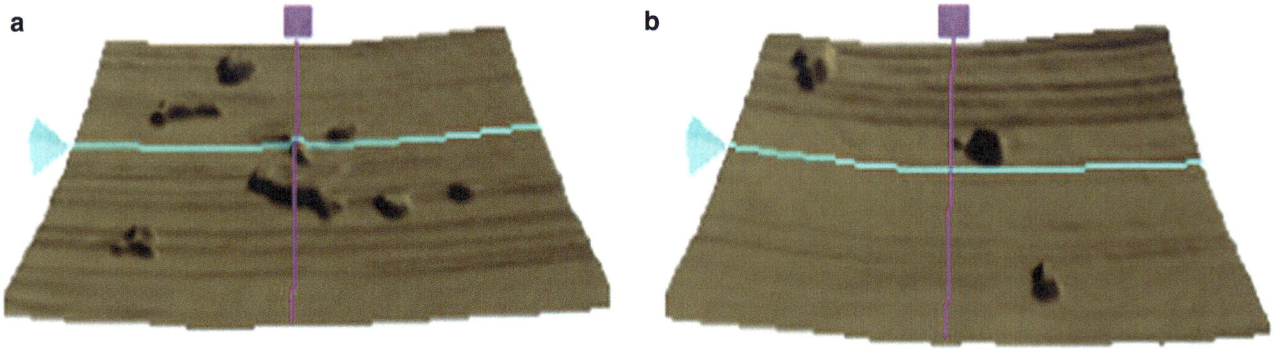

Fig. 9.5 (**a**) Retinal pigment epithelium (RPE) single-layer map prior to anti-VEGF injection with alterations in all quadrants. (**b**) Reduction of RPE alterations

of the photoreceptors [94–96]. Hence, RPE is essential for both developments of retinal structures and visual function.

As stated earlier, RPE is a major secretor of VEGF. In a cell culture model, VEGF secretion has been found to be associated with proliferation of RPE. Hypoxia stimulates the secretion of VEGF in bovine RPE cells, which in turn causes proliferation of RPE. A significant association has been observed between the concentration of VEGF and proliferation of RPE cells [97]. In another study done on human ARPE-19 cells and primary porcine RPE cells, Ablonczy et al. also concluded that an increase in RPE permeability is initiated by an upsurge in intraocular levels of VEGF [98].

Retinal topography maps are used for providing imaging of the spatial distribution of cell densities across the retina.

Traditionally, cell densities have been visualized as retinal cell topography. Retinal topography maps are generated from cell counts measured across a systematic sampling grid using a number of stereology software. Such a sampling method is considered efficient and less predisposed to bias [99]. On SD-OCT single-layer (SL)-RPE map, RPE alterations are well established in DME.

VEGF causes biochemical changes in the retina through increased expression of AGEs, and oxidative and nitrosative stress resulting in an increase in CAT in DME [51, 100]. Several trials have reported a significant reduction of CAT in patients of DME after anti-VEGF treatment [75]. A significant decrease in CAT was also observed after anti-VEGF therapy. An increase in VEGF level is associated with RPE proliferation. This implies that as VEGF levels increase in DR, RPE alteration also increase. Anti-VEGF therapy leads to a sequential decrease in grades of RPE alterations and a decrease in CAT which is associated with a decrease in logMAR VA.

9.8 Conclusion

SD-OCT provides us with unparalleled detailed in vivo histology of the retinal layers which helps us in understanding of the morphological changes taking place in each layer in DME. Diabetic macular edema causes complex pathomorphological changes like DRIL, EZ, and ELM disruption and RPE alterations which result in decrease in VA. Anti-VEGF treatment restores all these layers and thus improves visual functions.

References

1. Lee R, Wong TY, Sabanayagam C. Epidemiology of diabetic retinopathy, diabetic macular edema and related vision loss. Eye Vis (Lond). 2015;2:17.
2. Klein R, Knudtson MD, Lee KE, Gangnon R, Klein BE. The Wisconsin epidemiologic study of diabetic retinopathy XXIII: the twenty-five-year incidence of macular edema in persons with type 1 diabetes. Ophthalmology. 2009;116(3):497–503. https://doi.org/10.1016/j.ophtha.2008.10.016.
3. Gardner TW, Antonetti DA, Barber AJ, LaNoue KF, Levison SW. Diabetic retinopathy: more than meets the eye. Surv Ophthalmol. 2002;47(supplement 2):S253–62.
4. Mohamed Q, Gillies MC, Wong TY. Management of diabetic retinopathy: a systematic review. JAMA. 2007;298(8):902–16.
5. Antonetti DA, Klein R, Gardner TW. Diabetic retinopathy. N Engl J Med. 2012;366(13):1227–39.
6. Prasad K, Mishra M. AGE-RAGE stress, stressors, and antistressors in health and disease. Int J Angiol. 2018;27:1–12.
7. Lu M, Kuroki M, Amano S, Tolentino M, Keough K, et al. Advanced glycation end products increase retinal vascular endothelial growth factor expression. J Clin Invest. 1998;101:1219–24.
8. Yamagishi S, Inagaki Y, Amano S, Okamoto T, Takeuchi M, Makita Z. Pigment epithelium-derived factor protects cultured retinal pericytes from advanced glycation end product-induced injury through its antioxidative properties. Biochem Biophys Res Commun. 2002;296(4):877.
9. Simó R, Carrasco E, García-Ramírez M, Hernández C. Angiogenic and antiangiogenic factors in proliferative diabetic retinopathy. Curr Diabetes Rev. 2006;2:71–98.
10. Ferrara N, Houck K, Jakeman L, et al. Molecular and biological properties of the vascular endothelial growth factor family of proteins. Endocr Rev. 1992;13:18–32.
11. Senger DR, Galli SJ, Dvorak AM, Perruzzi CA, Harvey VS, Dvorak HF. Tumor cells secrete a vascular permeability factor that promotes accumulation of ascites fluid. Science. 1983;219(45):983–5.
12. Marneros AG, Fan J, Yokoyama Y, et al. Vascular endothelial growth factor expression in the retinal pigment epithelium is essential for choriocapillaris development and visual function. Am J Pathol. 2005;167:1451–9.
13. Stefánsson E. Ocular oxygenation and the treatment of diabetic retinopathy. Surv Ophthalmol. 2006;51:364–80.
14. Stefansson E, Geirsdottir A, Sigurdsson H. Metabolic physiology in age related macular degeneration. Prog Retin Eye Res. 2011;30:72–80.
15. Hui-Zhuo X, Song Z, et al. RPE barrier breakdown in diabetic retinopathy: seeing is believing. J Ocul Biol Dis Inform. 2011;4:83–92.
16. Lund-Andersen H. Mechanisms for monitoring changes in retinal status following therapeutic intervention in diabetic retinopathy. Surv Ophthalmol. 2002;47(Suppl 2):S270–7.
17. Ghassemifar R, Lai CM, Rakoczy PE. VEGF differentially regulates transcription and translation of ZO-1α+ and ZO-1α− and mediates trans-epithelial resistance in cultured endothelial and epithelial cells. Cell Tissue Res. 2006;323(1):117–25.
18. Hartnett ME, Lappas A, Darland D, McColm JR, Lovejoy S, D'Amore PA. Retinal pigment epithelium and endothelial cell interaction causes retinal pigment epithelial barrier dysfunction via a soluble VEGF-dependent mechanism. Exp Eye Res. 2003;77:593–9.
19. Fine BS, Brucker AJ. Macular edema and cystoid macular edema. Am J Ophthalmol. 1981;92(4):466–81.
20. Tso MOM. Pathology of cystoid macular edema. Ophthalmology. 1982;89(8):902–15.
21. Yanoff M, Fine BS, Brucker AJ, Eagle RC Jr. Pathology of human cystoid macular edema. Surv Ophthalmol. 1984;28(supplement):505–11.
22. Otani T, Kishi S, Maruyama Y. Patterns of diabetic macular edema with optical coherence tomography. Am J Ophthalmol. 1999;127(6):688–93.
23. Otani T, Kishi S. Correlation between optical coherence tomography and fluorescein angiography findings in diabetic macular edema. Ophthalmology. 2007;114(1):104–7.
24. Bolz M, Ritter M, Schneider M, Simader C, Scholda C, Schmidt-Erfurth U. A systematic correlation of angiography and high-resolution optical coherence tomography in diabetic macular edema. Ophthalmology. 2009;116(1):66–72.
25. Gandorfer A, Rohleder M, Grosselfinger S, Haritoglou C, Ulbig M, Kampik A. Epiretinal pathology of diffuse diabetic macular edema associated with vitreomacular traction. Am J Ophthalmol. 2005;139(4):638–52.
26. Gaucher D, Tadayoni R, Erginay A, Haouchine B, Gaudric A, Massin P. Optical coherence tomography assessment of the vitreoretinal relationship in diabetic macular edema. Am J Ophthalmol. 2005;139(5):807–13.
27. Ophir A, Martinez MR. Epiretinal membranes and incomplete posterior vitreous detachment in diabetic macular edema, detected by spectral-domain optical coherence tomography. Invest Ophthalmol Vis Sci. 2011;52(9):6414–20.

28. Kaiser PK, Riemann CD, Sears JE, Lewis H. Macular traction detachment and diabetic macular edema associated with posterior hyaloidal traction. Am J Ophthalmol. 2001;131(1):44–9.
29. Hangai M, Ojima Y, Gotoh N, et al. Three-dimensional imaging of macular holes with high-speed optical coherence tomography. Ophthalmology. 2007;114(4):763–73.
30. Takahashi A, Nagaoka T, Ishiko S, Kameyama D, Yoshida A. Foveal anatomic changes in a progressing stage 1 macular hole documented by spectral-domain optical coherence tomography. Ophthalmology. 2010;117(4):806–10.
31. MacKinnon JR, O'Brien C, Swa K, Aspinall P, Butt Z, Cameron D. Pulsatile ocular blood flow in untreated diabetic retinopathy. Acta Ophthalmol. 1997;75:661–4.
32. Bude RO, Rubin JM. Relationship between the resistive index and vascular compliance and resistance. Radiology. 1999;211:411–7.
33. Basturk T, Albayrak R, Ulas T, Akcay M, Unsal A, Toksoy M, Koc Y. Evaluation of resistive index by color Doppler imaging of orbital arteries in type II diabetes mellitus patients with microalbuminuria. Ren Fail. 2012;34:708–12.
34. Mendivil A, Cuartero V, Mendivil MP. Ocular blood flow velocities in patients with proliferative diabetic retinopathy and healthy volunteers: a prospective study. Br J Ophthalmol. 1995;1(79):413–6.
35. Patz A. Retinal neovascularization: early contributions of Professor Michaelson and recent observations. Br J Ophthalmol. 1984;68:42–6.
36. Crawford TN, Alfaro DV, Kerrison JB, Jablon EP. Diabetic retinopathy and angiogenesis. Curr Diabetes Rev. 2009;5:8–13.
37. Funatsu H, Yamashita H, Noma H, Shimizu E, Yamashita T, Hori S. Stimulation and inhibition of angiogenesis in diabetic retinopathy. Jpn J Ophthalmol. 2001;45:577–84.
38. Khuu LA, Tayyari F, Sivak JM, Flanagan JG, Singer S, Brent MH, Huang D, Tan O, Hudson C. Aqueous humour concentrations of TGF-β, PLGF and FGF-1 and total retinal blood flow in patients with early non-proliferative diabetic retinopathy. Acta Ophthalmol. 2017;95:e206–11.
39. Birol G, Wang S, Budzynski E, Wangsa-Wirawan ND, Linsenmeier RA. Oxygen distribution and consumption in the macaque retina. Am J Physiol Heart Circ Physiol. 2007;293:H1696–704.
40. Delaey C, Van De Voorde J. Regulatory mechanisms in the retinal and choroidal circulation. Ophthalmic Res. 2000;32(6):249–56.
41. Yi J, Liu W, Chen S, Backman V, Sheibani N, Sorenson CM, Fawzi AA, Linsenmeier RA, Zhang HF. Visible light optical coherence tomography measures retinal oxygen metabolic response to systemic oxygenation. Light Sci Appl. 2015;4(9):e334.
42. Scarinci F, Jampol LM, Linsenmeier RA, Fawzi AA. Association of diabetic macular non-perfusion with outer retinal disruption on optical coherence tomography. JAMA Ophthalmol. 2015;133:1036–44.
43. Maheshwary AS, Oster SF, Yuson RM, Cheng L, Mojana F, Freeman WR. The association between percent disruption of the photoreceptor inner segment-outer segment junction and visual acuity in diabetic macular edema. Am J Ophthalmol. 2010;150:63–7.
44. Khatri M, Saxena S, Kumar M, Chabbra AK, Bhasker S, et al. Resistive index of ophthalmic artery as a bioimaging biomarker for the severity of diabetic retinopathy. Biom J. 2017;3:16. https://doi.org/10.21767/2472-1646.100038.
45. Khatri M, Saxena S, Kaur A, Bhasker SK, Kumar M, Meyer CH. Resistive index of ophthalmic artery correlates with retinal pigment epithelial alterations on spectral domain optical coherence tomography in diabetic retinopathy. Int J Retina Vitreous. 2018;4:12. PMID: 29657836; PMCID: PMC5890348. https://doi.org/10.1186/s40942-018-0116-0.
46. Soliman AZ, Radwan SH, Prager SG, et al. Spectral domain optical coherence tomography parameters associated with visual acuity in patients with resolved center-involved diabetic macular edema. Invest Ophthalmol Vis Sci. 2012; ARVO E-Abstract 1338.
47. Pelosini L, Hull CC, Boyce JF, McHugh D, Stanford MR, Marshall J. Optical coherence tomography may be used to predict visual acuity in patients with macular edema. Invest Ophthalmol Vis Sci. 2011;52(5):2741–8.
48. Kollias AN, Ulbig MW. Diabetic retinopathy: Early diagnosis and effective treatment. Dtsch Arztebl Int. 2010;107(5):75–83; quiz 84. Epub 2010 Feb 5. PMID: 20186318; PMCID: PMC2828250. https://doi.org/10.3238/arztebl.2010.0075.
49. Xu J, Chen LJ, Yu J, et al. Involvement of advanced glycation end products in the pathogenesis of diabetic retinopathy. Cell Physiol Biochem. 2018;48(2):705–17. Epub 2018 Jul 19. https://doi.org/10.1159/000491897.
50. Yamagishi S, Amano S, Inagaki Y. Advanced glycation end products induced apoptosis and overexpression of vascular endothelial growth factor in bovine retinal pericytes. Biochem Biophys Res Commun. 2002;290:973–8.
51. Jain A, Saxena S, Khanna VK, et al. Status of serum VEGF and ICAM-1 and its association with external limiting membrane and inner segment-outer segment junction disruption in type 2 diabetes mellitus. Mol Vis. 2013;19:1760–8.
52. Sharma SR, Saxena S, Mishra N, et al. The association of grades of photoreceptor inner segment-ellipsoid band disruption with severity of retinopathy in type 2 diabetes mellitus. J Case Rep Stud. 2014;2:502–8.
53. Saxena S, Ruia S, Prasad S, et al. Increased serum levels of urea and creatinine are surrogate markers for disruption of retinal photoreceptor external limiting membrane and inner segment ellipsoid zone in type 2 diabetes mellitus. Retina. 2017;37:344–9.
54. Omri S, Omri B, Savoldelli M, et al. The outer limiting membrane (OLM) revisited: clinical implications. Clin Ophthalmol. 2010;4:183–95.
55. Murukami T, Felinski EA, Antonetti DA. Occludin phosphorylation and ubiquitination regulate tight junction trafficking and vascular endothelial growth factor (VEGF)-induced permeability. J Biol Chem. 2009;284:21036–46.
56. Mori Y, Suzuma K, Uji A, et al. Restoration of foveal photoreceptors after intravitreal ranibizumab injections for diabetic macular edema. Sci Rep. 2016;6(39161):3–5.
57. Decanini A, Karunadharma PR, Nordgaard CL, et al. Human retinal pigment epithelium proteome changes in early diabetes. Diabetologia. 2008;51(6):1051–61.
58. van Reyk DM, Gillies MC, Davies MJ. The retina: oxidative stress and diabetes. Redox Rep. 2003;8:187–92.
59. Sharma S, Saxena S, Srivastav K, et al. Nitric oxide and oxidative stress is associated with severity of diabetic retinopathy and retinal structural alterations. Clin Experiment Ophthalmol. 2015;43(5):429–36.
60. Hartnett ME, Lappas A, Darland D, et al. Retinal pigment epithelium and endothelial cell interaction causes retinal pigment epithelial barrier dysfunction via a soluble VEGF-dependent mechanism. Exp Eye Res. 2003;77:593–9.
61. Vlassara H, Cai W, Crandall J, et al. Inflammatory mediators are induced by dietary glycotoxins, a major risk factor for diabetic angiopathy. Proc Natl Acad Sci U S A. 2002;99:15596–601.
62. Yamagishi S, Maeda S, Matsui T, et al. Role of advanced glycation end products (AGEs) and oxidative stress in vascular complications in diabetes. Biochim Biophys Acta. 2012;1820(5):663–71. Epub 2011 Apr 2. PMID: 21440603. https://doi.org/10.1016/j.bbagen.2011.03.014.
63. Sinha S, Saxena S, Prasad S, et al. Association of serum levels of anti-myeloperoxidase antibody with retinal photoreceptor ellipsoid zone disruption in diabetic retinopathy. J Diabetes Complications. 2017;31(5):864–8. Epub 2017 Feb 28. PMID: 28279572. https://doi.org/10.1016/j.jdiacomp.2017.02.011.

64. Nadri G, Saxena S, Kaur A, et al. Correlation between vitamin D serum levels and severity of diabetic retinopathy in patients with type 2 diabetes mellitus. J Endocrinol Metabol Diabetes S Afr. Published online: 27 Apr 2021.
65. Ankita SJ, Saxena S, et al. Hyperglycemia potentiates the effect of ionic calcium in photoreceptor ellipsoid zone disruption in diabetic retinopathy. Int Ophthalmol. 2019;39(10):2237–43. Epub 2019 Jan 9. PMID: 30628026. https://doi.org/10.1007/s10792-018-01063-8.
66. Andrade GC, Dias JR, Maia A, Farah ME, Meyer CH, Rodrigues EB, et al. Intravitreal injections of ziv-aflibercept for diabetic macular edema: a pilot study. Retina. 2016;36:1640–5.
67. de Oliveira Dias JR, Badaró E, Novais EA, Colicchio D, Chiarantin GM, Matioli MM, et al. Preclinical investigations of intravitreal ziv-aflibercept. Ophthalmic Surg Lasers Imaging Retina. 2014;45:577–84.
68. Wells JA, Glassman AR, Ayala AR, Jampol LM, Aiello LP, et al. Diabetic retinopathy clinical research network. Aflibercept, bevacizumab, or ranibizumab for diabetic macular edema. N Engl J Med. 2015;372:1193–203.
69. de Andrade GC, de Oliveira Dias JR, Maia A, Farah ME, Meyer CH, Rodrigues EB, et al. Intravitreal ziv-aflibercept for diabetic macular edema: 48-week outcomes. Ophthalmic Surg Lasers Imaging Retina. 2018;49:245–50.
70. Cunningham ET Jr, Adamis AP, Altaweel M, Aiello LP, Bressler NM, D'Amico DJ. A phase II randomized double-masked trial of pegaptanib, an anti-vascular endothelial growth factor aptamer, for diabetic macular edema. Ophthalmology. 2005;112:1747–57.
71. Rajendram R, Fraser-Bell S, Kaines A, Michaelides M, Hamilton RD, Esposti SD, et al. A 2-year prospective randomized controlled trial of intravitreal bevacizumab or laser therapy (BOLT) in the management of diabetic macular edema: 24-month data: report 3. Arch Ophthalmol. 2012;130:972–9.
72. Nguyen QD, Brown DM, Marcus DM, Boyer DS, Patel S, Feiner L, et al. Ranibizumab for diabetic macular edema: results from 2 phase III randomized trials: RISE and RIDE. Ophthalmology. 2012;119:789–801.
73. Brown DM, Schmidt-Erfurth U, Do DV, Holz FG, Boyer DS, Midena E, et al. Intravitreal aflibercept for diabetic macular edema: 100-week results from the VISTA and VIVID studies. Ophthalmology. 2015;122:2044–52.
74. Wells JA, Glassman AR, Ayala AR, Jampol LM, Bressler NM, Bressler SB, et al. Aflibercept, bevacizumab, or ranibizumab for diabetic macular edema: two-year results from a comparative effectiveness randomized clinical trial. Ophthalmology. 2016;123:1351–9.
75. Comyn O, Sivaprasad S, Peto T, Neveu MM, Holder GE, Xing W, et al. A randomized trial to assess functional and structural effects of ranibizumab versus laser in diabetic macular edema (the LUCIDATE study). Am J Ophthalmol. 2014;157:960–70.
76. Wells JA, Glassman AR, Ayala AR, Jampol LM, Aiello LP, Antoszyk AN, et al. Aflibercept, bevacizumab, or ranibizumab for diabetic macular edema. N Engl J Med. 2015;372:1193–203.
77. Aiello LP, Edwards AR, Beck RW, Bressler NM, Davis MD, Ferris F, et al. Diabetic retinopathy clinical research network factors associated with improvement and worsening of visual acuity 2 years after focal/grid photocoagulation for diabetic macular edema. Ophthalmology. 2010;117:946–95.
78. Nguyen QD, Brown DM, Marcus DM, Boyer DS, Patel S, Feiner L, et al. RISE and RIDE research group Ranibizumab for diabetic macular edema: results from 2 phase III randomized trials: RISE and RIDE. Ophthalmology. 2012;119:789–801.
79. Saxena S, Srivastav K, Cheung CM, Ng JY, Lai TY. Photoreceptor inner segment ellipsoid band integrity on spectral domain optical coherence tomography. Clin Ophthalmol. 2014;8:2507–22.
80. Theodossiadis PG, Theodossiadis GP, Charonis A, Emfietzoglou I, Grigoropoulos VG, Liarakos VS. The photoreceptor layer as a prognostic factor for visual acuity in the secondary epiretinal membrane after retinal detachment surgery: imaging analysis by spectral-domain optical coherence tomography. Am J Ophthalmol. 2011;151:973–80.
81. Kwon Y, Lee D, Kim H, Kwon O. Predictive findings of visual outcome in spectral domain optical coherence tomography after ranibizumab treatment in age-related macular degeneration. Korean J Ophthalmol. 2014;28:386–92.
82. Uji A, Murakami T, Nishijima K, Akagi T, Horii T, Arakawa N, et al. Association between hyperreflective foci in the outer retina, status of photoreceptor layer, and visual acuity in diabetic macular edema. Am J Ophthalmol. 2012;153:710–7.
83. Kang HM, Chung EJ, Kim YM, Koh HJ. Spectral-domain optical coherence tomography (SD-OCT) patterns and response to intravitreal bevacizumab therapy in macular edema associated with branch retinal vein occlusion. Graefes Arch Clin Exp Ophthalmol. 2013;251:501–8.
84. Hareedy NH, Gaafar AA, El-Dayem HK, El-Shinawy RF. The relation between inner segment/outer segment junction and visual acuity before and after ranibizumab in diabetic macular edema. J Egypt Ophthalmol Soc. 2018;111:102–7.
85. Achiron A, Kydyrbaeva A, Man V, et al. Photoreceptor integrity predicts response to anti-VEGF treatment. Ophthalmic Res. 2017;57:37–41.
86. Chatziralli I, Theodossiadis G, Dimitriou E, Kazantzis D, Theodossiadis P. Association between the patterns of diabetic macular edema and photoreceptors' response after intravitreal ranibizumab treatment: a spectral-domain optical coherence tomography study. Int Ophthalmol. 2020;40:2441. https://doi.org/10.1007/s10792-020-01423-3.
87. De S, Saxena S, Kaur A, Mahdi AA, Misra A, Singh M, Meyer CH, Akduman L. Sequential restoration of external limiting membrane and ellipsoid zone after intravitreal anti-VEGF therapy in diabetic macular oedema. Eye (Lond). 2021;35(5):1490–5. Epub 2020 Jul 20. PMID: 32690922; PMCID: PMC8182796. https://doi.org/10.1038/s41433-020-1100-0.
88. Marmor MF. Mechanisms of fluid accumulation in retinal edema. Doc Ophthalmol. 1999;97(3–4):239–49. https://doi.org/10.1023/a:1002192829817.
89. Adamis AP, Shima DT, Yeo KT, Yeo TK, Brown LF, Berse B, D'Amore PA, Folkman J. Synthesis and secretion of vascular permeability factor/vascular endothelial growth factor by human retinal pigment epithelial cells. Biochem Biophys Res Commun. 1993;193(2):631–8. https://doi.org/10.1006/bbrc.1993.1671.
90. Jablonski MM, Tombran-Tink J, Mrazek DA, Iannaccone A. Pigment epithelium-derived factor supports normal development of photoreceptor neurons and opsin expression after retinal pigment epithelium removal. J Neurosci. 2000;20(19):7149–57. https://doi.org/10.1523/JNEUROSCI.20-19-07149.2000.
91. King GL, Suzuma K. Pigment-epithelium-derived factor—a key coordinator of retinal neuronal and vascular functions. N Engl J Med. 2000;342(5):349–51. https://doi.org/10.1056/NEJM200002033420511.
92. Dornonville de la Cour M. Ion transport in the retinal pigment epithelium. A study with double barrelled ion-selective microelectrodes. Acta Ophthalmol Suppl. 1993;209:1–32.
93. Steinberg RH. Interactions between the retinal pigment epithelium and the neural retina. Doc Ophthalmol. 1985;60:327–46. https://doi.org/10.1007/BF00158922.
94. Bok D. The retinal pigment epithelium: a versatile partner in vision. J Cell Sci Suppl. 1993;17:189–95. https://doi.org/10.1242/jcs.1993.supplement_17.27.

95. Finnemann SC. Focal adhesion kinase signaling promotes phagocytosis of integrin-bound photoreceptors. EMBO J. 2003;22(16):4143–54. https://doi.org/10.1093/emboj/cdg416.
96. Strauss O, Stumpff F, Mergler S, Wienrich M, Wiederholt M. The Royal College of surgeons rat: an animal model for inherited retinal degeneration with a still unknown genetic defect. Acta Anat. 1998;162(2–3):101–11. https://doi.org/10.1159/000046474.
97. Li Y, Tang L, Jia S. Yan ke xue bao = Eye Sci. 2003;19(4):248–52.
98. Ablonczy Z, Crosson CE. VEGF modulation of retinal pigment epithelium resistance. Exp Eye Res. 2007;85(6):762–71. https://doi.org/10.1016/j.exer.2007.08.010.
99. Cohn BA, Collin SP, Wainwright PC, Schmitz L. Retinal topography maps in R: new tools for the analysis and visualization of spatial retinal data. J Vis. 2015;15(9):19. https://doi.org/10.1167/15.9.19.
100. Mishra N, Saxena S, Shukla RK, Singh V, Meyer CH, Kruzliak P, Khanna VK. Association of serum N(ε)-Carboxy methyl lysine with severity of diabetic retinopathy. J Diabetes Complications. 2016;30(3):511–7.

Diabetic Macular Ischemia and Anti-VEGF Therapy

10

Gemmy Cheung, Majid Al-Shaaibi, and Kelvin Teo

10.1 Introduction

Reduction in retinal blood flow and capillary non-perfusion have been demonstrated in eyes with diabetic microvasculopathy [1–4]. In the macula, occlusion and/or loss of retinal capillaries with narrowing or obliteration of precapillary arterioles lead to macular ischemia. Diabetic macular ischemia (DMI) is traditionally diagnosed on fluorescein angiography (FA) as an enlargement of the foveal avascular zone (FAZ) with irregular borders, leading to a moth-eaten appearance. The true prevalence of DMI is underestimated as FA is not routinely performed as part of clinical assessment unless there is significant visual impairment.

The FAZ area has been shown to increase with increasing severity of DR [5]. Severe DMI has been associated with poor vision, although the correlation between FAZ measurements and functional losses has been variable and of modest degree.

With the recent advances in OCT-angiography (OCTA), the diagnosis and monitoring of DMI is much more accessible and can be performed noninvasively. A key improvement in clinical interpretation with the use of OCTA is the ability to evaluate DMI across the retina layers by independently analyzing the superficial and deep retinal plexus. This allows us to recognize different phenotypes of DMI and quantify the severity to allow for precise assessment of progression longitudinally. Different phenotypes of DMI, in turn, may explain the variability in the functional deficit between individuals. In addition to assessing the FAZ, quantification of perfusion/vessel density and vessel length density offers additional parameters to evaluate macular perfusion. Cross-sectional OCTA studies have found that the FAZ area and vessel density in the deep plexus correlated more closely with visual acuity than similar changes in the superficial vascular plexus [6, 7]. The changes in the FAZ area and circularity on OCTA are also precursors to the development of DR, suggesting that these alterations are potential early biomarkers [8, 9].

10.2 DMI

10.2.1 Pathogenesis

In diabetes, key processes affecting the retinal vasculature include oxidative stress, hypoxia, and inflammation. These induce endothelial cell apoptosis and pericyte loss which contribute to the clinical findings of microaneurysms, leakage, capillary non-perfusion, and intraretinal microvascular abnormalities [10–12]. Leukostasis can act as a further trigger for retinal capillary non-perfusion [13]. Concurrently, VEGF overexpression results in endothelial cell hypertrophy and narrowing of the vascular lumen [14]. VEGF further promotes leukocyte plugging through promoting in ICAM-1 expression in the retinal capillary endothelial cells [15–18]. In addition to VEGF, other cytokines, including TNF-α and inducible nitric oxide synthase, have been proposed to mediate tissue injury due to ischemia through inflammation and neurotoxicity [19].

10.2.2 Diagnosis: FA

Until recently, the gold standard for the diagnosis of DMI is based on FAZ size, outline, and capillary loss in the central subfield as detected on FA [5, 20]. In the Early Treatment for Diabetic Retinopathy Study (ETDRS), DMI was classified as none, questionable, mild, moderate, or severe based on the assessment of FAZ size, outline, and capillary loss in the central subfield. Eyes with a regular capillary outline were

G. Cheung (✉) · K. Teo
Duke-NUS Medical School, National University of Singapore, Singapore, Singapore
e-mail: gemmy.cheung.c.m@singhealth.com.sg; kelvin.teo.y.c@singhealth.com.sg

M. Al-Shaaibi
Singapore National Eye Centre, Singapore, Singapore

S. Saxena et al. (eds.), *Diabetic Macular Edema*, https://doi.org/10.1007/978-981-19-7307-9_10

graded based on the area of the FAZ compared to a reference circle with a radius of 300 μm. An enlarged FAZ size was defined as any FAZ area larger than the reference circle of radius 300 μm, equating to 0.28 mm^2. In eyes with an irregular outline, DMI was graded into Grade 0 (normal), Grade 1 (relatively round or oval outline but visible irregularities were noted), Grade 2 (destroyed outline for less than half of the original circumference), Grade 3 (destroyed outline for half or more of the original circumference), Grade 4 (completely destroyed capillary outline). The grading of capillary loss had five levels: 0 (absent), 1 (questionable), 2 (definitely present), 3 (moderate), 4 (severe) [21, 22].

In addition to the potential risk of allergic reactions due to the invasive nature of the procedure FA also confers imaging limitations. These include the obscuration of capillary details due to dye leakage and the inability to differentiate the three capillary networks within the retina with alterations in FA image corresponding mainly to the superficial capillary network [23–25].

10.2.3 Diagnosis: OCTA

OCTA can diagnose DMI through a similar assessment of FAZ parameters like area and perimeter and circularity as FA. However, the cut-off value for defining DMI has not been established. Studies of normal eyes suggest that the upper range of the FAZ size was about 0.5 mm^2 [26, 27]. However, a number of characteristics unrelated to diabetes such as ethnicity, axial length, age, and gender are known to affect FAZ size [28, 29].

Enlarged FAZ has been reported in diabetic patients compared to control [30]. Furthermore, FAZ area has been reported to correlate with visual acuity in patients with DR. With the high resolution of OCTA, the capillary network immediately adjacent to the FAZ can also be assessed to provide further markers of non-perfusion such as intercapillary area and the percentage of the area of non-perfusion (PAN) [31–33].

In addition to quantifying areas in which perfusion was not present, several novel OCTA-based metrics used to quantify perfusion have been proposed as useful biomarkers for evaluating DMI. These metrics include perfusion density (PD) (ratio of perfused area to total scanned area), and vessel length density (VLD) (ratio of pixels after skeletonization to total scanned area). A number of studies have reported a decrease in perfusion density in diabetics compared to controls. Among diabetics, a decrease in perfusion density was observed with increasing DR severity levels [34–38].

In addition to the evaluation of perfusion, alteration in vascular patterns can be assessed by evaluating vascular tortuosity and fractal dimension (FD). Reduced fractal dimension has been hypothesized to result from ischemia which also leads reduction in vessel density. FD has been associated with progression of DR [39].

OCTA also offers the ability to analyze the superficial and deep retinal plexuses separately. Most commercially available OCTA instruments automatically segment the SCP and the DCP. Several studies have reported the importance of differentiating the SCP and DCP in DMI (see section below).

10.2.4 Visual Prognosis

Multiple studies have found that visual function is affected in DMI [40–45]. When DMI is present with concomitant DME or neuronal loss, the functional impact may be more significant [33, 46]. In addition to the severity of DMI, the phenotype of DMI may also affect the level of functional impairment. The relative involvement of the SCP and the DCP may explain various structure-function phenotypes [47]. Eyes that have perfusion deficits in both the SCP and DCP appear to have a more functional loss, probably due to both inner and outer retina disturbance [48–50]. Several reports have shown that the visual loss in diabetic eyes correlated more with the alterations in the DCP than in the SCP [51, 52].

One scheme to differentiate the DMI phenotypes categories DMI into i) generalized, ii) predominant DCP, and iii) predominant SCP. Eyes with generalized DMI exhibit reduction of vessel density in both the SCP and DCP and consequent reduction in vision [53]. This pattern may be accompanied by structural OCT changes such as disorganization of retinal inner layers (DRIL) or outer retinal atrophy [54] (Fig. 10.1). Eyes with predominant DCP ischemia have a greater reduction in the vessel density of the DCP compared to the SCP. This phenotype has been shown to correlate closely with visual loss and reduced retinal sensitivity due to DCP contribution of blood supply to the outer retina and photoreceptor. This phenotype has also been associated with recurrent or persistent DME, as disruption of DCP can impair the outflow of fluid accumulation within the retina [55–59]. In contrast, eyes with predominant SCP ischemia may represent a milder phenotype. Ischemia of the SCP may affect the inner retina preferentially and manifest as loss of neuronal cells and the development of DRIL (Fig. 10.2).

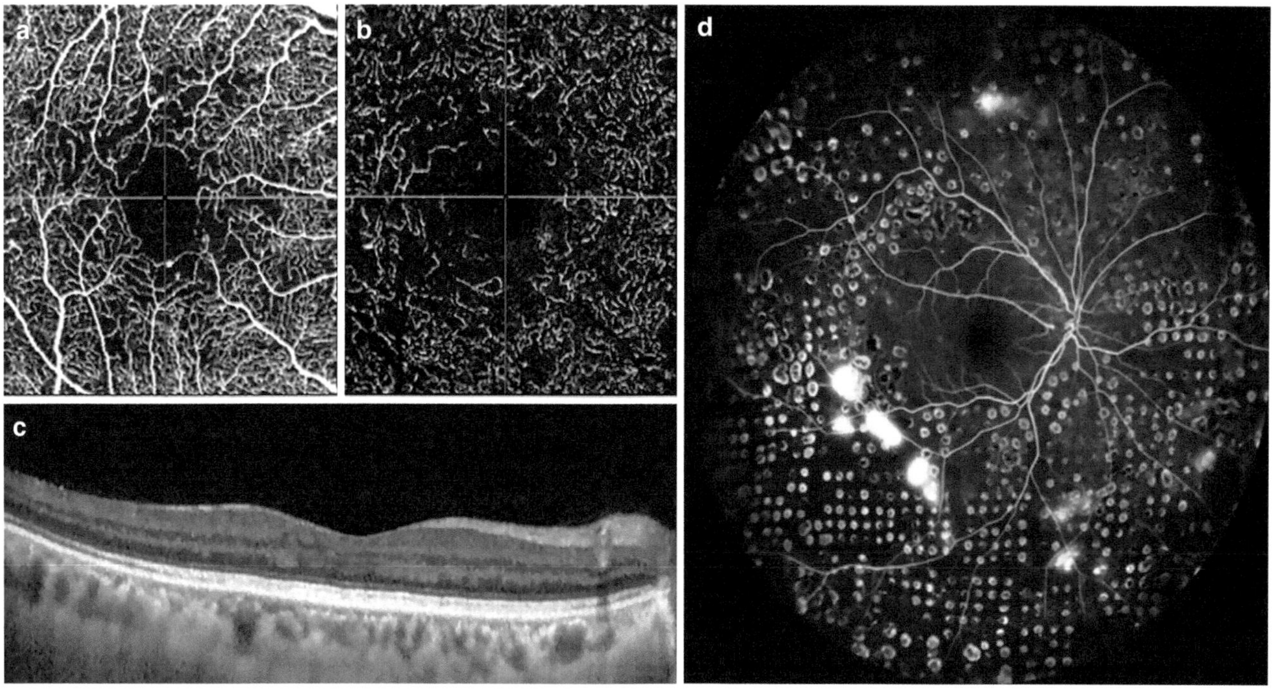

Fig. 10.1 OCTA images (**a**) and (**b**) show decrease vessel density of both SCP and DCP at the perifoveal area. Structural OCT (**c**) shows dry retina with some DRILL, and the FFA image (**d**) shows hyperfluorescent areas corresponding to NVEs

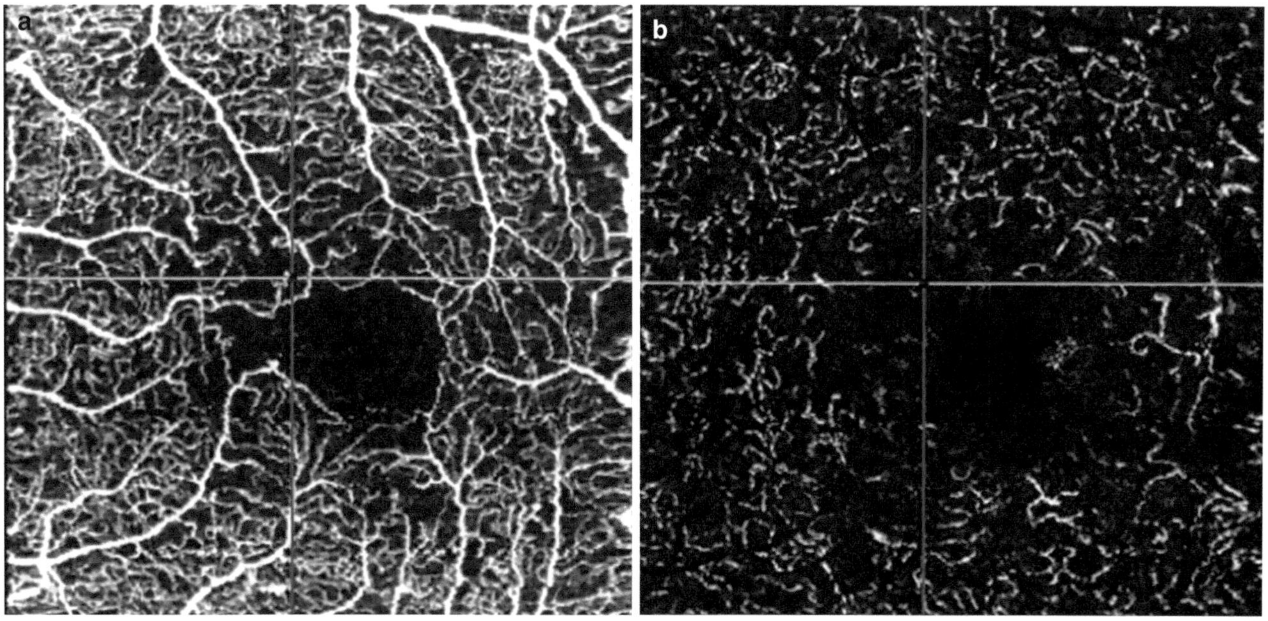

Fig. 10.2 OCTA images (**a**) and (**b**) show an enlarged FAZ with irregular borders more at SCP compared to DCP. (**c**) Centre of Cross line in Enface image and (**d**) Structural OCT shows some intraretinal cysts which may appear as dark and erroneously be interpreted as capillary loss in OCTA

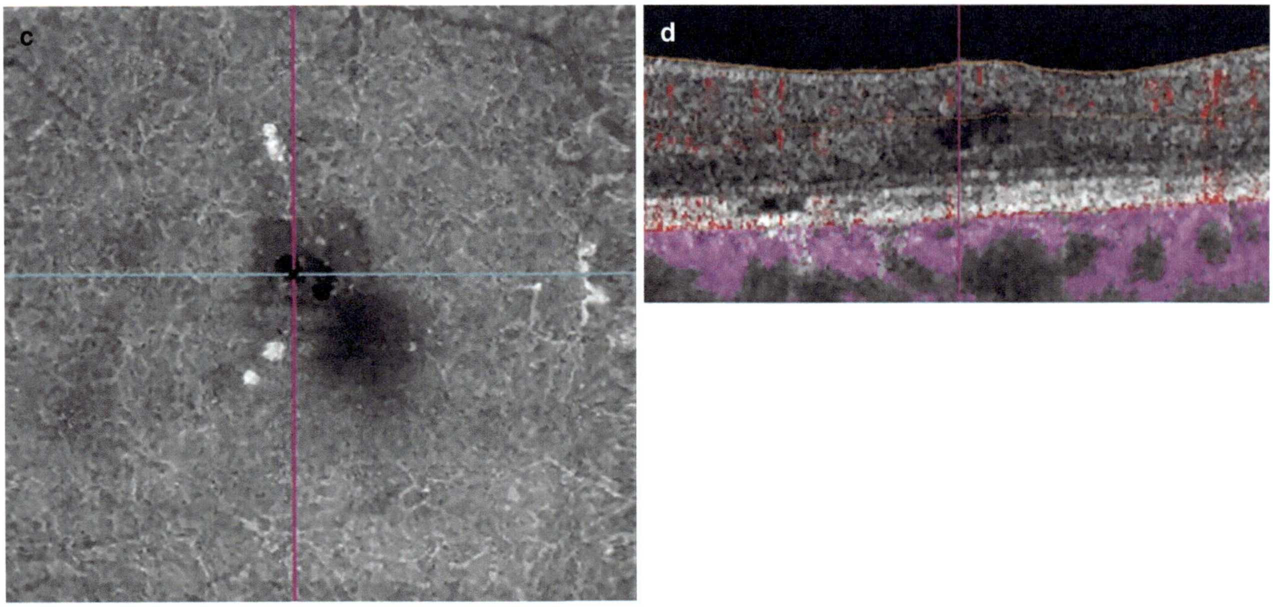

Fig. 10.2 (continued)

10.3 DMI and Anti-VEGF

Current anti-VEGF therapy is mainly targeted at DME. Many studies have examined the relationship between vascular endothelial growth factors (VEGF) and macular ischemia. An experiment on monkey eyes has demonstrated retinal vascular endothelial cell hypertrophy in response to VEGF, resulting in narrowing of the capillary lumen and in subsequent retinal ischemia. Pan Retinal Photocoagulation (PRP) reduces the VEGF drive in eyes with proliferative diabetic retinopathy, and this results in improved perfusion of the posterior pole [60].

The relationship between DMI and DME has not been clearly elucidated. It has been proposed that DMI may be partly responsible for recurrent DME. Alternatively, whether DME triggers DMI and whether anti-VEGF further influences the development or progression of DMI remain important clinical questions.

10.3.1 Influence of DMI on Anti-VEGF Therapy in Eyes with DME

DME response to anti-VEGF treatment is variable. The degree of underlying DMI has been proposed to influence this variability. In addition, the persistence of DMI despite the resolution of edema may limit the visual improvement that can be achieved with anti-VEGF therapy.

The RESTORE study compared ranibizumab alone or combined with laser versus laser alone in eyes with DME. Eyes were classified according to their macular ischemia status based on FA. This study did not find a clear association between reduced treatment effect and increasing DMI. However, those observations were based on simplified schemes for grading DMI on FA [61].

A number of case series comparing good and poor responders to anti-VEGF therapy for DME have reported a larger baseline FAZ area in poor responders. Usui-Ouchi et al. evaluated potential factors affecting short-term response to anti-VEGF in 102 eyes with DME. At 1 month, 65.9% of the cohort were classified as good responders (defined as >20% reduction in central macular thickness). The authors identified higher HbA1c, larger FAZ, and higher number of microaneurysms as features associated with poor response [62]. Chung et al. reported macular ischemia had a negative effect on the outcome of 3 monthly intravitreal bevacizumab treatments for DME [63]. Eighteen of 59 participants in the series had macular ischemia (defined as FAZ > 1000 μm, or a broken capillary ring at the border of the FAZ). At 3 months, mean visual acuity improved in the non-ischemic group but decreased in the ischemic group. They observed a reduction in foveal thickness in the ischemic group, but this did not correlate with improvement in vision. A negative impact from macular ischemia was also reported by Douvali et al. Following 6 months of ranibizumab treatment for DME, non-ischemic eyes experienced a statistically significant improvement in vision and retinal thickness, while ischemic eyes had no significant improvement in vision despite significant retinal thickness reduction. Potential limitations from these reports include the relatively short follow-up period and the variation in definition of FAZ and treatment response.

More recent studies have used OCTA to define macular ischemia and evaluate the potential influence of macular ischemia on response to anti-VEGF. Lee et al. compared the OCTA features between eyes with good response (defined as <50 μm reduction in central retinal thickness after three consecutive anti-VEGF injections) and those with poor response [64, 65]. The features evaluated included vascular density, FAZ area, and number of microaneurysms in each layer. A larger FAZ area and higher number of microaneurysms in the DCP were found in the poor responder group. No difference in the SCP was observed between groups. Hsieh et al. also reported baseline macular ischemia may influence treatment response following three consecutive ranibizumab injections. They defined response based on visual gain and found parafoveal vessel density in the SCP as an important predictor. Larger FAZ area in the DCP was also reported in the poor visual improvement group, but the difference was not statistically significant.

Technical aspects of OCTA should be considered when interpreting these results. Accurate quantification of the DCP is more challenging than the SCP as this layer is particularly susceptible to the decay of image signals, especially in the presence of macular edema. In addition, projection artifacts may also introduce flow signals from the overlying layers.

Evidence regarding the efficacy of anti-VEGF therapy on DME in eyes with severe macular ischemia is limited, as severe macular ischemia was excluded in many randomized controlled trials evaluating the efficacy of anti-VEGF on DME. For example, patients with a FAZ of >1000 μm at baseline were not included into the BOLT study (BOLT). Similarly, retinal ischemia >500 μm located within 500 μm from the center of the macula was an exclusion criterion in the RESOLVE study (Mitchell). Few small case series have specifically evaluated the outcome of anti-VEGF therapy in this group of eyes. In contrast, another case series comprising 10 eyes with DME and severe capillary loss, mean improvement at 54 weeks following intravitreal bevacizumab therapy was 2.28 ETDRS lines [66].

10.3.2 Influence of Anti-VEGF on DMI

The potential of worsening retinal ischemia with anti-VEGF therapy remains a concern and evidence to-date remains inconsistent. VEGF upregulation has been shown to contribute to leukostasis, venous plugging and the development of retinal ischemia. Therefore, anti-VEGF therapy has the potential to alleviate retinal ischemia. On the other hand, VEGF plays an important role in maintaining the retinal vasculature under normal physiological conditions. Following this line of reasoning, chronic inhibition of VEGF may lead to worsening of retinal ischemia. In addition, peripheral ischemia and macular ischemia may show different responses to anti-VEGF treatment.

A number of reports have investigated the effect of anti-VEGF therapy on peripheral ischemia. Most of these studies found no significant improvement in areas of peripheral nonperfusion, despite the clinical observation of resolution of retinal hemorrhages and venous beading [67, 68]. A few studies have shown that areas of peripheral capillary fallouts have re-perfused following monthly ranibizumab and aflibercept injection [68, 69]. This chapter will focus on macular ischemia.

The majority of reports suggest there is no effect from anti-VEGF therapy on macular ischemia, while some investigators have reported worsening of macular ischemia [70]. These variations may arise from differences in the anti-VEGF exposure, follow-up periods and methods used to assess macular ischemia. It is also important to note that macular ischemia was not included as an endpoint in the pivotal anti-VEGF trials for DME. Hence, most of the published reports consisted of case series with limited sample sizes.

The RISE/RIDE studies evaluated ranibizumab vs. sham for DME over 24 months. In a post hoc analysis using FA to evaluate macular ischemia in 666 eyes, the authors reported an increase in the proportion of eyes with an increase in posterior retinal non-perfusion increased in all groups, but at a slower rate in the ranibizumab-treated group than sham (16.1 vs. 37.6%, $p < 0.001$). These findings suggest that ranibizumab treatment may slow the progression of macular ischemia. To further support this hypothesis, patients initially randomized to the sham arm were switched to ranibizumab at month 24. Evaluation at months 30 and 36 showed a reduction in the proportion of patients exhibiting an increase in retinal non-perfusion.

In the BOLT study which compared the effect of bevacizumab against laser for DME in 80 participants, no worsening of macular ischemia on FA was observed in either group over 4 months (Michaelides). In the LUCIDATE study which prospectively assessed the functional and structural effects of ranibizumab versus laser in DME, a small increase in FAZ area was observed on FA, but the difference was not significant. Many other case series with smaller sample sizes reported no significant change in macular ischemia evaluated with FA following anti-VEGF therapy [71].

Worsening of macular ischemia following anti-VEGF therapy has been reported by a few investigators. Several groups have observed an enlarged foveal avascular zone on FA after anti-VEGF injections [72, 73]. Erol et al. reported an increase in FAZ area on FA by 13% in 29 eyes after three bevacizumb injections. Similarly, Feucht reported 19.7% increase in FAZ area on FA after a single bevacizumab injection in 28 eyes. A consideration when interpreting these reports is the lack of control group. Progression of macular ischemia may reflect the natural history of DR. In addition, macula ischemia at baseline may be under-estimated on FA due to leakage in the presence of DME. As DME improved with treatment and leakage progressively resolved, the effect of masking likely led to a more accurate appreciation of the true degree of macular ischemia. The lack of a control group in which DME improved without anti-VEGF treatment further limits the conclusions that can be drawn from these case series.

A number of investigators have evaluated the effect of anti-VEGF on macular ischemia using OCTA. Conflicting results have been reported, with several groups reporting no change in macular ischemia following anti-VEGF therapy, and others reporting worsening of macular ischemia [74]. In addition to variations in study design and anti-VEGF exposure mentioned above, variations in OCTA instrument and analytic methods may further contribute to some of the different results reported.

A sub-analysis of the RESTORE (Extension) study which included 240 eyes found that repeated injections of ranibizumab did not result in impaired macular perfusion [75]. Over 36 months, no change in FAZ area on OCTA and no difference in capillary loss was observed across the three treatment groups.

Moon et al. evaluated macular ischemia on OCTA based on FAZ area and vessel density (VD) in 97 eyes with DME treated with anti-VEGF agents. Over 12 months, they observed no significant difference in FAZ area and VD in the SCP. There was also no difference in DCP FAZ area although increase in DCP VD was observed.

A few case series have reported worsening of macular perfusion following anti-VEGF therapy. Elnahry et al. prospectively evaluated 40 eyes of 26 patients who received 3 monthly bevacizumab and reported increase in FAZ area and decrease in vessel density in both the SCP and DCP [76]. Golshani et al. reported reduction in vessel density by 5.2% (SCP) and 6.3% (DCP) following 12 months of aflibercept treatment in 20 eyes [77]. Similarly, Statler et al. also reported reduction in vessel density by 5.3% (SCP) and 4.4% (DCP) as well as increase in FAZ area following 24 months of aflibercept treatment in 16 eyes [78].

To add to the complexity, some investigators have reported conflicting effects of anti-VEGF therapy on the SCP and DCP. Busch et al. reported FAZ area increased in the SCP but reduced in the DCP in 20 eyes following aflibercept treatment for DME.

While OCTA is not affected by masking from leakage, other sources of artefacts should be considered. In eyes with DME, the retinal capillary system may be displaced in the presence of intraretinal cysts and subretinal fluid. This can result in failure of the pre-set segmentation of the SCP and DCP to capture the flow signal despite presence of the vasculature. As the retinal architecture is restored with resolution of DME, apparent improvement of flow may be observed, but this may simply reflect the return of these retinal capillaries to a more physiological location.

In conclusion, a substantial proportion of eyes with DME have concomitant DMI. OCTA and FA are complementary methods to evaluate and quantify DMI. Understanding the strengths and weaknesses of each modality is important when interpreting results. Variation in the definition of DMI may also lead to differences in reports regarding the relationship between DMI and anti-VEGF therapy. The current body of evidence suggest DMI does not preclude improvement in vision and retinal anatomy with anti-VEGF therapy, although evidence regarding eyes with severe DMI are limited. Conversely, there are conflicting reports of whether anti-VEGF therapy may worsen DMI. These studies are limited by small sample size, retrospective nature and short follow-up. Given the increased accessibility of assessing DMI, this entity should be incorporated as part of DR assessment.

References

1. Grunwald JE, Piltz J, Patel N, Bose S, Riva CE. Effect of aging on retinal macular microcirculation: a blue field simulation study. Invest Ophthalmol Vis Sci. 1993;34:3609–13.
2. Kohner EM. The retinal blood flow in diabetes. Diabete Metab. 1993;19:401–4.
3. Nagaoka T, Sato E, Takahashi A, Yokota H, Sogawa K, Yoshida A. Impaired retinal circulation in patients with type 2 diabetes mellitus: retinal laser Doppler velocimetry study. Invest Ophthalmol Vis Sci. 2010;51:6729–34.
4. Srinivas S, Tan O, Nittala MG, Wu JL, Fawzi AA, Huang D, Sadda SR. Assessment of retinal blood flow in diabetic retinopathy using doppler Fourier-domain optical coherence tomography. Retina. 2017;37:2001–7.
5. Mansour AM, Schachat A, Bodiford G, Haymond R. Foveal avascular zone in diabetes mellitus. Retina. 1993;13:125–8.
6. Dupas B, Minvielle W, Bonnin S, Couturier A, Erginay A, Massin P, Gaudric A, Tadayoni R. Association between vessel density and visual acuity in patients with diabetic retinopathy and poorly controlled type 1 diabetes. JAMA Ophthalmol. 2018;136:721–8.
7. Samara WA, Shahlaee A, Adam MK, Khan MA, Chiang A, Maguire JI, Hsu J, Ho AC. Quantification of diabetic macular ischemia using optical coherence tomography angiography and its relationship with visual acuity. Ophthalmology. 2017;124:235–44.
8. de Carlo TE, Chin AT, Bonini Filho MA, Adhi M, Branchini L, Salz DA, Baumal CR, Crawford C, Reichel E, Witkin AJ, Duker JS, Waheed NK. Detection of microvascular changes in eyes of patients with diabetes but not clinical diabetic retinopathy using optical coherence tomography angiography. Retina. 2015;35:2364–70.
9. Durbin MK, An L, Shemonski ND, Soares M, Santos T, Lopes M, Neves C, Cunha-Vaz J. Quantification of retinal microvascular density in optical coherence tomographic angiography images in diabetic retinopathy. JAMA Ophthalmol. 2017;135:370–6.
10. Cogan DG, Kuwabara T. Capillary shunts in the pathogenesis of diabetic retinopathy. Diabetes. 1963;12:293–300.
11. Cogan DG, Toussaint D, Kuwabara T. Retinal vascular patterns. IV. Diabetic retinopathy. Arch Ophthalmol. 1961;66:366–78.
12. Hammes HP, Feng Y, Pfister F, Brownlee M. Diabetic retinopathy: targeting vasoregression. Diabetes. 2011;60:9–16.
13. Campochiaro PA. Molecular pathogenesis of retinal and choroidal vascular diseases. Prog Retin Eye Res. 2015;49:67–81.

14. Hofman P. Endothelial cell hypertrophy induced by vascular endothelial growth factor in the retina. Arch Ophthalmol. 2001;119:861.
15. Zheng L, Gong B, Hatala DA, Kern TS. Retinal ischemia and reperfusion causes capillary degeneration: similarities to diabetes. Invest Ophthalmol Vis Sci. 2007;48:361–7.
16. Joussen AM, Poulaki V, Qin W, Kirchhof B, Mitsiades N, Wiegand SJ, Rudge J, Yancopoulos GD, Adamis AP. Retinal vascular endothelial growth factor induces intercellular adhesion molecule-1 and endothelial nitric oxide synthase expression and initiates early diabetic retinal leukocyte adhesion in vivo. Am J Pathol. 2002;160:501–9.
17. Miyamoto K, Khosrof S, Bursell SE, Moromizato Y, Aiello LP, Ogura Y, Adamis AP. Vascular endothelial growth factor (VEGF)-induced retinal vascular permeability is mediated by intercellular adhesion molecule-1 (ICAM-1). Am J Pathol. 2000;156:1733–9.
18. Nishiwaki A, Ueda T, Ugawa S, Shimada S, Ogura Y. Upregulation of P-selectin and intercellular adhesion molecule-1 after retinal ischemia-reperfusion injury. Invest Ophthalmol Vis Sci. 2003;44:4931–5.
19. Lam TT, Abler AS, Tso M. Apoptosis and caspases after ischemia-reperfusion injury in rat retina. Invest Ophthalmol Vis Sci. 1999;40:967–75.
20. Bresnick GH, Condit R, Syrjala S, Palta M, Groo A, Korth K. Abnormalities of the foveal avascular zone in diabetic retinopathy. Arch Ophthalmol. 1984;102:1286–93.
21. ETDRS Research Group. Early photocoagulation for diabetic retinopathy. ETDRS report 9. Ophthalmology. 1991:5(suppl);766–85.
22. ETDRS Research Group. Classification of diabetic retinopathy from fluorescein angiograms. ETDRS report 11. Ophthalmology. 1991:98(5);807–22.
23. Mendis KR, Balaratnasingam C, Yu P, Barry CJ, McAllister IL, Cringle SJ, Yu DY. Correlation of histologic and clinical images to determine the diagnostic value of fluorescein angiography for studying retinal capillary detail. Invest Ophthalmol Vis Sci. 2010;51:5864–9.
24. Spaide RF, Klancnik JM Jr, Cooney MJ. Retinal vascular layers in macular telangiectasia type 2 imaged by optical coherence tomographic angiography. JAMA Ophthalmol. 2015b;133:66–73.
25. Weinhaus RS, Burke JM, Delori FC, Snodderly DM. Comparison of fluorescein angiography with microvascular anatomy of macaque retinas. Exp Eye Res. 1995;61:1–16.
26. Magrath GN, Say EAT, Sioufi K, Ferenczy S, Samara WA, Shields CL. Variability in foveal avascular zone and capillary density using optical coherence tomography angiography machines in healthy eyes. Retina. 2017;37:2102–11.
27. Samara WA, Say EA, Khoo CT, Higgins TP, Magrath G, Ferenczy S, Shields CL. Correlation of foveal avascular zone size with foveal morphology in Normal eyes using optical coherence tomography angiography. Retina. 2015a;35:2188–95.
28. Iafe NA, Phasukkijwatana N, Chen X, Sarraf D. Retinal capillary density and foveal avascular zone area are age-dependent: quantitative analysis using optical coherence tomography angiography. Invest Ophthalmol Vis Sci. 2016;57:5780–7.
29. Sampson DM, Gong P, An D, Menghini M, Hansen A, Mackey DA, Sampson DD, Chen FK. Axial length variation impacts on superficial retinal vessel density and foveal avascular zone area measurements using optical coherence tomography angiography. Invest Ophthalmol Vis Sci. 2017;58:3065–72.
30. Takase N, Nozaki M, Kato A, Ozeki H, Yoshida M, Ogura Y. Enlargement of foveal avascular zone in diabetic eyes evaluated by en face optical coherence tomography angiography. Retina. 2015b;35:2377–83.
31. Balaratnasingam C, Inoue M, Ahn S, McCann J, Dhrami-Gavazi E, Yannuzzi LA, Freund KB. Visual acuity is correlated with the area of the foveal avascular zone in diabetic retinopathy and retinal vein occlusion. Ophthalmology. 2016;123:2352–67.
32. Schottenhamml J, Moult EM, Ploner S, Lee B, Novais EA, Cole E, Dang S, Lu CD, Husvogt L, Waheed NK. An automatic, intercapillary area based algorithm for quantifying diabetes related capillary dropout using OCT angiography. Retina. 2016;36:S93.
33. Nesper PL, Roberts PK, Onishi AC, Chai H, Liu L, Jampol LM, Fawzi AA. Quantifying microvascular abnormalities with increasing severity of diabetic retinopathy using optical coherence tomography angiography. Invest Ophthalmol Vis Sci. 2017a;58:BIO307–15.
34. Agemy SA, Scripsema NK, Shah CM, Chui T, Garcia PM, Lee JG, Gentile RC, Hsiao Y-S, Zhou Q, Ko T. Retinal vascular perfusion density mapping using optical coherence tomography angiography in normals and diabetic retinopathy patients. Retina. 2015a;35:2353–63.
35. Al-Sheikh M, Akil H, Pfau M, Sadda SR. Swept-source OCT angiography imaging of the foveal avascular zone and macular capillary network density in diabetic retinopathy. Invest Ophthalmol Vis Sci. 2016;57:3907–13.
36. Kim AY, Chu Z, Shahidzadeh A, Wang RK, Puliafito CA, Kashani AH. Quantifying microvascular density and morphology in diabetic retinopathy using spectral-domain optical coherence tomography angiography. Invest Ophthalmol Vis Sci. 2016a;57:OCT362–70.
37. Salz DA, Talisa E, Adhi M, Moult E, Choi W, Baumal CR, Witkin AJ, Duker JS, Fujimoto JG, Waheed NK. Select features of diabetic retinopathy on swept-source optical coherence tomographic angiography compared with fluorescein angiography and normal eyes. JAMA Ophthalmol. 2016;134:644–50.
38. Zahid S, Dolz-Marco R, Freund KB, Balaratnasingam C, Dansingani K, Gilani F, Mehta N, Young E, Klifto MR, Chae B. Fractal dimensional analysis of optical coherence tomography angiography in eyes with diabetic retinopathy. Invest Ophthalmol Vis Sci. 2016;57:4940–7.
39. Fayed AE, Abdelbaki AM, El Zawahry OM, Fawzi AA. Optical coherence tomography angiography reveals progressive worsening of retinal vascular geometry in diabetic retinopathy and improved geometry after panretinal photocoagulation. PLoS One. 2019;14:e0226629.
40. Arend O, Remky A, Evans D, Stuber R, Harris A. Contrast sensitivity loss is coupled with capillary dropout in patients with diabetes. Invest Ophthalmol Vis Sci. 1997;38:1819–24.
41. Arend O, Wolf S, Harris A, Reim M. The relationship of macular microcirculation to visual acuity in diabetic patients. Arch Ophthalmol. 1995;113:610–4.
42. Bresnick GH, De Venecia G, Myers FL, Harris JA, Davis MD. Retinal ischemia in diabetic retinopathy. Arch Ophthalmol. 1975;93:1300–10.
43. Onishi AC, Nesper PL, Roberts PK, Moharram GA, Chai H, Liu L, Jampol LM, Fawzi AA. Importance of considering the middle capillary plexus on OCT angiography in diabetic retinopathy. Invest Ophthalmol Vis Sci. 2018;59:2167–76.
44. Tyrberg M, Ponjavic V, Lovestam-Adrian M. Multifocal electroretinogram (mfERG) in patients with diabetes mellitus and an enlarged foveal avascular zone (FAZ). Doc Ophthalmol. 2008;117:185–9.
45. Unoki N, Nishijima K, Sakamoto A, Kita M, Watanabe D, Hangai M, Kimura T, Kawagoe N, Ohta M, Yoshimura N. Retinal sensitivity loss and structural disturbance in areas of capillary nonperfusion of eyes with diabetic retinopathy. Am J Ophthalmol. 2007;144:755–60.
46. Dmuchowska DA, Krasnicki P, Mariak Z. Can optical coherence tomography replace fluorescein angiography in detection of ischemic diabetic maculopathy? Graefes Arch Clin Exp Ophthalmol = Albrecht von Graefes Archiv fur klinische und experimentelle Ophthalmologie. 2014;252:731–8.

47. Abdelshafy M, Abdelshafy A. Correlations between optical coherence tomography angiography parameters and the visual acuity in patients with diabetic retinopathy. Clin Ophthalmol. 2020;14:1107–15.
48. Hsiao CC, Yang CM, Yang CH, Ho TC, Lai TT, Hsieh YT. Correlations between visual acuity and macular microvasculature quantified with optical coherence tomography angiography in diabetic macular oedema. Eye (Lond). 2020;34:544–52.
49. Moein HR, Novais EA, Rebhun CB, Cole ED, Louzada RN, Witkin AJ, Baumal CR, Duker JS, Waheed NK. Optical coherence tomography angiography to detect macular capillary ischemia in patients with inner retinal changes after resolved diabetic macular edema. Retina. 2018;38:2277–84.
50. Lavia C, Couturier A, Erginay A, Dupas B, Tadayoni R, Gaudric A. Reduced vessel density in the superficial and deep plexuses in diabetic retinopathy is associated with structural changes in corresponding retinal layers. PLoS One. 2019;14:e0219164.
51. DaCosta J, Bhatia D, Talks J. The use of optical coherence tomography angiography and optical coherence tomography to predict visual acuity in diabetic retinopathy. Eye (Lond). 2020;34:942–7.
52. Gill A, Cole ED, Novais EA, Louzada RN, de Carlo T, Duker JS, Waheed NK, Baumal CR, Witkin AJ. Visualization of changes in the foveal avascular zone in both observed and treated diabetic macular edema using optical coherence tomography angiography. Int J Retina Vitreous. 2017;3:19.
53. Freiberg FJ, Pfau M, Wons J, Wirth MA, Becker MD, Michels S. Optical coherence tomography angiography of the foveal avascular zone in diabetic retinopathy. Graefes Arch Clin Exp Ophthalmol. 2016;254:1051–8.
54. Spaide RF. Volume-rendered optical coherence tomography of diabetic retinopathy pilot study. Am J Ophthalmol. 2015;160:1200–10.
55. Pereira F, Godoy BR, Maia M, Regatieri CV. Microperimetry and OCT angiography evaluation of patients with ischemic diabetic macular edema treated with monthly intravitreal bevacizumab: a pilot study. Int J Retina Vitreous. 2019;5:24.
56. Tsai ASH, Gan ATL, Ting DSW, Wong CW, Teo KYC, Tan ACS, Lee SY, Wong TY, Tan GSW, Gemmy Cheung CM. Diabetic macular ischemia: correlation of retinal vasculature changes by optical coherence tomography angiography and functional deficit. Retina. 2020;40:2184–90.
57. Bhardwaj S, Tsui E, Zahid S, Young E, Mehta N, Agemy S, Garcia P, Rosen RB, Young JA. Value of fractal analysis of optical coherence tomography angiography in various stages of diabetic retinopathy. Retina. 2018;38:1816–23.
58. Carnevali A, Sacconi R, Corbelli E, Tomasso L, Querques L, Zerbini G, Scorcia V, Bandello F, Querques G. Optical coherence tomography angiography analysis of retinal vascular plexuses and choriocapillaris in patients with type 1 diabetes without diabetic retinopathy. Acta Diabetol. 2017;54:695–702.
59. Chen Q, Ma Q, Wu C, Tan F, Chen F, Wu Q, Zhou R, Zhuang X, Lu F, Qu J, Shen M. Macular vascular fractal dimension in the deep capillary layer as an early indicator of microvascular loss for retinopathy in type 2 diabetic patients. Invest Ophthalmol Vis Sci. 2017;58:3785–94.
60. Fawzi AA, Fayed AE, Linsenmeier RA, Gao J, Yu F. Improved macular capillary flow on optical coherence tomography angiography after Panretinal photocoagulation for proliferative diabetic retinopathy. Am J Ophthalmol. 2019;206:217–27.
61. Mitchell P, Bandello F, Schmidt-Erfurth U, Lang GE, Massin P, Schlingemann RO, Sutter F, Simader C, Burian G, Gerstner O, Weichselberger A, Group RS. The RESTORE study: ranibizumab monotherapy or combined with laser versus laser monotherapy for diabetic macular edema. Ophthalmology. 2011;118:615–25.
62. Usui Y, Westenskow PD, Kurihara T, Aguilar E, Sakimoto S, Paris LP, Wittgrove C, Feitelberg D, Friedlander MS, Moreno SK, Dorrell MI, Friedlander M. Neurovascular crosstalk between interneurons and capillaries is required for vision. J Clin Invest. 2015;125:2335–46.
63. Chung EJ, Roh MI, Kwon OW, Koh HJ. Effects of macular ischemia on the outcome of intravitreal bevacizumab therapy for diabetic macular edema. Retina. 2008;28:957–63.
64. Lee DH, Kim JT, Jung DW, Joe SG, Yoon YH. The relationship between foveal ischemia and spectral-domain optical coherence tomography findings in ischemic diabetic macular edema. Invest Ophthalmol Vis Sci. 2013;54:1080–5.
65. Lee H, Lee M, Chung H, Kim HC. Quantification of retinal vessel tortuosity in diabetic retinopathy using optical coherence tomography angiography. Retina. 2018;38:976–85.
66. Bonini-Filho M, Costa RA, Calucci D, Jorge R, Melo LAS, Scott IU. Intravitreal bevacizumab for diabetic macular edema associated with severe capillary loss: one-year results of a pilot study. Am J Ophthalmol. 2009;147:1022–1030.e5.
67. Chatziralli I, Touhami S, Cicinelli MV, Agapitou C, Dimitriou E, Theodossiadis G, Theodossiadis P. Disentangling the association between retinal non-perfusion and anti-VEGF agents in diabetic retinopathy. Eye. 2021;36:692.
68. Campochiaro PA, Wykoff CC, Shapiro H, Rubio RG, Ehrlich JS. Neutralization of vascular endothelial growth factor slows progression of retinal nonperfusion in patients with diabetic macular edema. Ophthalmology. 2014;121:1783–9.
69. Levin A, Rusu I, Orlin A, Gupta M, Coombs P, D'Amico D, Kiss S. Retinal reperfusion in diabetic retinopathy following treatment with anti-VEGF intravitreal injections. Clin Ophthalmol. 2017;11:193–200.
70. Manousaridis K, Talks J. Macular ischaemia: a contraindication for anti-VEGF treatment in retinal vascular disease? Br J Ophthalmol. 2012a;96:179–84.
71. Nicholson L, Ramu J, Triantafyllopoulou I, Patrao NV, Comyn O, Hykin P, Sivaprasad S. Diagnostic accuracy of disorganization of the retinal inner layers in detecting macular capillary non-perfusion in diabetic retinopathy. Clin Experiment Ophthalmol. 2015;43:735–41.
72. Goel N, Kumar V, Ghosh B. Ischemic maculopathy following intravitreal bevacizumab for refractory diabetic macular edema. Int Ophthalmol. 2011;31:39–42.
73. Chen E, Hsu J, Park CH. Acute visual acuity loss following intravitreal bevacizumab for diabetic macular edema. Ophthalmic Surg Lasers Imaging Retina. 2009;40:68–70.
74. Elnahry AG, Elnahry GA. Optical Coherence Tomography Angiography of Macular Perfusion Changes after Anti-VEGF Therapy for Diabetic Macular Edema: A Systematic Review. J Diabetes Res. 2021;2021:6634637.
75. Karst SG, Deak GG, Gerendas BS, Waldstein SM, Lammer J, Simader C, Guerin T, Schmidt-Erfurth UM. Association of Changes in macular perfusion with Ranibizumab treatment for diabetic macular edema. JAMA Ophthalmol. 2018;136:315.
76. Elnahry AG, Abdel-Kader AA, Raafat KA, Elrakhawy K. Evaluation of changes in macular perfusion detected by optical coherence tomography angiography following 3 intravitreal monthly bevacizumab injections for diabetic macular edema in the IMPACT study. J Ophthalmol. 2020;2020:5814165. PMID: 32411431; PMCID: PMC7201518. https://doi.org/10.1155/2020/5814165.
77. Golshani C, Conti TF, Conti FF, et al. Diabetic macular edema treated with intravitreal Aflibercept injection after treatment with other anti-VEGF agents (SWAP-TWO study)—12-month analysis. J Vitreo Retinal Dis. 2020;4(5):364–71. https://doi.org/10.1177/2474126420916074.
78. Statler B, Conti TF, Conti FF, Silva FQ, Rachitskaya A, Yuan A, Schachat A, Kaiser PK, Singh RP, Babiuch A. Twenty-four-month OCTA assessment in diabetic patients undergoing fixed-interval intravitreal Aflibercept therapy. Ophthalmic Surg Lasers Imaging Retina. 2020;51(8):448–55. PMID: 32818277. https://doi.org/10.3928/23258160-20200804-05.

Dexamethasone Implant in Diabetic Macular Edema

11

Atul Arora, Nikita Gupta, and Vishali Gupta

11.1 Introduction

Diabetic macular edema (DME) is the most common cause of moderate vision loss in patients with diabetes mellitus. The prevalence of DME in various population-based studies has been reported to be between 1.4% and 12.8% and is more common in type 2 diabetics [1]. DME can occur at any stage of retinopathy, i.e., from early non-proliferative diabetic retinopathy (NPDR) to proliferative diabetic retinopathy (PDR). Clinically DME is seen as presence of hard exudates with retinal thickening characterized by the presence of intraretinal or subretinal fluid involving the macula. These changes result from breakdown of blood–retinal barrier and alteration of vascular permeability mediated by VEGF and inflammatory cytokines. Hyperglycemia, hypertension, dyslipidemia, duration of diabetes, HbA1c levels, and diabetic nephropathy are known risk factors for development of DME. Besides these, novel risk factors being evaluated in the pathophysiology of DME are role of inflammation, genetics, and oxidative stress. The etiology of DME is multifactorial, and thus the treatment too needs to be customized depending upon the possible etiology. Since inflammation may be playing a major role in causation of DME in a subset of patients, it is important to identify these patients so that intravitreal steroids can be initiated at the earliest to avoid visual loss due to long-standing edema as well as to avoid financial burden due to multiple anti-VEGF injections. In the following sections, we shall discuss the possible role of inflammation in DME as well as possible role of dexamethasone implant in the management of DME.

A. Arora · N. Gupta · V. Gupta (✉)
Department of Ophthalmology, Postgraduate Institute of Medical Education and Research (PGIMER), Advanced Eye Centre, Chandigarh, India
e-mail: gupta.vishali@pgimer.edu.in

11.2 Role of Inflammation in DME

Inflammation plays an important role in the pathogenesis of DME. Hyperglycemia leads to increased expression of inflammatory cytokines like interleukin-1β (IL-1β), nuclear factor-κB (NF-κB), vascular endothelial growth factor (VEGF), tumor necrosis factor-α (TNF-α), transforming growth factor-beta, and intracellular adhesion molecule-1 (ICAM-1) in retinal pericytes and Muller cells [2]. The molecular pathways activated in diabetic retinopathy have been shown in Fig. 11.1. The pericytes enveloping the retinal endothelial cells play a vital role in maintaining the inner blood–retinal barrier. The tight junctions or the zonula occludens form the main constituent of blood–retinal barrier allowing only selective transport of water and solutes across the vascular endothelium. Chronic hyperglycemia causes loss of pericytes and retinal endothelial cell tight junctions that causes release of VEGF and other inflammatory mediators including IL-1, IL-6, IL-8, TNF-α, MMP, Kallikrin-kinin, and MCP-1. These inflammatory mediators along with VEGF cause further weakening of cell tight junctions. VEGF has been shown to cause phosphorylation of tight junction protein occludin which correlates with increased vascular permeability. Other growth factors released in response to hyperglycemia also cause change in morphology of tight junction causing its disassembly and increased paracellular permeability [3]. Similarly, vascular permeability has been shown to increase by TNF-α via protein kinase C zeta [4]. VEGF along with NF-κB in response to oxidative stress causes upregulation of ICAM-1 on retinal endothelial cells, which mediates leukocyte adhesion to the vascular endothelium. These molecular changes during inflammation cause microvascular damage by release of cytokines and superoxide radicals. Mechanical occlusion of capillaries secondary to leucostasis results in ischemia of retinal tissue supplied by them. Leucostasis has been shown to be associated with diabetic retinopathy in studies on animal models [5] with deletion of mediators responsible for WBC adherence to vascular endothelium protecting against diabetes induced capillary

S. Saxena et al. (eds.), *Diabetic Macular Edema*, https://doi.org/10.1007/978-981-19-7307-9_11

Fig. 11.1 The molecular pathways activated in diabetic retinopathy

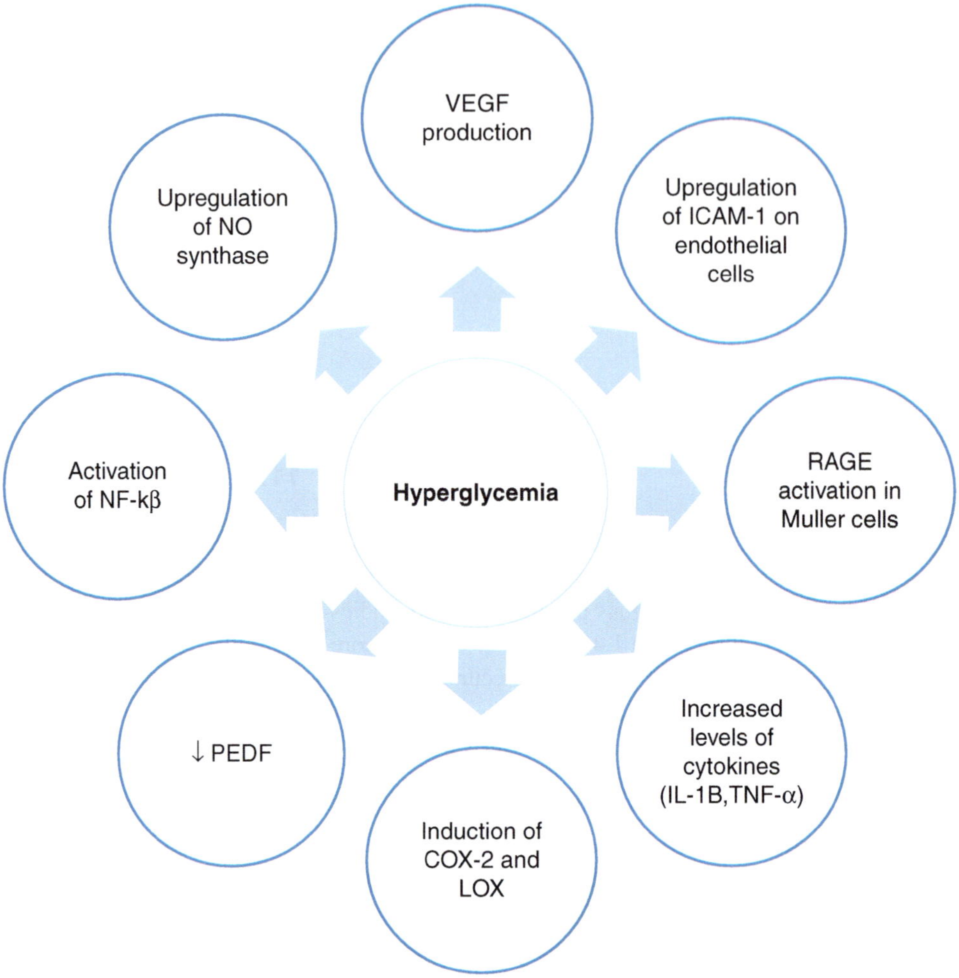

damage [6]. All these events lead to in breakdown of blood–retinal barrier and extravasation of fluid, proteins, and lipids resulting in DME (Fig. 11.2).

Besides these, the breakdown of outer blood–retinal barrier causing serous retinal detachment secondary to RPE dysfunction is also seen in one third of DME patients [7]. This occurs secondary to release of proinflammatory mediators, mostly cytokines, NF-κB activation, VEGF-mediated increased vascular permeability, and MMP activation [8, 9].

Studies have shown that retinal macroglia (Muller cells and astrocytes) undergo changes in diabetic retinopathy with increased population of Muller cells leading to greater expression of VEGF molecule [10, 11]. Not just the macroglia, the microglial cells are also one of the prime cells which sense the inflammatory environment in diabetes and get activated in response to the inflammatory cytokines that leak from retinal vasculature [12]. These activated microglial cells in turn lead to the production of more proinflammatory and neurotoxic cytokines like TNF-α, IL-1β, and nitric oxide along with increased production of vascular endothelial growth factor. These substances on their release may propagate the inflammatory response within the retina leading to a vicious cycle of inflammation, neuronal cell death, and microvascular damage [10].

Intravitreal corticosteroids ameliorate the above-mentioned inflammatory cascade and therefore find role in management of DME.

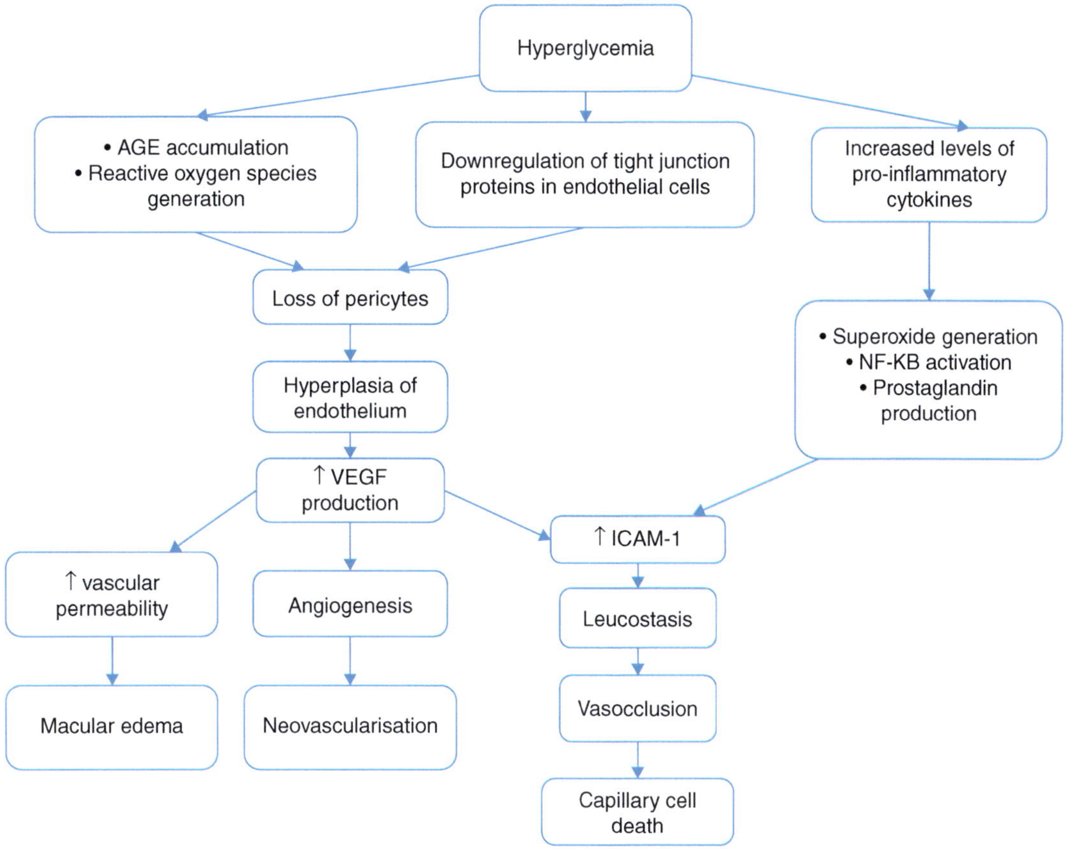

Fig. 11.2 Flowchart depicting the activation of inflammatory cascade and its role in pathophysiology of diabetic macular edema

11.3 Cataract Surgery and DME

Cataract surgery is a known risk factor for progression of diabetic retinopathy with a 5–13% risk of development of treatment requiring DME post surgery in diabetic patients [13]. This incidence is higher in patients with preexisting macular edema at the time of cataract surgery. The highest risk has been shown to be between 3 and 6 months after surgery [13]. It has been postulated that cataract surgery increases the levels of inflammatory mediators like prostaglandin, thromboxane A2, nitric oxide, and VEGF secondary to the tissue manipulation during surgery. Corticosteroids can help counteract this inflammation by inhibiting COX-2-mediated production of prostaglandins and downregulating other inflammatory mediators like TNF-α, IFN-γ, IL-6, chemokines (CXCL-10, CCL5), and metalloproteinases (MMP-1, MMP-2, MMP-3, MMP-9) [13–15]. A recent retrospective study compared results of combining phacoemulsification with dexamethasone implant in patients with DME with cataract with phacoemulsification alone. The anatomical and functional results at 3 months favored administration of dexamethasone implant at the end of phacoemulsification proving it to be an effective and safe treatment option in patients with visually significant cataract along with DME [16, 17].

11.4 Steroids as Therapeutic Option in DME

Intravitreal anti-VEGF agents are the current gold standard for treating center involving DME. However, not all patients respond to anti-VEGF. Results from two major randomized trials RISE and RIDE failed to show ≥15 letter gain in over 50% patients who received monthly 0.5 mg intravitreal ranibizumab for a period of 2 years [18]. Besides, there is a subset of patients referred as non-responder or recalcitrant DME, who show persistence of macular edema even after three doses of intravitreal anti-VEGF. Up to 40% of patients being treated with anti-VEGF may have recalcitrant

DME. Intravitreal corticosteroids provide a useful treatment alternative for such patients [19]. In some patients, anti-VEGF therapy maybe contraindicated due to recent history of vascular events like stroke and myocardial infarction. The need for frequent hospital visits for monthly VEGF injections too adds to the costs involved in the monthly treatment but also causes great inconvenience to the caregivers.

Intravitreal corticosteroids form an important armamentarium for the treatment of DME. In addition to suppressing VEGF levels, they work by counteracting the inflammatory mediators involved in the pathogenesis of DME as elucidated above. Common concerns with use of intravitreal steroids are cataract formation and increase of intraocular pressure. Available corticosteroids for intravitreal use include triamcinolone acetonide (TA), fluocinolone acetonide, and dexamethasone with variable glucocorticoid receptor binding properties and different potencies. It is interesting to note that although systemic half-life of these three potent steroids may vary, all three are rapidly eliminated from the vitreous in 2–3 h (based on observation in monkeys and rabbits) [15]. This will require repeated administration of these drugs with potential adverse effects. For this reason, sustained drug delivery devices in the form of drug suspensions and implants have been developed in order to reduce treatment burden. Upon intravitreal injection or delivery of these implants, the glucocorticosteroid slowly diffuses along a gradient from the depot to posterior pole with minimal systemic exposure. The drug gets eliminated either via diffusion through the retina, diffusion anteriorly into the anterior chamber, and elimination via aqueous outflow pathways.

11.5 Dexamethasone Implant: Introduction

Dexamethasone is a more potent anti-inflammatory agent compared to TA with fewer side effects. The recently developed sustained release dexamethasone implant (Ozurdex®; Allergan, Inc., Irvine, CA, United States) provides long-acting anti-inflammatory action, thereby reducing the frequency of injections needed. It is a sustained release biodegradable copolymer which degrades into lactic acid and glycolic acid, which are subsequently metabolized to carbon dioxide and water. The implant contains 0.7 mg of dexamethasone and provides long-lasting effect up to 6 months. Ozurdex was FDA approved in September 2014 for the treatment of DME after the results of MEAD study which showed long-term results favoring dexamethasone in DME [20]. The drug delivery system is a single-use device which uses a 22 G needle to insert the implant intravitreally, leaving a self-sealing sutureless wound.

11.6 Role of Dexamethasone Implant in Current Clinical Practice: An Evidence-Based Approach

As per the EURETINA guidelines, steroids maybe considered as second-line treatment option in patients refractory to anti-VEGF injections (after 3–6 injections) or as primary treatment option in those who have a contraindication to anti VEGF agents (history of major cardiovascular event in recent past or pregnant females) or are not willing to come for monthly injections [21].

PLACID trial was the first randomized multicentric trial evaluating Ozurdex® in DME [22]. It randomized patients into two arms: Ozurdex plus laser at 1 month vs. laser monotherapy alone. The proportion of patients with 10 or more letter gain in visual acuity was significantly higher in the Ozurdex plus laser arm at 9 months. Also, the combination of Ozurdex implant with laser was shown to improve central retinal thickness and in patients with diffuse macular edema compared to laser alone. Raised intraocular pressure (IOP) was seen in 16% patients, which was managed by IOP lowering medications. Around 20% had cataract-related adverse events in phakic eyes.

The major landmark trials evaluating the efficacy and safety of Ozurdex in DME that ultimately led to FDA approval of Ozurdex were the MEAD trials [20]. MEAD were two large, randomized, multicentric, phase 3 clinical trials with identical protocols. A total of 1048 patients with center-involving DME were randomized into three arms (Ozurdex 0.7 mg, 0.35 mg, and sham) and followed for a 3-year period. Retreatment criteria were predefined, and injections were to be repeated after a minimum duration of 6 months. The average number of injections required over 3 years were 4.1, 4.4, and 3.3 with DEX implant 0.7 mg, DEX implant 0.35 mg, and sham, respectively. At the end of study period, proportion of patients who gained ≥15-letter improvement in BCVA from baseline were significantly greater with DEX implant 0.7 mg (22.2%) and DEX implant 0.35 mg (18.4%) compared to sham (12.0%; $P \leq 0.018$). Average reduction in central retinal thickness from baseline was also greater with DEX implant 0.7 mg (−111.6 μm) and DEX implant 0.35 mg (−107.9 μm) than sham (−41.9 μm; $P < 0.001$). Cataract and raised IOP were important side effects. Cataract-related adverse events were as high as 65% in phakic eyes who received the DEX implant versus only 20% in the sham group. Around 40% patients in the Ozurdex groups required IOP-lowering medications while this percentage was low in the sham group (10%).

Following FDA approval and commercial availability of DEX implant, a number of studies evaluating its efficacy and safety profile have been published. Table 11.1 summarizes

Table 11.1 Brief summary of important studies on the role of intravitreal dexamethasone implant in diabetic macular edema

Study	Study design	Intervention in DME eyes	Follow-up	Results
PLACID Study Group Callanan et al. [22]	Multicentric randomized phase 2	Ozurdex plus laser vs. laser	9 months	Statistically significant greater number of patients in Ozurdex with laser group had ≥10 letter gain in vision Combined group had greater CRT reduction
MEAD Study Group Boyer et al. [20]	Multicentric randomized phase 3	Ozurdex 0.7 mg, 0.35 mg vs. sham	3 years	Statistically significant improvement in BCVA and greater CMT reduction with Dex implant compared to sham
MOZART Guigou et al. [23]	Multicentric retrospective	Ozurdex 0.7 mg	6 months	Decrease in mean CMT: 135 μm at 6 months Increase in BCVA from baseline: 7.6 l at 6 months
CHAMPLAIN Boyer et al. [24]	Multicentric prospective open label phase 2	Single Ozurdex implant in refractory DME in vitrectomised eyes	6 months	Significant improvement in BCVA at month 2 and 6 (3 letters) from baseline Significant decrease in CMT at months 2 and 6 after injection
BEVORDEX Study Group Gillies et al. [25]	Multicenter, prospective, randomized, phase 2 study	Intravitreal bevacizumab monthly vs. Dex implant every 4 monthly	12 months	Greater mean CMT reduction in the DEX group than in bevacizumab (187 μm vs. 122 μm) No difference in percentage of patients with ≥10-letter improvement in BCVA
RELDEX Study Malcles et al. [26]	Bicentric retrospective study	Ozurdex 0.7 mg	3 years	Significantly decreased CMT and improved BCVA at 3 years from baseline Proportion of eyes achieving ≥15-letter improvement from baseline was 25.4% at month 36 Mean number of injections over 3-year follow-up: 3.6
ARTES Study Group Rosenblatt et al. [27]	Multicenter, retrospective, cohort study	Ozurdex 0.7 mg	1.7 years	Statistically significant CMT reduction was obtained throughout the first 6 months though this effect diminished after month 3. Mean change in CMT: −174 μm Significant improvement in BCVA during the first 6 months Treatment naïve patients had greater visual acuity improvement than previously treated patients

CMT central macular thickness, *CRT* central retinal thickness, *BCVA* best corrected visual acuity

important studies on the role of intravitreal dexamethasone implant in diabetic macular edema.

Use of DEX implant in special conditions like vitrectomized eyes, DME refractory to treatment by anti-VEGF agents too has been evaluated.

The MOZART (Multicenter Ozurdex® assessment for DME) study was a small retrospective study evaluating the efficacy and safety of 0.7 mg DEX implant in DME patients with visual impairment. The study established that dexamethasone gives favorable anatomical and functional outcomes with single injection. The side effects are rare and manageable in accordance with previous studies. The authors concluded that favorable anatomical and functional outcomes were obtained with an acceptable and manageable side effect profile as previously published studies [23].

CHROME study was a retrospective real-world study which included patients with retinal diseases with macular edema including DME, retinal vascular occlusion, and uveitis. For DME cohort, it showed that the reduction in CRT was not reflected in significant visual acuity improvement. The visual acuity gains were more pronounced in pseudophakic eyes compared to phakic eyes. The mean retreatment interval was 2.3–4.9 months being longest in DME eyes, i.e., 5.8 ± 0.5 months [28].

The CHAMPLAIN study evaluated the safety and efficacy of DEX implant in vitrectomized eyes. The faster clearance of anti-VEGF agents in vitrectomized eyes leading to suboptimal concentrations and lower efficacy prompted to evaluate the need for a sustained release implant in these eyes. This was a prospective 6 month, open label, phase 2 clinical study where a single Ozurdex implant was administered to treatment refractory diabetic eyes who had undergone pars plana vitrectomy in the past. A six-letter gain in BCVA was observed at 8 weeks while a gain of three letters was maintained at week 26. About 30% patients had gained 10 letters in BCVA at 2 months after the injection. Around 16% patients reported cataract progression, and a similar number had increase in IOP; however, no patient required filtration surgery.

The very recent ARTES study group extensively evaluated efficacy of dexamethasone in real-life setting in DME by dividing study population based on previous treatment history, duration of diabetes, and measure of control of diabetes. It was a retrospective study which compared results between treatment naïve group and previously treated group, early DME (<6 months of documentation of DME) and late DME, well-controlled diabetes (HbA1c lower than 8 mg%) versus uncontrolled diabetes. BCVA was found to be better in treatment naive eyes at baseline and remained so at the end of study period; however, there was no significant difference. Treatment outcomes were evaluated in early and late DME, and it was concluded that visual acuity outcomes were worse in late DME group, stressing the fact that duration of diabetes is an important prognostic marker. Patients with uncontrolled diabetes had poorer baseline visual acuity and higher risk of visual loss, which may be related to higher prevalence of complications like vitreous hemorrhage and recurrent DME with poor glycemic control. Although the official product label in Europe recommends retreatment after a minimal interval of 6 months, this collaborative study concluded that shorter treatment intervals would be more practical as peak effect was seen at 3 months after which it attenuated [27]. The treatment interval between repeat dexamethasone injections is still debatable and depends heavily on treatment response and needs to be decided on an individual basis.

Several real-life studies have shown the efficacy of DEX implant in previously treated patients of DME refractory to other treatment although visual improvement was more pronounced in naïve eyes [26, 29, 30].

Diabetic Retinopathy Clinical Research Network (DRCR.net) protocol U was a phase 2 randomized clinical trial which evaluated utility of adding intravitreal dexamethasone implant in persistent DME after three monthly intravitreal ranibizumab injections [31]. A total of 116 patients were randomized to receive either combination therapy with intravitreal ranibizumab and dexamethasone implant (to be given within 0–8 days of ranibizumab) or intravitreal ranibizumab alone. The patients were followed up monthly and received intravitreal ranibizumab based on a strict retreatment protocol. Although there was no difference in visual acuity outcomes at 24 weeks, combination therapy with dexamethasone implant did show a significant reduction in central foveal thickness in eyes with persistent DME despite anti-VEGF agents.

A meta-analysis on efficacy and safety of single-dose dexamethasone implantation for patients with persistent diabetic macular edema refractory to anti-VEGF therapy showed switching to a dexamethasone implant could achieve significant anatomical and functional improvement among patients with refractory DME [32].

A head-to-head comparison between an anti-VEGF agent and corticosteroid was done in the phase 2 prospective clinical trial BEVORDEX. A total of 88 eyes with center involving DME were randomized to receive intravitreal bevacizumab monthly and dexamethasone implant every 4 monthly on a pro re nata basis. At the end of 1 year, the functional outcomes were similar in both the groups; however, the reduction in CRT was significantly higher in dexamethasone group with reduced number of injections (2.7 vs. 8.6) [25].

In clinical trial setting, therapeutic effect of Ozurdex was propagated to last for at least 6 months. But in real-life practice, it has been seen that the effect may wean off early and thus more frequent dosing in prn may be required in some patients.

Systematic review on long-term efficacy and safety profile of multiple injections of intravitreal dexamethasone implant to manage diabetic macular edema by Bukolo et al. [33] provides interesting information. In 21 peer-reviewed publications about 1/3 of the eyes were retreated before 6 months from first injection of DEX implant (mean retreatment average time: 5.3 ± 0.9 months). This reinforces the need for shorter treatment intervals based on *prn*. The study found overall good tolerance of long-term DEX implant.

Recently there have been discussions among treating physicians to form consensus about uniform guidelines for use of DEX implant given varied opinions among experts. In a consensus congregation by a group of Spanish experts on the use of DEX implant by Delphi approach, the panelists agreed that DEX implants were preferred as first-line therapy for DME in specific group of patients (pseudophakic, poor-adherents, vitrectomized, candidates for cataract surgery, and with a history of cardiovascular events). Additionally, DEX implants were recommended in patients who inadequately respond to anti-VEGF therapy, after a maximum of three injections [34].

11.7 Dexamethasone Implant and Imaging Biomarkers of DME

Recently, there has been interest in identifying imaging biomarkers of DME and correlate these with response to intravitreal therapy. Optical coherence tomography (OCT) biomarkers like subfoveal serous retinal detachment (SSRD), hyper-reflective foci (HRF), hard exudates, etc. are shown to indicate possible inflammatory pathophysiology of DME and respond better with intravitreal corticosteroids.

11.7.1 Subretinal Fluid (SRF)/Subfoveal Serous Retinal Detachment (SSRD)

DME eyes with SRF have been shown to respond significantly with dexamethasone implants (Fig. 11.3) in various studies [35, 36]. The efficacy of steroids in eyes with serous retinal detachment on OCT along with DME has also been shown in a prospective case series comparing intravitreal ranibizumab and intravitreal triamcinolone acetonide. Superior visual acuity and greater CRT reduction was seen at 24 weeks with intravitreal steroid injection [37]. In another study by Vujosevic et al. [38], subfoveal neuroretinal detachment resolved in 85.7% dexamethasone-treated eyes ($p = 0.014$) and in 50% ranibizumab-treated eyes ($p = 0.025$). Mean IFAF area decreased in both groups ($p < 0.0001$, for both). A significantly higher decrease in CMT was observed in dexamethasone- versus ranibizumab-treated eyes ($p = 0.032$).

A prospective study correlating aqueous inflammatory cytokine levels with different morphological OCT patterns in DME showed that IL-6 levels were raised in patients with serous retinal detachment [39]. This could provide possible explanation for better results with use of Ozurdex as an anti-inflammatory agent in these patients.

11.7.2 Hyperreflective Foci (HRF)

Recently, hyperreflective foci (HRF) in the retina have been considered active inflammatory cells, especially microglia and macrophages, when examined with optical coherence tomography (OCT) (Fig. 11.4), indicating inflammation also plays an important role in the pathogenesis of DME [40].

Corticosteroid implants have been shown to have better outcomes compared with anti-VEGF agents in subjects with DME in the presence of HRF [41, 42].

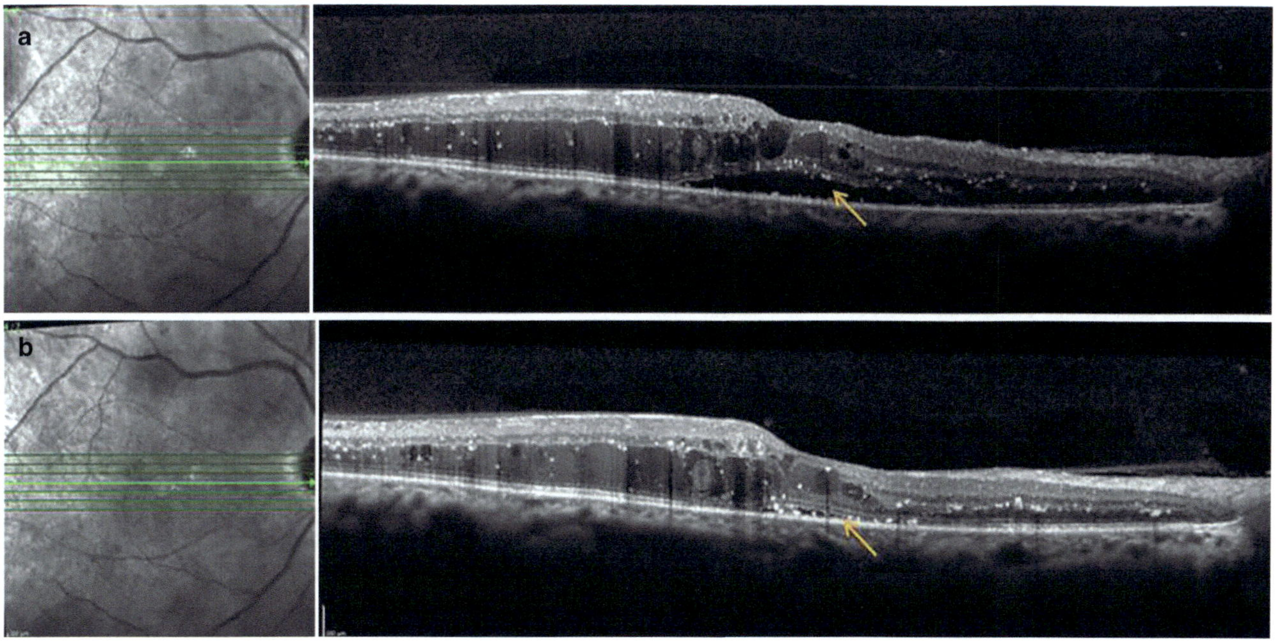

Fig. 11.3 Spectral domain optical coherence tomography (Heidelberg Engineering GmbH, Spectralis®) line scan passing through the foveal center showing subfoveal serous retinal detachment (SSRD) in a patient with diabetic macular edema (**a**). Marked resolution of SSRD was observed 3 weeks (**b**) following treatment with intravitreal dexamethasone implant. (Ozurdex®; Allergan, Inc., Irvine, CA, United States)

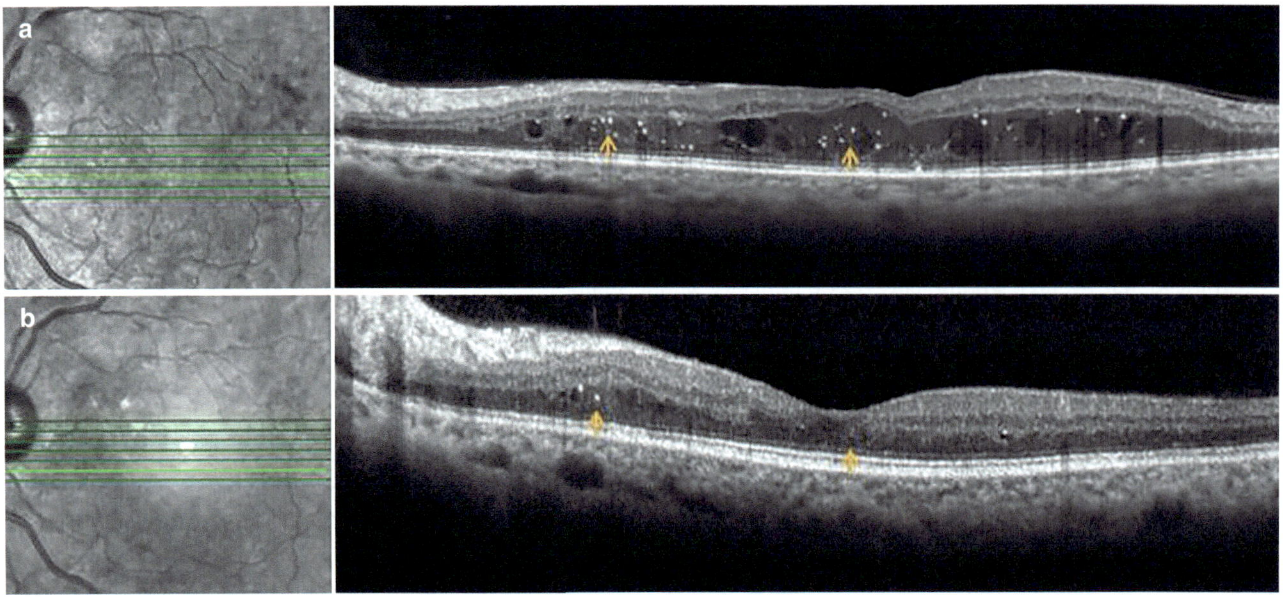

Fig. 11.4 Spectral domain optical coherence tomography (Heidelberg Engineering GmbH, Spectralis®) line scan showing hyper-reflective foci (HRF) in a patient with diabetic macular edema (**a**). The HRF show marked resolution (**b**) following treatment with intravitreal dexamethasone implant. (Ozurdex®; Allergan, Inc., Irvine, CA, United States)

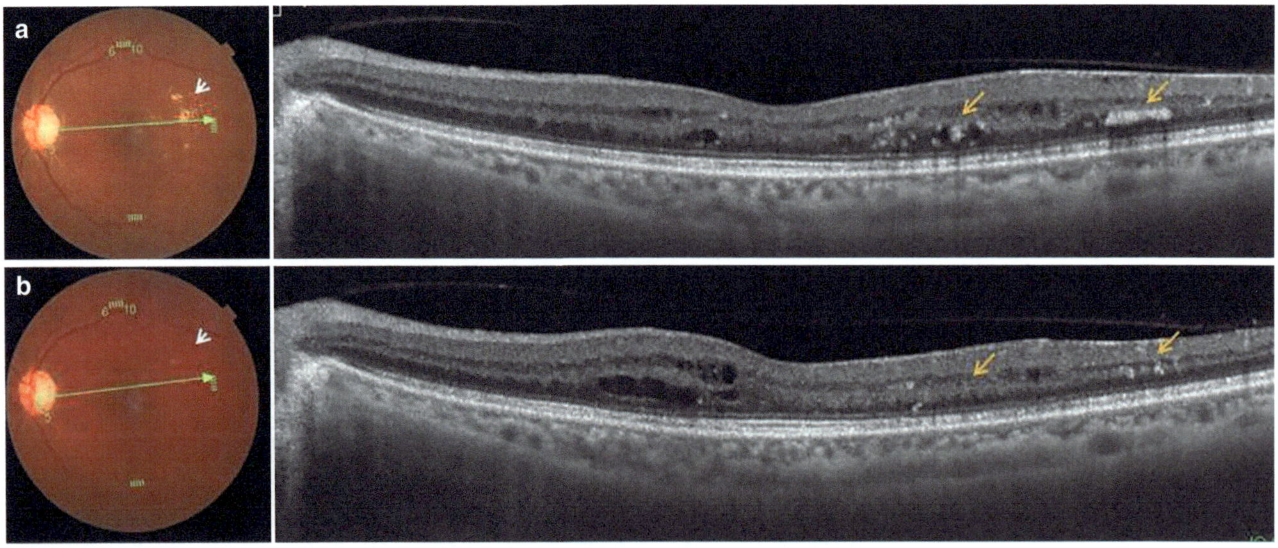

Fig. 11.5 Swept-source optical coherence tomography (DRI SS-OCT; Topcon) line scan passing through the foveal center in a patient with diabetic macular edema (**a**). Hard exudates can be seen temporal to the foveal center (white arrow head). Corresponding OCT B scan shows hyperreflective spots with back-shadowing present in the outer retinal layers. Marked resolution of hard exudates is observed (**b**) 6 weeks after intravitreal dexamethasone implant. (Ozurdex®; Allergan, Inc., Irvine, CA, United States)

11.7.3 Hard Exudates

Extravasation of lipids and lipoproteins due to breach of blood–retinal barrier results in the development of hard exudates in DME eyes. On OCT, these appear as hyperreflective spots which are larger than 30 μm, associated with back-shadowing (Fig. 11.5), present in the outer retinal layers, having reflectivity similar to RPE–Bruch's complex [43].

Intravitreal dexamethasone implant has been shown more effective in reducing hard exudates in patients with DME compared with anti-VEGF agents, especially when the exudates are subfoveal [44].

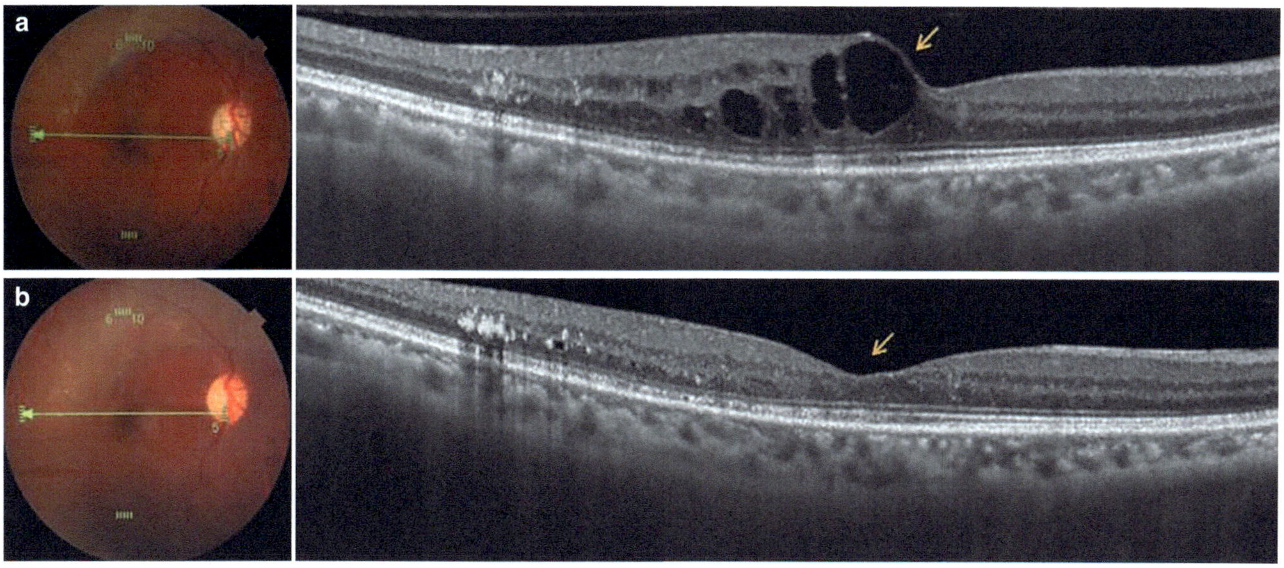

Fig. 11.6 Swept-source optical coherence tomography (DRI SS-OCT; Topcon) line scan passing through the foveal center in a patient with diabetic macular edema showing cystoid spaces 6 weeks following cataract surgery (**a**). Resolution of cystoid spaces can be observed following treatment with intravitreal dexamethasone implant (**b**). (Ozurdex®; Allergan, Inc., Irvine, CA, United States)

11.7.4 Disorganization of Retinal Inner Layers (DRIL)

Disorganization of retinal inner layers (DRIL) essentially describes the inability to delineate the inner retinal layer boundaries within the central retina [45]. DRIL has been associated with poor visual acuity outcomes after treatment in DME eyes [46] and has also been shown to be associated with increasing severity of diabetic retinopathy [47]. In a multicentric, retrospective series by Zur et al., DEX implant could ameliorate DRIL in 75% of eyes [48] (Fig. 11.6).

11.8 Contraindications of DEX Implant

Besides the usual conditions where intravitreal injections are contraindicated, the prescription manual for Ozurdex implant contradicts its use in glaucoma patients with a cup-to-disk ratio > 0.8, patients with a torn or ruptured posterior lens capsule and patients with known hypersensitivity to any component of the implant. Patients with history of viral or fungal infection should also be excluded before injecting steroid in the vitreous cavity in order to avoid a reactivation of infection.

11.9 Summary

Anti-VEGF agents remain gold standard and are the first-line treatment of diabetic macular edema. DEX implant has been shown to provide a favorable anatomical and functional outcome in DME randomized-controlled studies but has a relatively higher ocular side effect profile such as increased risk of cataract formation and raised intraocular pressure when compared to the gold standard anti-VEGF agents. Thus, DEX implant becomes the second-line treatment option in patients with DME. However, it can be preferred as the first-line treatment in where anti-VEGF agents are contra-indicated, e.g., pregnancy, in patients with recent history of a major cardiovascular or cerebrovascular event. It can also be considered as first-line agent in vitrectomized and pseudophakic eyes. DEX implant can also be useful in patients with refractory/recalcitrant macular edema. The ease of injection, similar cost as compared to other anti-VEGF injections, longer periods of remission, and the need for decreased number of injections resulting in decreasing risk of injection-related side effects and reducing number of hospital visits are potential advantages of DEX implants over anti-VEGF agents.

The choice of DME therapy must be individualized for each patient and broad therapeutic access for patients is critical to maximize outcomes.

Disclosures Any of the authors do not have any conflict of interest.

Funding Source None.

References

1. Lee R, Wong TY, Sabanayagam C. Epidemiology of diabetic retinopathy, diabetic macular edema and related vision loss. Eye Vis. 2015;2:17.
2. Kowluru RA, Zhong Q, Kanwar M. Metabolic memory and diabetic retinopathy: role of inflammatory mediators in retinal pericytes. Exp Eye Res. 2010;90(5):617–23.
3. Antonetti DA, Lieth E, Barber AJ, Gardner TW. Molecular mechanisms of vascular permeability in diabetic retinopathy. Semin Ophthalmol. 1999;14:240–8.
4. Aveleira CA, Lin C-M, Abcouwer SF, Ambrósio AF, Antonetti DA. TNF-α signals through PKCζ/NF-κB to alter the tight junction complex and increase retinal endothelial cell permeability. Diabetes. 2010;59(11):2872–82.
5. Kim SY, Johnson MA, McLeod DS, Alexander T, Hansen BC, Lutty GA. Neutrophils are associated with capillary closure in spontaneously diabetic monkey retinas. Diabetes. 2005;54(5):1534–42.
6. Joussen AM, Poulaki V, Le ML, Koizumi K, Esser C, Janicki H, et al. A central role for inflammation in the pathogenesis of diabetic retinopathy. FASEB J. 2004;18(12):1450–2.
7. Shereef H, Comyn O, Sivaprasad S, Hykin P, Cheung G, Narendran N, et al. Differences in the topographic profiles of retinal thickening in eyes with and without serous macular detachment associated with diabetic macular oedema. Br J Ophthalmol. 2014;98(2):182–7.
8. Daruich A, Matet A, Moulin A, Kowalczuk L, Nicolas M, Sellam A, et al. Mechanisms of macular edema: beyond the surface. Prog Retin Eye Res. 2018;63:20–68.
9. Ţălu Ş, Nicoara SD. Malfunction of outer retinal barrier and choroid in the occurrence and progression of diabetic macular edema. World J Diabetes. 2021;12(4):437–52.
10. Zeng H, Green WR, Tso MOM. Microglial activation in human diabetic retinopathy. Arch Ophthalmol. 2008;126(2):227–32.
11. Rungger-Brändle E, Dosso AA, Leuenberger PM. Glial reactivity, an early feature of diabetic retinopathy. Invest Ophthalmol Vis Sci. 2000;41(7):1971–80.
12. Krady JK, Basu A, Allen CM, Xu Y, LaNoue KF, Gardner TW, et al. Minocycline reduces proinflammatory cytokine expression, microglial activation, and caspase-3 activation in a rodent model of diabetic retinopathy. Diabetes. 2005;54(5):1559–65.
13. Denniston AK, Chakravarthy U, Zhu H, Lee AY, Crabb DP, Tufail A, et al. The UK diabetic retinopathy electronic medical record (UK DR EMR) users group, report 2: real-world data for the impact of cataract surgery on diabetic macular oedema. Br J Ophthalmol. 2017;101(12):1673–8.
14. Masferrer JL, Kulkarni PS. Cyclooxygenase-2 inhibitors: a new approach to the therapy of ocular inflammation. Surv Ophthalmol. 1997;41(Suppl 2):S35–40.
15. Shah TJ, Conway MD, Peyman GA. Intracameral dexamethasone injection in the treatment of cataract surgery induced inflammation: design, development, and place in therapy. Clin Ophthalmol Auckl NZ. 2018;12:2223–35.
16. Furino C, Boscia F, Niro A, D'Addario M, Grassi MO, Saglimbene V, et al. Diabetic macular edema and cataract surgery: phacoemulsification combined with dexamethasone intravitreal implant compared with standard phacoemulsification. Retina. 2021;41(5):1102.
17. Gupta G, Ram J, Gupta V, Singh R, Bansal R, Gupta PC, Gupta A. Efficacy of intravitreal dexamethasone implant in patients of uveitis undergoing cataract surgery. Ocul Immunol Inflamm. 2019;27(8):1330–8.
18. Nguyen QD, Brown DM, Marcus DM, Boyer DS, Patel S, Feiner L, et al. Ranibizumab for diabetic macular edema: results from 2 phase III randomized trials: RISE and RIDE. Ophthalmology. 2012;119(4):789–801.
19. Akıncıoğlu D, Küçükevcilioğlu M, Durukan AH, Aykaş S, Ayyıldız Ö, Erdurman FC. Outcomes of intravitreal dexamethasone implant in the treatment of recalcitrant diabetic macular edema. Turk J Ophthalmol. 2017;47(5):274–8.
20. Boyer DS, Yoon YH, Belfort R Jr, Bandello F, Maturi RK, Augustin AJ, Li XY, Cui H, Hashad Y, Whitcup SM, Ozurdex MEAD Study Group. Three-year, randomized, sham-controlled trial of dexamethasone intravitreal implant in patients with diabetic macular edema. Ophthalmology. 2014;121(10):1904–14.
21. Schmidt-Erfurth U, Garcia-Arumi J, Bandello F, Berg K, Chakravarthy U, Gerendas BS, et al. Guidelines for the Management of Diabetic Macular Edema by the European Society of Retina Specialists (EURETINA). Ophthalmol J Int Ophtalmol Int J Ophthalmol Z Augenheilkd. 2017;237(4):185–222.
22. Callanan DG, Gupta S, Boyer DS, Ciulla TA, Singer MA, Kuppermann BD, Liu CC, Li XY, Hollander DA, Schiffman RM, Whitcup SM. Dexamethasone intravitreal implant in combination with laser photocoagulation for the treatment of diffuse diabetic macular edema. Ophthalmology. 2013;120:1843–51.
23. Guigou S, Hajjar C, Parrat E, Merite PY, Pommier S, Matonti F, et al. Multicenter Ozurdex® assessment for diabetic macular edema: MOZART study. J Fr Ophtalmol. 2014;37(6):480–5.
24. Boyer DS, Faber D, Gupta S, Patel SS, Tabandeh H, Li XY, Liu CC, Lou J, Whitcup SM. Dexamethasone intravitreal implant for treatment of diabetic macular edema in vitrectomized patients. Retina. 2011;31:915–23.
25. Gillies MC, Lim LL, Campain A, Quin GJ, Salem W, Li J, et al. A randomized clinical trial of intravitreal bevacizumab versus intravitreal dexamethasone for diabetic macular edema: the BEVORDEX study. Ophthalmology. 2014;121(12):2473–81.
26. Malclès A, Dot C, Voirin N, Agard É, Vié AL, Bellocq D, Denis P, Kodjikian L. Real-life study in diabetic macular edema treated with dexamethasone implant: the Reldex Study. Retina. 2017;37:753–60.
27. Rosenblatt A, Udaondo P, Cunha-Vaz J, Sivaprasad S, Bandello F, Lanzetta P, et al. A collaborative retrospective study on the efficacy and safety of intravitreal dexamethasone implant (Ozurdex) in patients with diabetic macular edema: the European DME Registry Study. Ophthalmology. 2020 Mar;127(3):377–93.
28. Lam W-C, Albiani DA, Yoganathan P, Chen JC, Kherani A, Maberley DA, et al. Real-world assessment of intravitreal dexamethasone implant (0.7 mg) in patients with macular edema: the CHROME study. Clin Ophthalmol Auckl NZ. 2015;9:1255–68.
29. Escobar-Barranco JJ, Pina-Marín B, Fernández-Bonet M. Dexamethasone implants in patients with Naïve or refractory diffuse diabetic macular edema. Ophthalmologica. 2015;233(3–4):176–85.
30. Iglicki M, Busch C, Zur D, Okada M, Mariussi M, Chhablani JK, et al. Dexamethasone implant for diabetic macular edema in naive compared with refractory eyes: the International Retina Group Real-Life 24-Month Multicenter Study. The IRGREL-DEX Study. Retina. 2019;39(1):44–51.

31. Maturi RK, Glassman AR, Liu D, Beck RW, Bhavsar AR, Bressler NM, et al. Effect of adding dexamethasone to continued Ranibizumab treatment in patients with persistent diabetic macular edema: a DRCR Network phase 2 randomized clinical trial. JAMA Ophthalmol. 2018;136(1):29–38.
32. Yuan Q, Liu Y, Xu H, Gao Y, Qin L, Gou Y, Tao M, Zhang M. Efficacy and safety of single-dose dexamethasone implantation for patients with persistent diabetic macular edema: a systematic review and meta-analysis. Graefes Arch Clin Exp Ophthalmol. 2022;260(2):405–13.
33. Bucolo C, Gozzo L, Longo L, Mansueto S, Vitale DC, Drago F. Long-term efficacy and safety profile of multiple injections of intravitreal dexamethasone implant to manage diabetic macular edema: a systematic review of real-world studies. J Pharmacol Sci. 2018;138(4):219–32.
34. García Layana A, Adán A, Ascaso FJ, Cabrera F, Donate J, Escobar Barranco JJ, Peralta G, Reyes García R, Rodríguez Maqueda M, Ruiz-Moreno JM, Vinagre I, MOMENTUM-D Study Group. Use of intravitreal dexamethasone implants in the treatment of diabetic macular edema: expert recommendations using a Delphi approach. Eur J Ophthalmol. 2020;30(5):1042–52.
35. Moon BG, Lee JY, Yu HG, et al. Efficacy and safety of a dexamethasone implant in patients with diabetic macular edema at tertiary centers in Korea. J Ophthalmol. 2016;2016:9810270.
36. Zur D, Iglicki M, Busch C, Invernizzi A, Mariussi M, Loewenstein A. OCT biomarkers as functional outcome predictors in diabetic macular edema treated with dexamethasone implant. Ophthalmology. 2018;125(2):267–75.
37. Liu Q, Hu Y, Yu H, Yuan L, Hu J, Atik A, et al. Comparison of intravitreal triamcinolone acetonide versus intravitreal bevacizumab as the primary treatment of clinically significant macular edema. Retina. 2015;35(2):272–9.
38. Vujosevic S, Torresin T, Bini S, Convento E, Pilotto E, Parrozzani R, Midena E. Imaging retinal inflammatory biomarkers after intravitreal steroid and anti-VEGF treatment in diabetic macular oedema. Acta Ophthalmol. 2017;95(5):464–71.
39. Bandyopadhyay S, Bandyopadhyay SK, Saha M, Sinha A. Study of aqueous cytokines in patients with different patterns of diabetic macular edema based on optical coherence tomography. Int Ophthalmol. 2018;38(1):241–9.
40. Midena E, Pilotto E, Bini S. Hyperreflective Intraretinal foci as an OCT biomarker of retinal inflammation in diabetic macular edema. Invest Ophthalmol Vis Sci. 2018;59(13):5366.
41. Uji A, Murakami T, Nishijima K, Akagi T, Horii T, Arakawa N, et al. Association between hyperreflective foci in the outer retina, status of photoreceptor layer, and visual acuity in diabetic macular edema. Am J Ophthalmol. 2012;153:710–7.
42. Funatsu H, Noma H, Mimura T, Eguchi S, Hori S. Association of vitreous inflammatory factors with diabetic macular edema. Ophthalmology. 2009;116:73–9.
43. Vujosevic S, Bini S, Torresin T, et al. Hyperreflective retinal spots in normal and diabetic eyes: B-scan and en face spectral domain optical coherence tomography evaluation. Retina. 2017;37:1092–103.
44. Shin YU, Hong EH, Lim HW, Kang MH, Seong M, Cho H. Quantitative evaluation of hard exudates in diabetic macular edema after short-term intravitreal triamcinolone, dexamethasone implant or bevacizumab injections. BMC Ophthalmol. 2017;17(1):182.
45. Sun JK, Lin MM, Lammer J, Prager S, Sarangi R, Silva PS, Aiello LP. Disorganization of the retinal inner layers as a predictor of visual acuity in eyes with center-involved diabetic macular edema. JAMA Ophthalmol. 2014;132:1309–16.
46. Radwan SH, Soliman AZ, Tokarev J, Zhang L, Van Kuijk FJ, Koozekanani DD. Association of disorganization of retinal inner layers with vision after resolution of center-involved diabetic macular edema. JAMA Ophthalmol. 2015;133:820–5.
47. Das R, Spence G, Hogg RE, Stevenson M, Chakravarthy U. Disorganization of inner retina and outer retinal morphology in diabetic macular edema. JAMA Ophthalmol. 2018;136:202–8.
48. Zur D, Iglicki M, Sala-Puigdollers A, Chhablani J, Lupidi M, Fraser-Bell S, Mendes TS, Chaikitmongkol V, Cebeci Z, Dollberg D, Busch C, Invernizzi A, Habot-Wilner Z, Loewenstein A. International retina group (IRG). Disorganization of retinal inner layers as a biomarker in patients with diabetic macular oedema treated with dexamethasone implant. Acta Ophthalmol. 2020;98(2):e217–23.

Laser Photocoagulation for Diabetic Macular Edema

12

Chaitra Jayadev, Santosh Gopikrishna Gadde, and Aaditi Anil Kumar

12.1 Introduction

Diabetic retinopathy (DR) is a leading cause of preventable blindness globally. Up to 75% of patients with more than 20 years of diabetes mellitus (DM) will have some form of DR (WHO Report, 2005) [1]. Diabetic macular edema (DME) is a manifestation of DR that results from blood–retinal barrier breakdown leading to leakage from retinal capillaries and fluid accumulation within the retinal layers resulting in a thickened macula. This can lead to a compromised or loss of central vision due to the microvascular complications. The Wisconsin Epidemiologic Study of Diabetic Retinopathy estimated that with 15 years of diabetes, the prevalence of DME is approximately 20% in patients with Type 1 DM, 25% in Type 2 DM who are on insulin, and 14% in Type 2 DM who are not on insulin. Systemic factors associated with DME include a long duration of diabetes, higher systolic blood pressure, and a higher glycosylated hemoglobin value [2, 3].

12.2 Pathophysiology of DME

To understand how various treatment modalities work, it is important to know the pathophysiology of DME, which is complex and multifactorial. Prolonged hyperglycemia in DM leads to reduced retinal oxygen tension in the capillary plexuses of inner retina, venous dilation, leukocyte stasis, and dysregulated growth factor levels leading to increased exudation of serum out of the retinal vasculature and into the extracellular space due to endothelial cell damage and the inner blood–retinal barrier (BRB) breakdown [4]. The RPE pump is also overwhelmed leading to outer BRB breakdown which further contributes to DME [5]. This is in accordance with Starling's law, which explains increased intravascular pressure and vascular permeability result in a net flow of water, ions, and macromolecules from the intravascular space into the extravascular space [6].

Type 2 DM patients are found to have decreased subfoveal choroidal blood flow, especially in eyes with DME than eyes without DME, suggesting relative hypoxia of the RPE and outer retina, and consequent increased permeability of the outer blood–retinal barrier [7]. Vitreous due to its close proximity to the retina has a direct effect of traction causing leakage from blood vessels, localizing mediators of vessel permeability in proximity to macular capillaries and thus impede oxygenation of the retina, thereby causing venous dilation and increased edema via Starling's law and by upregulation of VEGF [8–10].

Many variables modulate the above pathological process. The duration of diabetes and elevated glycated hemoglobin (HbA1C) have a major influence. Increased inflammation, characterized by leucostasis, accumulation of macrophages, intercellular adhesion molecule-1 (ICAM-1) activation, and upregulation of vascular endothelial growth factor, interleukin-6, and prostacyclin, which are associated with capillary nonperfusion and breakdown of the blood–retina barrier is noted in DME (Fig. 12.1) [11, 12].

C. Jayadev (✉) · S. G. Gadde · A. A. Kumar
Narayana Nethralaya Eye Institute, Bangalore, Karnataka, India

S. Saxena et al. (eds.), *Diabetic Macular Edema*, https://doi.org/10.1007/978-981-19-7307-9_12

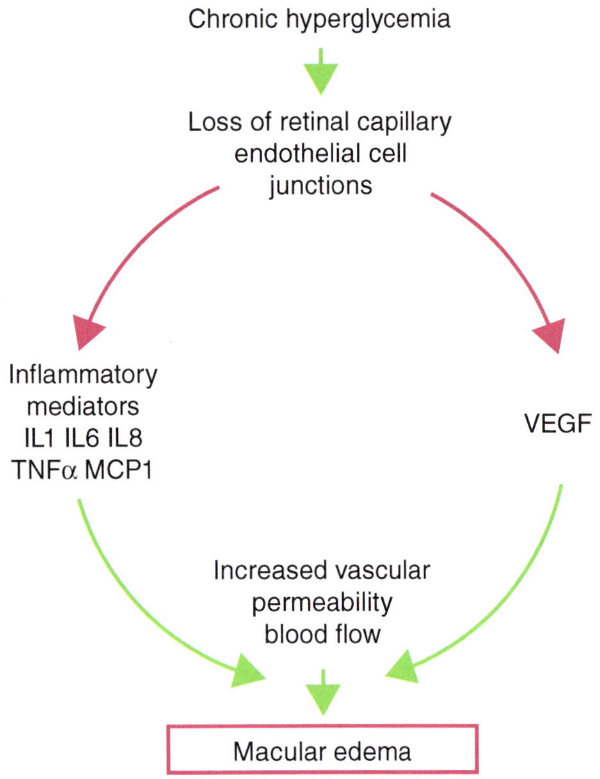

Fig. 12.1 Pathophysiology of diabetic macular edema

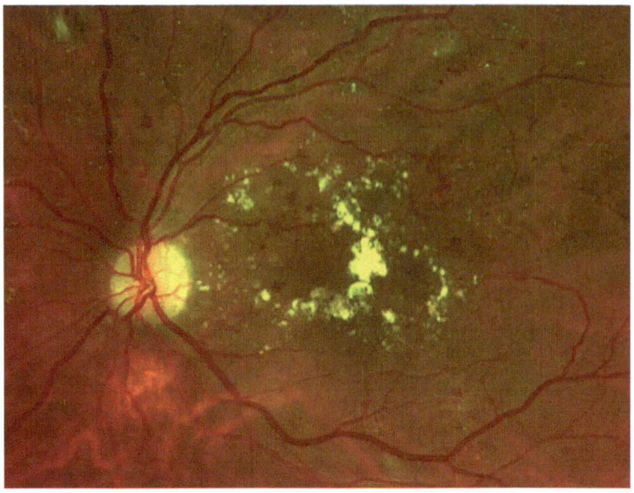

Fig. 12.2 Color fundus photo depicting diabetic macular edema with hard exudates

12.3 Clinical Diagnosis of DME

The diagnosis of DME is clinical, based on slit lamp biomicroscopy and indirect ophthalmoscopy and seen as a thickening at the macula with the presence of microaneurysms, hemorrhages, and/or hard exudates (Fig. 12.2). Optical coherence tomography (OCT) is an essential non-invasive and repeatable diagnostic modality to confirm the morphological pattern of DME and response to treatment and for follow-up (Fig. 12.3). Fundus fluorescein angiography (FFA) is an invasive dye-based test to further investigate the type of leakage, nonperfusion areas at the macula and periphery and to grade DR (Fig. 12.4). Optical coherence tomography angiography (OCTA) is a non-invasive imaging modality that allows assessment of the blood flow of each retinal capillary layer. Abnormalities in capillary flow density and microaneurysms from the deep capillary layer can be detected, which was not possible on the conventional FFA. Macular ischemia, a poor prognostic indicator in DME, can also be well appreciated on the OCTA (Fig. 12.5).

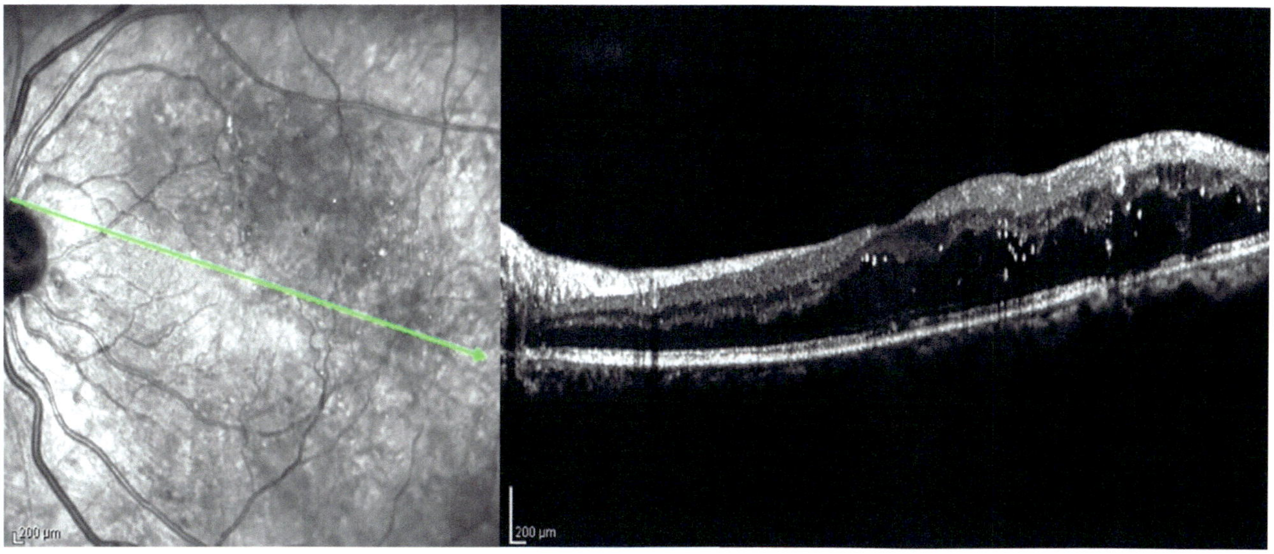

Fig. 12.3 An optical coherence tomography scan showing spongi form retinal thickening with intraretinal fluid in diabetic macular edema

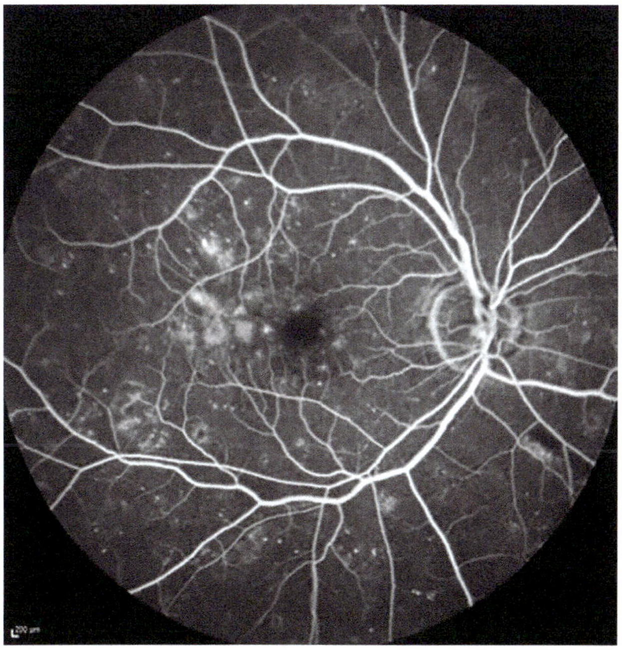

Fig. 12.4 Fundus fluorescein angiography of a patient with non-proliferative diabetic retinopathy with focal leak of microaneurysms close to the macula in diabetic macular edema

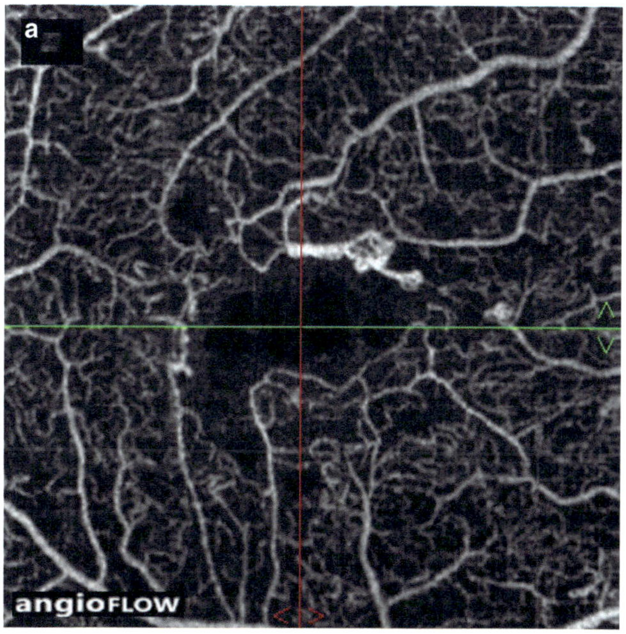

Fig. 12.5 Superficial capillary plexus (**a**) and deep capillary plexus (**b**) slab in an optical coherence tomography angiography showing enlargement of the foveal avascular zone in both the slabs. A telangiectatic and beaded vessel can be appreciated in the superficial capillary plexus with microaneurysms noted in the deep capillary plexus

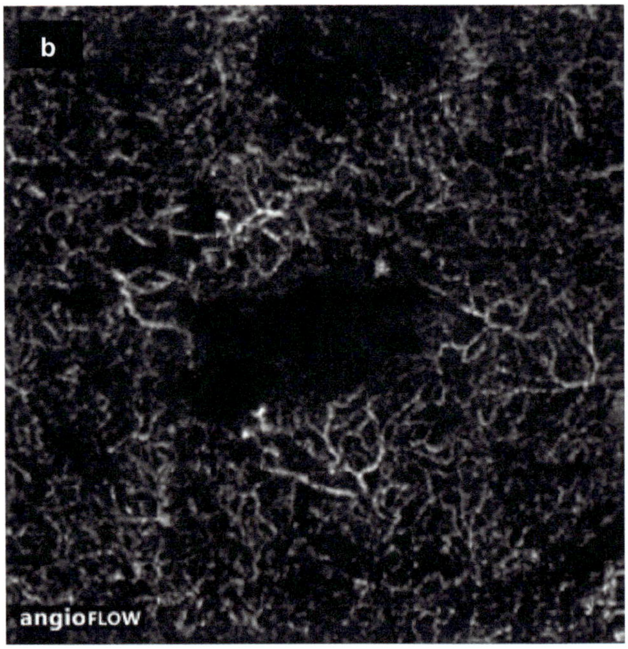

Fig. 12.5 (continued)

12.4 Definitions of DME

Diabetic macular edema can be classified as center involved, when the fovea is affected, or non-center involved. The Early treatment Diabetic Retinopathy Study (ETDRS) has classified DME as mild when there is some retinal thickening or hard exudates in the posterior pole away from the center of the macula, moderate when there is retinal thickening or hard exudates near the center of the macula but not involving the center, severe when there is retinal thickening or hard exudates involving the center of the macula and no edema when there is no apparent thickening [13]. Clinically significant macular edema (CSME) is defined as (Fig. 12.6).

- Thickening of the retina at or within 500 μm of the center of the macula.
- Hard exudates at or within 500 μm of the center of the macula, if associated with thickening of the adjacent retina (not residual hard exudates remaining after the disappearance of retinal thickening).
- A zone or zones of retinal thickening one-disc area or larger, any part of which is within one-disc diameter of the center of the macula [14].

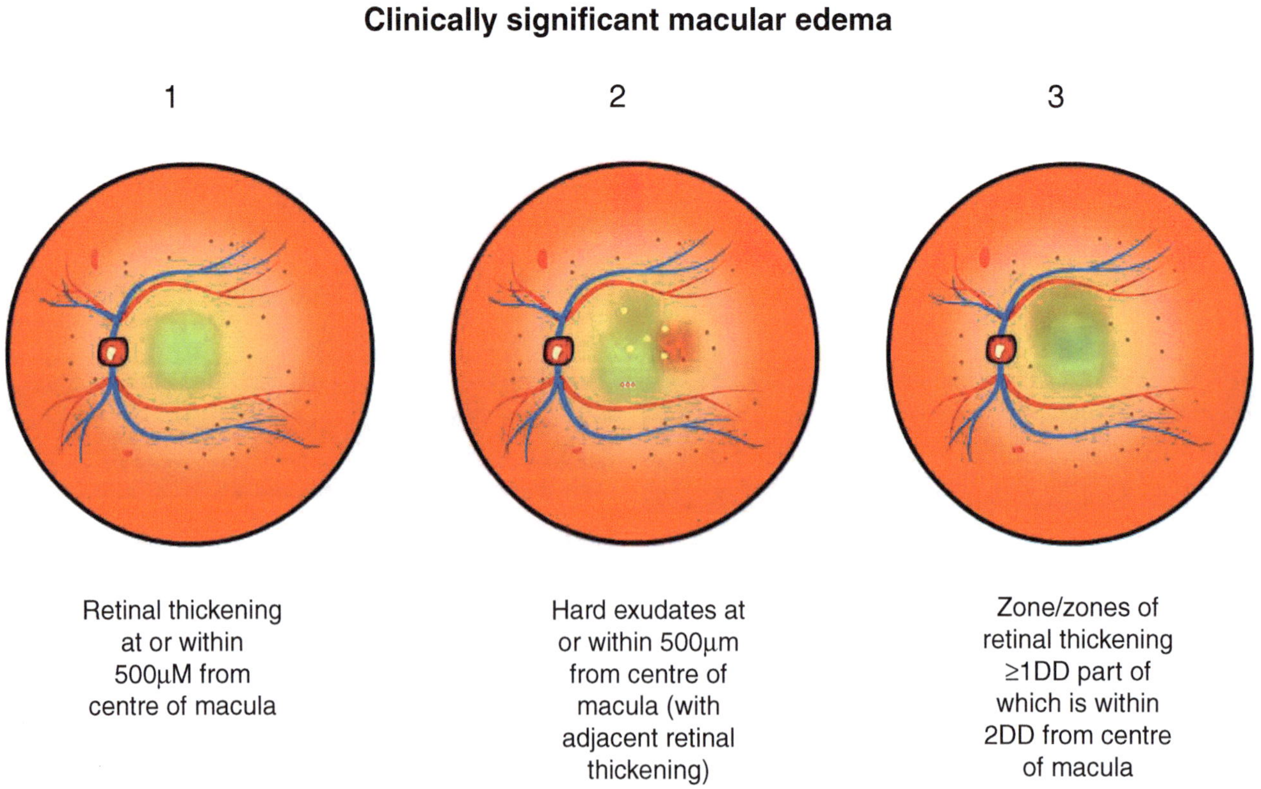

Fig. 12.6 A graphical representation of clinically significant macular edema

12.5 Laser Therapy for Diabetic Retinopathy

Since its development in mid-twentieth century, laser photocoagulation had been the mainstay of diabetic retinopathy treatment. In 1964, Bridges discovered and implemented the use of argon laser photocoagulation [15]. It had emissions in blue (488 nm) and green (514 nm) wavelengths. The resolution of hard exudates after xenon laser photocoagulation was first described by Spalter [16]. Subsequently, laser therapy has evolved over the years with reduced collateral damage to adjacent tissues, and fewer complications.

12.5.1 Types of Laser

Argon blue-green laser (514 nm)—absorbed selectively by xanthophyll and hemoglobin, it coagulates from choriocapillaris till inner nuclear layer. It has high intraocular scattering and may cause macular damage.

Infrared/Krypton red laser (647 nm)—produces deeper, less visible, and more painful burns [17].

Frequency-doubled Nd-YAG Laser (532 nm) green laser—highly absorbed by hemoglobin and melanin and safer for macular treatment. It can be used either continuously or in pulsed mode.

Yellow laser (577 nm)—requires less power to achieve the same degree of burn, less scattering by cataractous lenses, and less macular damage from heat absorption by the macula pigment, xanthophyll [18]. The yellow laser wavelength occurs outside the absorption spectrum of xanthophylls, potentially allowing for treatment closer to the fovea. It also has the highest oxyhemoglobin to melanin absorption ratio and therefore, is the most effective laser for vascular structures. The combined absorption by both melanin and oxyhemoglobin of 577 nm causes lesser scatter compared to 532 nm or other yellow wavelengths (561/568 nm). This leads to energy concentration to a smaller volume allowing for use of lower powers and shorter pulse durations.

12.5.2 Properties of Laser [19]

Monochromatic—single wavelength, eliminating chromatic aberration.

Coherent—all light is in the same phase and allows precise focusing of the laser beam width to as small as a few microns.

Polarized—all photons produced are in phase with each other with limited divergence allowing for a smoother passage through media.

Collimated—light moves in one direction and is non-spreading.

12.5.3 Laser Absorption Characteristics of Tissues

Melanin pigment universally absorbs light spectrum between 400 and 700 nm, whereas xanthophyll and hemoglobin pigments are selective absorbers.

Hemoglobin absorbs blue, green, and yellow light significantly and red light poorly. The shorter wavelength yellow light is more easily absorbed. The red and near infrared wavelength lights are totally nonabsorbable by hemoglobin.

Xanthophyll pigment is present in the inner and outer plexiform layers of retina of macular area and absorbs blue light maximally and green light poorly. Hence in macular photocoagulation argon green laser (514 nm) is preferred as it avoids unwanted inner retinal damage.

12.5.4 Laser Treatment of Macular Edema

For several decades, the only treatment option for DME had been laser photocoagulation Focal laser photocoagulation of "clinically significant" DME substantially reduced the risk of moderate visual loss by half, increased the chances of visual improvement, and decreased the frequency of persistent macular edema with only minor visual field losses [20]. Even ETDRS had also demonstrated the beneficial effect of macular laser photocoagulation with argon laser in combination with focal treatment of each leaking microaneurysms and grid treatment to areas of diffuse leakage and capillary nonperfusion [21, 22]. The ETDRS Report 19 (1995) recommended that focal photocoagulation should be considered for eyes with CSME, particularly when the center of the macula is involved or imminently threatened. A lesser thickening of the macula and when the center is not involved can be closely observed initially. This was said to be preferable to immediate treatment, particularly when most of the leakage to be treated arises close to the center of the macula, due to the risk of damage from direct treatment or subsequent migration of treatment scars [23].

ETDRS followed two macular laser treatment protocols: focal and grid, both performed between 500 and 3000 μm from the fovea but not within 500 μm from the papillary border. Focal laser was applied for focal lesions that not only included microaneurysms but also intraretinal microvascular abnormalities and small capillaries with focal leakage (Fig. 12.7). Grid laser was performed in non-center involving areas of macular thickening with diffuse leakage or capillary loss. Grid laser is done, two burns width apart, with a spot size of 50–200 μm for a duration of 0.05–0.5 s, not placed within 500 μm of the center of the macula or within 500 μm of the disc margin, the end point being grayish burns (Fig. 12.8) [20–23]. In cases where the laser needed to be closer to the fovea, a modified technique called modified

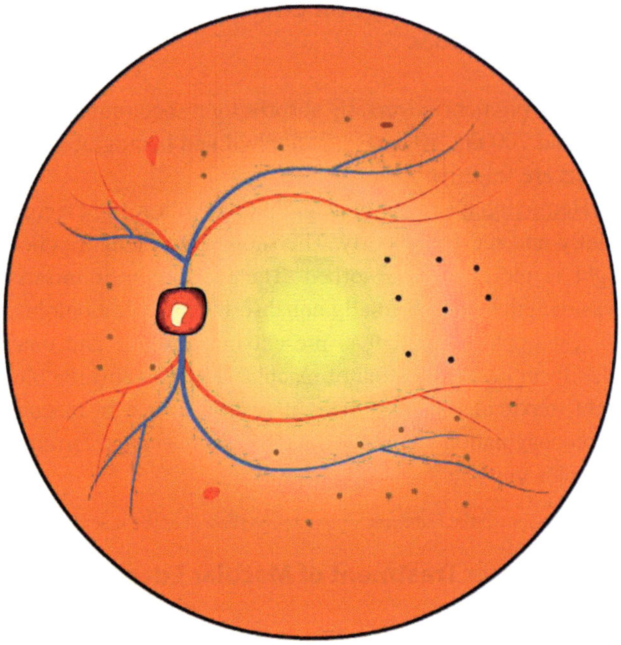

Fig. 12.7 A graphical representation of focal laser application to microaneurysms in a case of non-center involving diabetic macular edema

ETDRS technique was followed to avoid potential complications, wherein a smaller spot of 50 μm size and 50–100 milliseconds burn duration was performed (Fig. 12.9) [20–23].

12.5.5 Mechanism of Action

The therapeutic effects of laser depend on characteristics such as wavelength, pulse, power, duration, absorption spectrum of the intended tissue, and the pigment concentration in these tissues. When the absorption spectrum of the tissue coincides with the wavelength of the laser energy, it is converted into heat energy. Pigmented tissues that absorb laser energy in the macular area include the retinal pigment epithelium (RPE), choroid, hemoglobin within red blood cells, and the xanthophyll pigment [24].

In a conventional laser, a continuous wave is delivered to the tissue throughout the entire duration of the laser pulse. These pigments absorb the laser energy and converts it to heat, which leads to an increase in tissue temperature. The heat wave extends laterally and vertically. This can result in collateral damage depending on the duration and magnitude of the laser pulse. A visible burn was earlier believed to be necessary for a successful treatment. This concept has evolved to splitting the pulse and deliver sub threshold forms of laser to minimize the collateral damage [24].

It has been proposed that laser works by occlusion of the leaking microaneurysms in the retina. This is followed by RPE recovery and the stimulation of cytokine production, which leads to reabsorption of fluid in the macula. Another hypothesis is that laser photocoagulation causes autoregulation of retinal vasculature and induction of endothelial cell proliferation [25]. This in turn decreases the retinal blood flow and subsequently, the macular edema. Resolution of edema prevents the migration of fluid and hard exudates toward the fovea (Fig. 12.10) [26–28]. Reduction in retinal blood flow and macular edema post laser photocoagulation could also be due to improved oxygenation following destruction of RPE, which have a high oxygen demand [26–28].

12.5.6 Complications

Laser photocoagulation of the macula for DME is not without complications. Destruction of the RPE can affect the visual acuity due to apoptosis of the surrounding retinal cells and enlargement of laser scars [26]. This might threaten the visual prognosis if the laser is applied too close to the fovea (Fig. 12.11) [29]. With the photoreceptors being denser in the posterior pole, many more of them are destroyed despite using the same spot size that is used in the midperiphery [30]. Other concerns are macular laser scar enlargement, paracentral scotomas, choroidal neovascularization, and subretinal fibrosis [29]. Advances in laser technology have helped reduce these complications to a large extent.

12.5.7 Newer Forms of Laser Therapy

12.5.7.1 Selective Laser Therapy

Selective laser therapy (SRT) is a micropulse and short duration laser developed to treat various diseases with RPE dysfunction, including DME. The melanosomes in the RPE absorbs almost 50% of the incident laser light [31]. Hence it prevents damage to the photoreceptors, neurosensory retina, and choroid. Therefore, complications associated with conventional laser can be avoided. The laser burns are invisible in SRT and therefore difficult to assess the energy required for therapeutic RPE damage.

12.5.7.2 Subthreshold Diode Micropulse Laser

Subthreshold diode micropulse laser is another laser modality that uses a near infrared diode laser 810 nm to bring about selective RPE damage [32, 33]. It delivers laser energy in "micropulses" in submilliseconds, rather than in a continuous mode. The endpoint in subthreshold diode micropulse laser is invisible pre- or posttreatment and the appropriate laser dosing is still unclear. The mechanism of action of subthreshold laser is hypothesized to be alteration of the metabolic activity of RPE [33, 34].

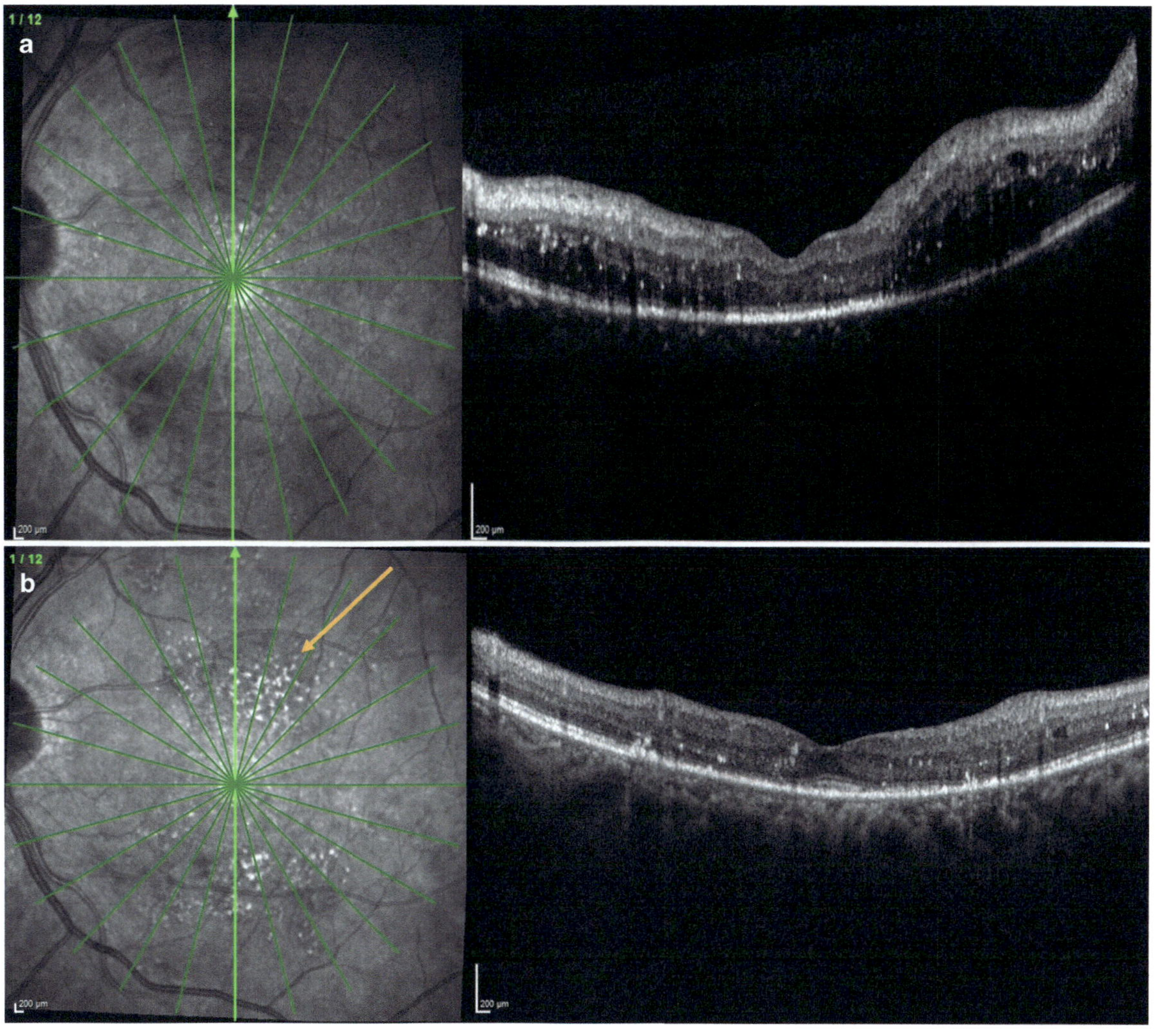

Fig. 12.8 Optical coherence tomography images of a case of non-center involving diabetic macular edema before (**a**) and after modified grid laser (**b**) showing resolution of macular edema. Grid laser spots are visible on the infrared images (yellow arrow)

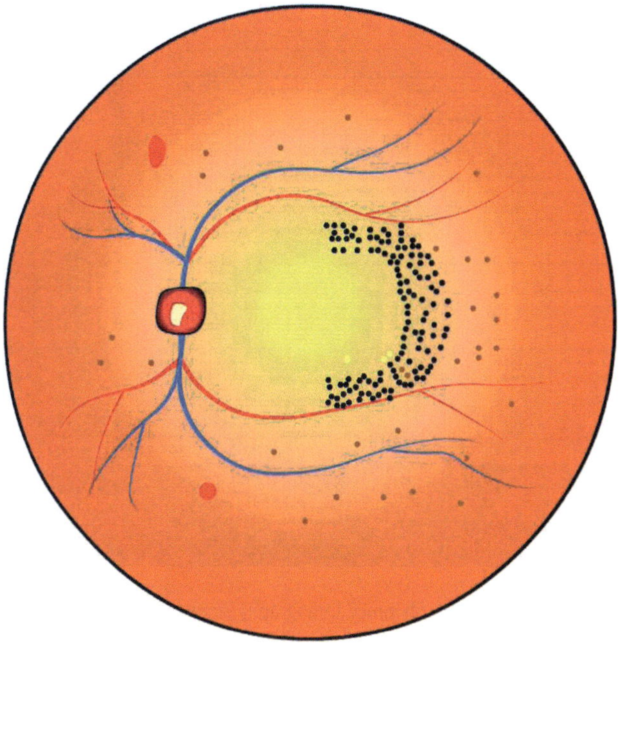

Fig. 12.9 A graphical representation of modified grid laser to the areas of edema in a case of non-center involving diabetic macular edema, sparing areas without edema, especially the papillomacular bundle to avoid collateral damage

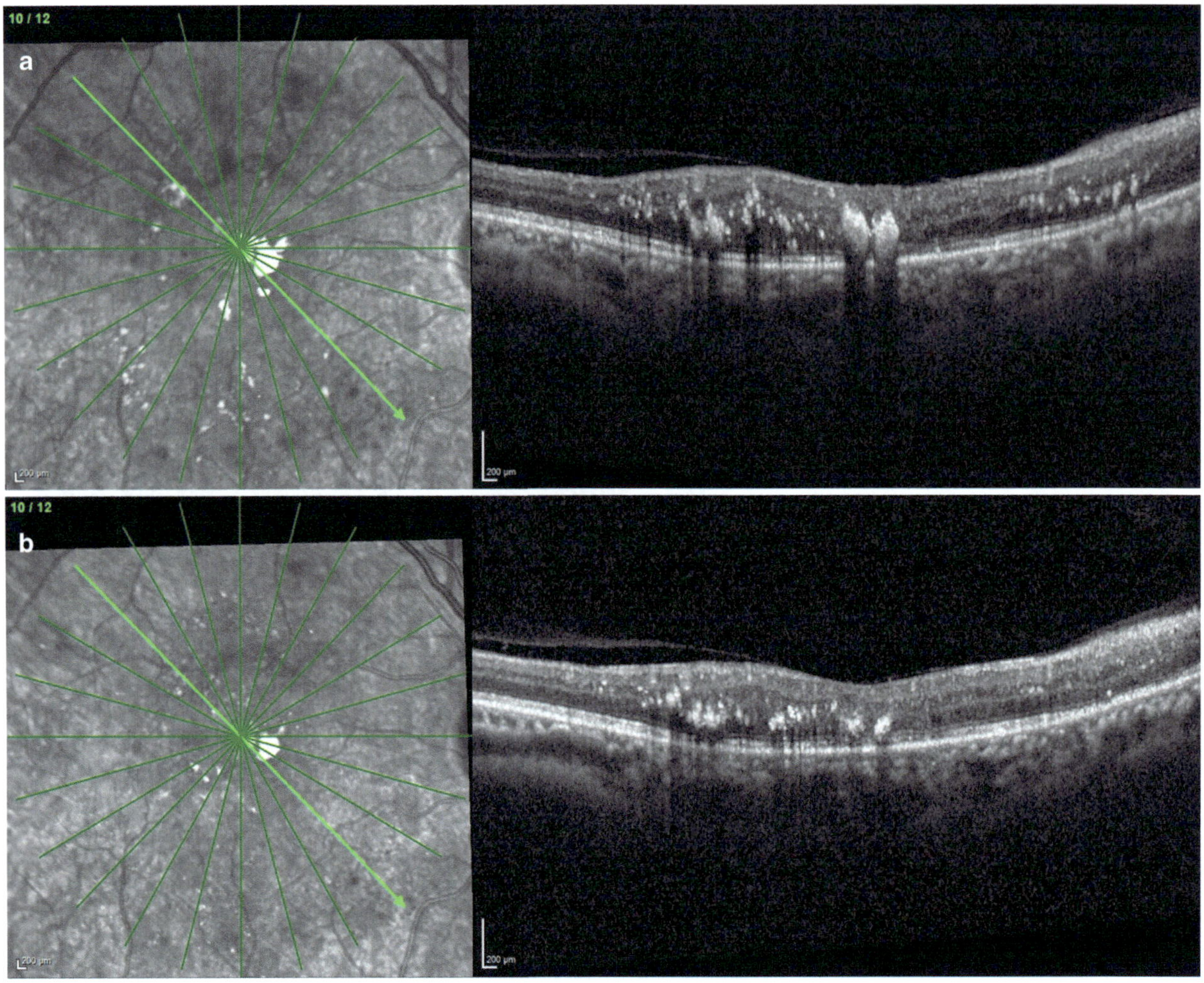

Fig. 12.10 Optical coherence tomography scans of spongy thickening with intraretinal hard exudates before modified grid laser (**a**). OCT image postgrid laser showing resolution of the intraretinal hard exudates even at the fovea (**b**)

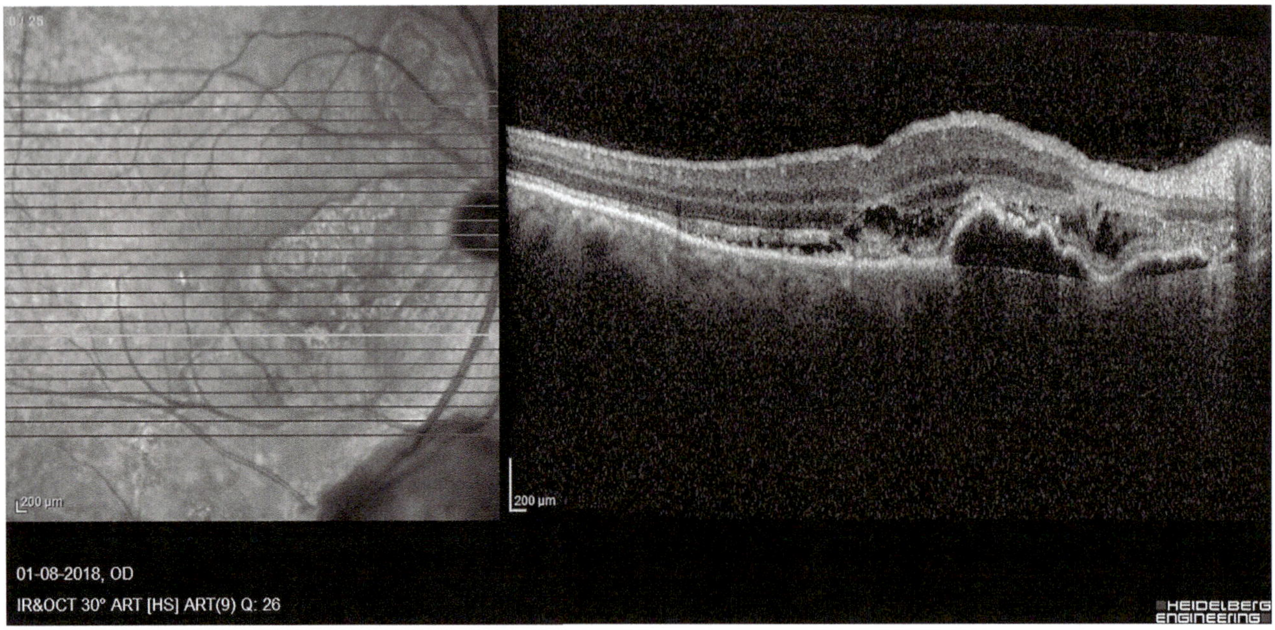

Fig. 12.11 Optical coherence tomography scans of postaccidental laser burns close to the fovea showing pigment epithelial detachments with subretinal fluid and subretinal hyperreflective material

12.5.7.3 Pattern Laser for DME

With pattern laser, application of multiple laser spots with a shorter pulse duration is possible (Fig. 12.12). Advantages include shorter treatment duration, increased safety, uniform and precise spot placement, accurate "subthreshold" grid-pattern placement, and reduced pain and visual field defect [35]. A shorter pulse duration allows for faster treatment with the total treatment time being reduced by several folds [35]. There is reduced collateral damage and pain due to the decrease in the width and axial extent of the retinal burns [36].

12.5.7.4 Image Guided Laser Therapy: Navigated Laser

Navigated laser combines imaging (infrared, color or fluorescein angiography) with integrated laser treatment of the retina, including pattern laser generation, fast retina tracking and target assistance systems, resulting in high precision of laser burns to complete the treatment plan with greater accuracy and success [37]. The preplanned treatment can be made based on color image, FFA, indocyanine green angiography, OCT, and/or OCTA [38].

12.5.8 Perspective of Intravitreal Pharmacotherapy

With the proven efficacy of intravitreal pharmacotherapy in the past few decades, the role of laser therapy appears to have diminished. Intravitreal anti-vascular endothelial growth factor (VEGF) and corticosteroid pharmacotherapy have revolutionized the treatment of center involved DME wherein focal laser has its limitations. Anti-VEGF drugs work by blocking the increased permeability and inflammation inducing effects of VEGF. Intravitreal corticosteroids have other non-VEGF-mediated effects, such as decreasing leukocyte recruitment and adhesion molecules, inhibiting collagenase induction expression and reduce expression of the VEGF gene and various VEGF receptors, that ultimately reduce the permeability of retinal microvessels [39, 40]. Several landmark trials, including the Diabetic Retinopathy Clinical Research network (DRCR.net), have compared the efficacy of monotherapy with laser and combined therapy with prompt or deferred laser in center involving DME to anti-VEGF alone.

The BOLT study which compared intravitreal bevacizumab with laser therapy in 2010 found that patients were 5.1 times more likely to gain 10 or greater ETDRS letters over 12 months with bevacizumab therapy [41]. The RESTORE study showed equal superiority of ranibizumab monotherapy and ranibizumab combined with laser therapy over standard laser therapy in patients with DME [42]. In a study of 854 eyes with DME, ranibizumab with prompt or deferred laser therapy showed greater visual acuity improvement compared to laser monotherapy [43].

12.5.9 Current Indications for Laser Therapy in DME

In patients with non-center involved CSME, focal and grid laser therapy offers relatively stable visual acuity, retinal thickness measurements, and decreased fluorescein leakage with reduced risk of moderate vision loss by 50% by 3 years

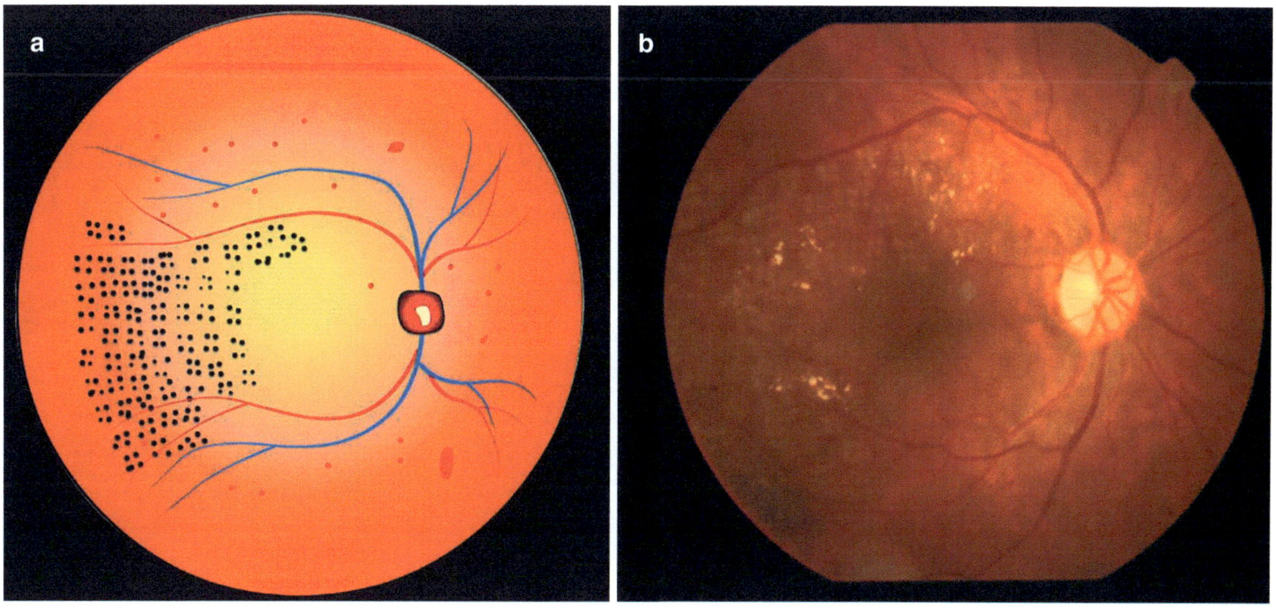

Fig. 12.12 A graphical representation (**a**) of pattern scan laser marks, which have covered the areas of thickening sparing the papillomacular bundle and fovea on the fundus photograph (**b**)

[20, 44]. Despite a clear advantage of anti-VEGF therapy for DME, there is still a role for combination therapy of anti-VEGF with laser photocoagulation. Some studies have shown that fewer injections are required and a reduced residual edema in those treated with a combination of both [45, 46]. Laser can provide similar outcomes in patients with a central macular thickness <300 μm compared to anti-VEGF monotherapy [42]. Even in center involving DME, the leakage can be caused by microaneurysms located outside the central subfield, which is amendable to laser treatment [42]. Focal extrafoveal DME, in which anti-VEGF therapy in not warranted, but when promptly treated with laser prevents encroachment of the fovea (Fig. 12.13). This has the advantage of preventing worsening of vision and saving the patient expensive intravitreal pharmacotherapy. Studies even encourage close observation for those with good visual acuity in spite of center involving DME [47, 48].

With the expenses being significant with pharmacotherapy, the cost-effectiveness of laser therapy for DME needs further exploration [49]. In low resource settings, laser photocoagulation for the treatment of DME has a continued role as an adjunct to intravitreal pharmacotherapy to reduce the burden of treatment costs. Diabetics with other co-morbidities may not be able to comply with the required pharmacotherapy follow-up visits. Hence, in patients with non-center involving DME or when anti-VEGF therapy is not accessible or affordable, macular laser treatment provides a viable treatment option to prevent vision loss [50]. In conclusion, laser photocoagulation for DME still has an important role to play. Its safety and long-term efficacy have been proven. A comprehensive outlook based on the severity and location of the edema, and patient-related factors including systemic control and affordability, will help take the optimal treatment decision.

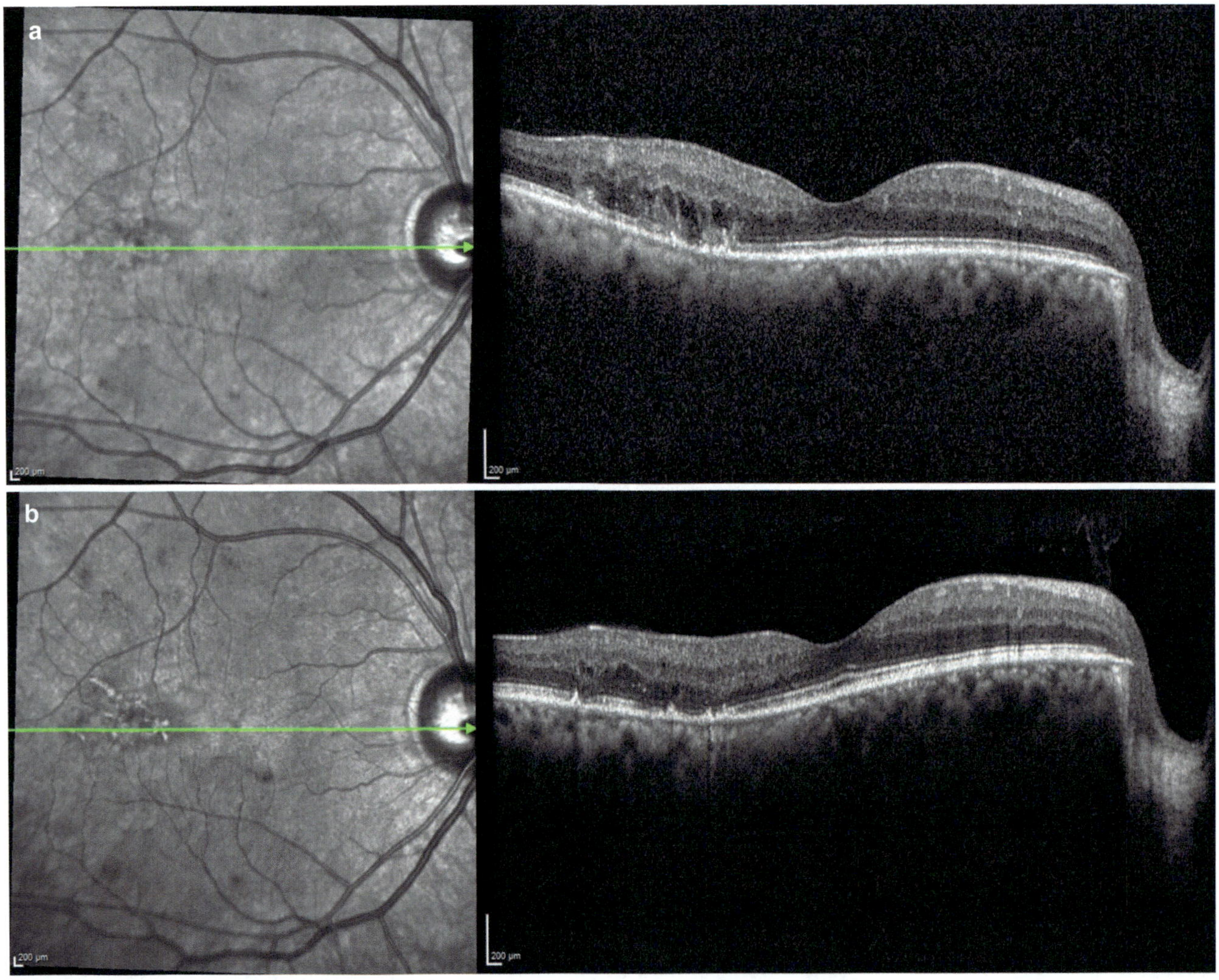

Fig. 12.13 Optical coherence tomography scans of a case of non-center involving diabetic macular edema. Figure **a** shows spongy thickening with intraretinal fluid and hyper reflective material. Figure **b** shows the resolution of spongy thickening after grid laser over the edematous macula prevent migration to the fovea

References

1. Report of the WHO consultation in Geneva, Switzerland 9–11 November 2005.
2. Klein R, Klein BE, Davis MD, DeMets DL. The Wisconsin Epidemiologic Study of Diabetic Retinopathy, IV: diabetic macular edema. Ophthalmology. 1984;91:1464–74.
3. Klein R, Moss SE, Klein BE, Davis MD, DeMets DL. The Wisconsin epidemiologic study of diabetic retinopathy. XI. The incidence of macular edema. Ophthalmology. 1989;96(10):1501–10.
4. Miyamoto K, Khosrof S, Bursell SE, Moromizato Y, Aiello LP, Ogura Y, et al. Vascular endothelial growth factor (VEGF)-induced retinal vascular permeability is mediated by intercellular adhesion molecule-1 (ICAM-1). Am J Pathol. 2000;156:1733–9.
5. Weinberger D, Fink-Cohen S, Gaton DD, Priel E, Yassur Y. Non-retinovascular leakage in diabetic maculopathy. Br J Ophthalmol. 1995;79(8):728–31.
6. Kristinsson JK, Gottfredsdóttir MS, Stefánsson E. Retinal vessel dilatation and elongation precedes diabetic macular oedema. Br J Ophthalmol. 1997;81(4):274–8.
7. Nagaoka T, Kitaya N, Sugawara R, Yokota H, Mori F, Hikichi T, Fujio N, Yoshida A. Alteration of choroidal circulation in the foveal region in patients with type 2 diabetes. Br J Ophthalmol. 2004;88(8):1060–3.
8. Sebag J, Balazs EA. Pathogenesis of cystoid macular edema: an anatomic consideration of vitreoretinal adhesions. Surv Ophthalmol. 1984;28(Suppl):493–8.
9. Otani T, Kishi S. A controlled study of vitrectomy for diabetic macular edema. Am J Ophthalmol. 2002;134(2):214–9.
10. Sebag J, Buckingham B, Charles MA, Reiser K. Biochemical abnormalities in vitreous of humans with proliferative diabetic retinopathy. Arch Ophthalmol. 1992;110(10):1472–6. https://doi.org/10.1001/archopht.1992.01080220134035.
11. Funatsu H, Noma H, Mimura T, Eguchi S, Hori S. Association of vitreous inflammatory factors with diabetic macular edema. Ophthalmology. 2009;116(1):73–9.
12. Kent D, Vinores SA, Campochiaro PA. Macular oedema: the role of soluble mediators. Br J Ophthalmol. 2000;84(5):542–5.
13. Early Treatment Diabetic Retinopathy Study Research Group. Ophthalmology. 1991;98(5 Suppl):786–806. PMID: 2062513.
14. Early Photocoagulation for Diabetic Retinopathy. ETDRS report number 9. Early treatment diabetic retinopathy study research group. Ophthalmology. 1991;98(5 Suppl):766–85.
15. Bridges WB. Laser oscillation in singly ionized argon in the visible spectrum. Appl Phys Lett. 1964;4(7):128–30.
16. Spalter HF. Photocoagulation of circinate maculopathy in diabetic retinopathy. Am J Ophthalmol. 1971;71(1 Pt 2):242–50.
17. Mainster MA. Decreasing retinal photocoagulation damage: principles and techniques. Semin Ophthalmol. 1999;14:200–9.
18. Castillejos-Rios D, Devenyi R, Moffat K, Yu E. Dye yellow vs. argon green laser in panretinal photocoagulation for proliferative diabetic retinopathy: a comparison of minimum power requirements. Can J Ophthalmol. 1992;27(5):243–4.
19. Ballal NV, Kundabala M, Bhat KS. Lasers general principles: a review. In: Clinical Dentistry Research Compendium. New York: Nova Science; 2013. p. 133–48.
20. Early Treatment Diabetic Retinopathy Study Research Group. Photocoagulation for diabetic macular edema. Early treatment diabetic retinopathy study report number 1. Arch Ophthalmol. 1985;103(12):1796–806.
21. Early Treatment Diabetic Retinopathy Study Research Group. Treatment techniques and clinical guidelines for photocoagulation of diabetic macular edema. Early treatment diabetic retinopathy study report number 2. Ophthalmology. 1987;94(7):761–74.
22. Early Treatment Diabetic Retinopathy Study Research Group. Photocoagulation for diabetic macular edema: Early Treatment Diabetic Retinopathy Study Report no. 4. Int Ophthalmol Clin. 1987;27:265–72.
23. Early Treatment Diabetic Retinopathy Study Research Group. Focal photocoagulation treatment of diabetic macular edema. Relationship of treatment effect to fluorescein angiographic and other retinal characteristics at baseline: ETDRS report no. 19. Arch Ophthalmol. 1995;113(9):1144–55.
24. Zas M, Cotic M, Wu M, Wu A, Wu L. Macular laser photocoagulation in the management of diabetic macular edema: still relevant in 2020? Taiwan J Ophthalmol. 2020;10(2):87–94.
25. Kim JW, Ai E. Diabetic retinopathy. In: Regillo CD, Brown GC, Flynn Jr HW, editors. Vitreoretinal disease: the essentials. New York: Thieme Medical; 1999. p. 133–59.
26. Romero-Aroca P, Reyes-Torres J, Baget-Bernaldiz M, Blasco-Suñe C. Laser treatment for diabetic macular edema in the 21st century. Curr Diabetes Rev. 2014;10(2):100–12.
27. Ogata N, Ando A, Uyama M, Matsumura M. Expression of cytokines and transcription factors in photocoagulated human retinal pigment epithelial cells. Graefes Arch Clin Exp Ophthalmol. 2001;239(2):87–95.
28. Wilson DJ, Finkelstein D, Quigley HA, Green WR. Macular grid photocoagulation. An experimental study on the primate retina. Arch Ophthalmol. 1988;106(1):100–5.
29. Schatz H, Madeira D, McDonald HR, Johnson RN. Progressive enlargement of laser scars following grid laser photocoagulation for diffuse diabetic macular edema. Arch Ophthalmol. 1991;109:1549–51.
30. Maeshima K, Utsugi-Sutoh N, Otani T, Kishi S. Progressive enlargement of scattered photocoagulation scars in diabetic retinopathy. Retina. 2004;24:507–11.
31. Gabel VP, Birngruber R, Hillenkamp F. Visible and near infrared light absorption in pigment epithelium and choroid. In: Shimizu K, editor. International congress series no.450, XXIII Concilium Ophthalmologicum, Kyoto. Princeton, NJ: Excerpta Medica; 1978. p. 658–62.
32. Paulus YM, Palanker D, Blumenkranz MS. Short-pulse laser treatment: redefining retinal therapy. Retin Physician. 2010;7:54–6.
33. Pankratov MP. Pulsed delivery of laser energy in experimental thermal retinal photocoagulation. In: Proceedings. Laser-tissue interaction; 1990.
34. Flaxel C, Bradle J, Acott T, Samples JR. Retinal pigment epithelium produces matrix metalloproteinases after laser treatment. Retina. 2007;27(5):629–34.
35. Blumenkranz MS, Yellachich D, Andersen DE, Wiltberger MW, Mordaunt D, Marcellino GR, Palanker D. Semiautomated patterned scanning laser for retinal photocoagulation. Retina. 2006;26(3):370–6.
36. Jain A, Blumenkranz MS, Paulus Y, Wiltberger MW, Andersen DE, Huie P, Palanker D. Effect of pulse duration on size and character of the lesion in retinal photocoagulation. Arch Ophthalmol. 2008;126(1):78–85.
37. Menzler J, Neubauer A, Ziemssen F. Navigated laser in diabetic macular edema: the impact of reduced injection burden on patients and physicians-who wins and who loses? Int J Ophthalmol. 2019;12(2):342–5.
38. Kato F, Nozaki M, Kato A, Hasegawa N, Morita H, Yoshida M, Ogura Y. Evaluation of navigated laser photocoagulation (Navilas 577+) for the treatment of refractory diabetic macular edema. J Ophthalmol. 2018;2018:3978514.
39. Faghihi H, Roohipoor R, Mohammadi SF, Hojat-Jalali K, Mirshahi A, Lashay A, Piri N, Faghihi S. Intravitreal bevacizumab versus combined bevacizumab-triamcinolone versus macular laser photocoagulation in diabetic macular edema. Eur J Ophthalmol. 2008;18(6):941–8.

patients leads to migration of fibrocytes and macrophages in the posterior hyaloid, which is often thickened and taut. Since the hyalocytes can transform in myofibroblasts, the hyaloid also acquires contractile properties, contributing to macular traction [1, 9]. A common finding in anomalous PVD is the persistence of vitreo-papillary adhesions. When associated with vitreoschisis, they may influence the vectors of forces on the macular interface, causing tangential epiretinal traction and intraretinal changes with cysts formation. In the presence of tractions causing DME, anti-VEGF injections may be poorly effective and induce metaplasia of the epiretinal cells causing an increase of fibrosis and tractional phenomena [8].

13.1.1 The Role of Epiretinal Membrane in Diabetic Macular Edema

It is known that the prevalence of epiretinal membranes (ERM) is higher in diabetic patients [11]. ERM formation is caused by a fibrocellular proliferation on ILM surface, followed by a cellular contraction [12]. Diabetic ERM is associated with reactive gliosis, fibrosis, and migration of the Müller cells, which proliferate and transdifferentiate showing a fibroblast-like phenotype. They also play a role in ERM contraction due to their ability to express a smooth muscle actin, involved in membrane contraction and in collagen production. Fibroblast are also involved in diabetic ERM, since they secrete contractile proteins, induce intracellular contraction, and deposit collagen [11]. Glial cells in ERM produce cytokines and growth factors, which stimulate pathological neovascularization mediated by VEGF. Its receptors are located on the ERM surface. VEGF also contributes to the progression of DME. ERM acts as a physical barrier and it decreases drug penetration after intravitreal injections of anti-VEGF or steroids used to treat DME. There is an unclear association between intravitreal injections and ERM formation. There are reports of increased incidence of secondary ERM formation after intravitreal anti-VEGF injections, probably due to the retinal tissue fibrosis caused by anti-VEGFs. Intravitreal injections of dexamethasone implants may be considered a risk factor for secondary ERM development, due to the drug delivery system, which may induce mechanical stress in the vitreous cavity and at the vitreomacular interface [12]. Also, the higher the number of intravitreal injections, the higher it is the risk of secondary ERM development [12]. Intravitreal injections for the treatment of DME have a significantly limited efficacy in reducing central retinal thickness (CRT) in eyes with ERM compared to patients without ERM. Also, when ERM is present, visual acuity (VA) does not significantly improve after injections [12].

13.2 History of Vitrectomy for the Treatment of Diabetic Macular Edema

The observation that spontaneous PVD could lead to reduction or resolution of DME suggested that the surgical induction of a vitreomacular separation could contribute to DME improvement [4, 13]. Remarkably, the idea of a surgical option for DME treatment emerged in an era when anti-VEGF and steroid intravitreal injections were not yet available [10]. Some of the patients included in the studies regarding the role of pars plana vitrectomy (PPV), in fact, had an inadequate response to macular laser for the treatment of DME, which was the standard treatment at that time. Moreover, focal photocoagulation was successful in avoiding further visual loss, but was associated with a very low rate of visual improvement [14].

The first report of vitrectomy for the treatment of DME dates back to 1992, when Lewis et al. reported performing PPV with the separation of the posterior hyaloid in ten eyes with DME and traction associated with a thickened and taut posterior hyaloid. The results were encouraging, showing visual improvement in nine eyes, and resolution (in eight eyes) or decrease (in two eyes) of macular traction and edema [15]. It was suggested that the attached posterior vitreous cortex might cause macular traction, which could be surgically released. Indeed, it was reported that, during a 1-year postoperative follow-up, DME resolved in all eyes and more than half of the patients experienced visual improvement [16]. Vitrectomy was also performed after failure of focal/grid laser on eyes with a taut posterior hyaloid adherent to the macula, often associated with shallow tractional macular detachment [17]. A prospective randomized study was performed, showing that PPV was superior to observation in eyes with a DME lasting 6–18 months, inadequate response to macular laser treatment, and posterior hyaloid attachment. The operation positively influenced visual acuity and the morphology of the edema [18]. Due to the positive results obtained, PPV shortly became the treatment of choice in cases with DME associated with a tractional component [19].

Due to the encouraging results, it was suggested to use early vitrectomy as a first-line therapy in order to avoid macular photocoagulation in selected patients with a rapid progression of visual loss associated with thickening of the posterior macular hyaloid and diffuse DME. Interestingly, it was observed that the best results in terms of visual outcomes occurred when the interval between the diagnosis of DME with thickened posterior hyaloid and vitrectomy was less than 1 month [20].

Later on, surgery was explored as a treatment for eyes with attached but not thickened and not taut hyaloid [17]. On this topic, however, results were controversial. Multiple studies showed a resolution of persistent DME and a visual improvement after PPV [21]. Visual improvement appeared to be higher in eyes without preoperative macular laser treatment, while DME resolution was not affected by a previous history of laser therapy [22]. When comparing the postoperative results according to the presence of vitreomacular tractions and/or alterations of the vitreomacular interface, a CRT improvement was observed following PPV after a 6-months follow-up in all the patient groups [19]. Other studies, on the opposite, showed anatomical and functional benefit following PPV in patients affected by diffuse DME with taut and thickened posterior hyaloid, but not in those with diffuse DME without thickened and taut posterior hyaloid [23]. Also other work groups showed a less relevant efficacy of vitrectomy for diffuse DME in absence of tractions. Indeed, despite an initial significant reduction in CRT, after a follow-up of 1 year the reduction in thickness was no more significant. No significant change in VA was noted [24].

A surgical approach was considered also for those eyes with an already present PVD, in the absence of epiretinal or fibrovascular membrane. Some authors reported promising results. In a study, partial or complete reduction of DME was reported in most cases, associated with VA improvement. This suggested that vitrectomy-related benefits were not only related to the detachment of the posterior hyaloid membrane, but also to the removal of factors increasing vascular permeability such as VEGF [25]. When comparing eyes with thickened and taut posterior vitreous membrane, eyes with adherent posterior vitreous, and eyes with PVD, visual acuity improvement was found to be similar. In an era when macular photocoagulation still represented the mainstay of DME treatment, these findings suggested the role of PPV for those eyes expected to have poor prognosis following laser treatment [26].

Terasaki and colleagues performed a compelling study evaluating the postoperative functional response following PPV for the treatment of DME without a tractional component in eyes with or without preoperative PVD. They observed that the CRT decreased shortly after the operation, while a significant visual improvement occurred only 12 months after PPV. They also performed multifocal electroretinogram, which showed an improved amplitude, evident after a 12-months follow-up. Interestingly, the amplitude increase was more marked when the PVD was realized during surgery. The amplitude improvement was found to be significantly correlated to the decreased foveal thickness [27].

Some authors have tried to compare the effectiveness of PPV and of macular laser treatment, with contrasting results. The aim of the comparison was to define the role of vitrectomy as a potential first-line therapy for those eyes with severe edema and important visual loss at presentation [17]. A study showed an association between PPV and an improvement of both macular structure and visual acuity, when compared to the natural history of the disease. Even if vitrectomy was superior to laser for the reduction of foveal thickness after 6 months, the benefit was not maintained after 12 months. Concerning visual acuity outcomes, vitrectomy was not superior to laser after 6 months and had a trend towards inferior outcomes at 12 months [28]. Even if it was evident that PPV produced both structural and functional benefit in the treatment of DME, the functional benefit was not significantly better than after macular laser. The doubt was raised that the structural benefit might decline or possibly reverse over time [29].

13.2.1 Limits of Early Studies

It is not easy to compare the studies performed on the subject, since there are some major differences regarding inclusion criteria, postoperative variables, and surgical techniques. It is also difficult to evaluate VA changes, due to the different lens status of the patients, even in the same study [30, 31]. Also, the patients involved in the studies are usually not stratified according to their glycemic control. However, it is known that poor diabetic control is associated with lower visual gains [31]. Moreover, many patients undergo PPV after a long history of DME, refractory to multiple treatments [32, 33]. For example, a study demonstrated a persistent anatomical improvement 1 year after PPV, not accompanied by an amelioration of visual acuity, in eyes affected by DME, without vitreomacular traction, and resistant to laser treatment and anti-VEGF injections. A possible explanation for this finding is that PPV was performed in eyes with a prolonged history of cystoid DME, which may impair the functional outcomes [19].

Long-standing DME may cause damage to photoreceptors and inner retina. Nevertheless, there is evidence that PPV leads to significant reduction of DME and improvement of VA also in treatment-naïve eyes, with a history of DME lasting between 3 and 12 months prior to surgery. Once again, results are not easy to interpret due to the presence of both tractional and non-tractional macular edema in the study eyes [32, 33]. Finally, most studies exploring the role of vitrectomy for the treatment of DME were performed before the advent of anti-VEGF therapies. In the current era, it would be useful to understand if there is a change on anti-VEGF effectiveness postoperatively. However, no major trials on the subject have been conducted [31].

It must also be remarked that in the oldest studies OCT was not performed since it was not widely available yet [31, 34]. Later on, low-resolution time-domain OCT was used to evaluate the vitreomacular interface of the patients. Modern spectral-domain OCT (SD-OCT) is in fact a quite recent acquisition, allowing for a more precise identification of anomalies which were previously undetectable. Therefore, it is likely that not only mild interface anomalies but also vitreomacular tractions and epiretinal membranes were misdiagnosed in some cases. This observation may explain the heterogeneity of anatomical and functional results of the reported studies. Also, in the studies which evaluated the OCT in order to compare the effectiveness of the various treatments, CRT is considered as the main outcome. However, nowadays it is recognized that other OCT markers may be more predictive of visual outcomes, such as the disorganization of retinal inner layers and the integrity of the external limiting membrane and of the junction between inner and outer segments of the photoreceptors. However, there are currently no studies evaluating the role of these factors on the prognosis of DME following PPV [31].

13.3 Present Knowledge and Adequate Surgical Indications

Even if several studies have been conducted over time in order to establish the role of vitrectomy in the treatment of DME, guidelines on the topic are not available. High quality evidence is unfortunately lacking. This is due to the absence of randomized clinical trials and to the heterogeneous nature of the studies. Indeed, there are many small reports with a lack of common methodology. The patient populations are extremely heterogeneous. Moreover, PPV is often compared to laser treatment, but a large trial comparing results of vitrectomy and anti-VEGF injections is needed [29, 33].

Some clinical trials have been performed in order to define the benefits of PPV in selected cases of DME [35]. The European Vitreo-Retinal Society conducted a non-randomized multicenter study to evaluate the appropriacy of different treatments for DME. Remarkably, at baseline VA in the group of patients treated with vitrectomy was lower than in groups treated with other therapies. In this study PPV with ILM peeling demonstrated a visual recovery at least 2–3 times higher than other therapies, i.e. anti-VEGF injections, triamcinolone acetonide injections, macular laser. Visual acuity continued to improve 12–24 months after surgery. PPV with ILM peeling was superior also to combination treatment of PPV, ILM peeling, intraoperative triamcinolone acetonide injection. Treatment with PPV and ILM peeling resulted in better visual outcomes than other therapies, including intravitreal triamcinolone monotherapy, macular laser, and intravitreal anti-VEGF monotherapy [36].

In certain scenarios, PPV plays a major role in the management of DME, in order to reduce macular thickness and promote visual acuity gain by removing retinal traction exerted by the posterior hyaloid or an epiretinal membrane [17, 35]. At present, in the absence of evident macular traction, pharmacotherapy with injections of anti-VEGF and steroids is the first line of treatment for DME, since they counteract the breakdown of the blood–retinal barrier and the inflammation [37].

13.3.1 Vitreomacular Interface Alterations

The main indication for vitrectomy is represented by the concomitant presence of ERM and/or VMT [38]. It is crucial to correctly identify the vectors of forces exerted on the macular interface. The exact detection of antero-posterior and tangential tractions is fundamental in order to prevent misdiagnosis of tractional and refractory DME, and to avoid poor treatment outcomes as well. It is important to understand that tangential tractions play a major role in the context of anomalous PVD. Since it is not easy to clinically detect the tractions, en-face SD-OCT may be useful, both preoperatively and postoperatively [8]. When a tractional DME is present, with evident ERM or VMT, it has been suggested to perform at first one intravitreal anti-VEGF injection, and subsequent surgery in case of inadequate response [39]. PPV appears to be useful when vitreoretinal interface abnormalities impede DME resolution, since it reduces the tangential and anterior-posterior tractions at the macula [8, 28, 40]. In fact, there is consensus that eyes with DME with vitreomacular interface anomalies such as an evident traction over the macula benefit from a surgical approach [33, 41, 42]. It is reasonable to perform PPV early in these patients, in order to relieve the tractions before damage of the foveal photoreceptors occur [43]. ERM removal is associated with a VA improvement, without association with degree of retinal thickness reduction, potentially reflecting resolution of distorted vision from ERM in addition to DME resolution [44].

The efficacy and safety of PPV for the treatment of DME associated with VMT were reported by a prospective observational study performed by DRCR.net [1]. A study has compared the results of vitrectomy in patients with DME and either VMT or ERM. It showed that the greatest VA improvements were seen in patients with a VMT, causing antero-posterior traction. However, the highest final VA was observed in cases with ERM, causing tangential traction. The most important CRT reduction was noted in patients with VMT, reflecting a higher grade of macular atrophy, related to a preoperative irreversible damage of the retinal layers. This finding may explain the reduced improvement in terms of VA [41]. It has been observed that, while in patients affected by idiopathic ERMs the main reduction in CRT takes place within 6 months after PPV and ERM removal, after diabetic ERM removal the CRT progressively and slowly reduces during the first year after the operation [45].

The preoperative evaluation of ERM appears to be a useful predictor of visual improvement in cases of resistant DME treated with PPV [46]. However, it must be noted that pathologic fibrocellular changes at the vitreomacular interface are present in all eyes with DME irrespective of the presence of an ERM [37].

13.3.2 Diffuse DME Without a Clinically Evident Tractional Component

There is more debate regarding the efficacy of vitrectomy for the treatment of diffuse DME without a tractional component [24]. There is evidence that PPV is likely to be more effective in terms of VA improvement in eyes with vitreomacular traction than in patients without traction. Other studies, on the opposite, show a similar VA improvement in patients with or without traction [30, 47]. A study has showed the same postoperative results after a 3 years follow-up, in terms of anatomical and visual improvement, both in eyes with tractional DME and in eyes without VMT but with DME resistant to laser photocoagulation or triamcinolone acetonide intravitreal injection [48]. A study on vitrectomy for the treatment of non-tractional DME showed a sustained VA improvement, maintained up to 80 months following PPV [34]. Some studies show that vitrectomy provides long-term benefits also for diffuse DME, not associated with a thickened posterior hyaloid. These studies claim that ILM peeling removes the tangential tractions exerted by the residual cortical vitreous and ILM and prevents postoperative ERM formation [9]. Also, the inflammatory mediators present in the pathological vitreous cause persistent edema [8]. Moreover, since the vitreous in diabetic eyes is rich in VEGF and inflammatory cytokines, vitreous removal leads to an antiangiogenic shift in eyes with proliferative diabetic retinopathy (PDR) [9]. It has been shown that the removal of the majority of the vitreous body along with the hyaloid membrane increases intraocular cytokine turnover and removes mechanical barriers to the egress of fluid and metabolites [40]. PPV also increases the oxygenation of the inner retinal layers by removing the diffusion barrier represented by a thickened ILM when present. There is evidence that increased oxygenation can reduce DME [1, 8, 9, 40]. This appears to be especially important since DME itself exacerbates retinal hypoxia, creating a vicious cycle, which can be interrupted by reducing CRT. The improved oxygenation may also lead to visual acuity improvement, especially in patients with recent-onset macular edema [49]. Moreover, it has been demonstrated that macular blood flow is higher in eyes affected by DME, and that it is reduced after resolution of DME, 12 weeks after vitrectomy. This appears to be relevant since the alterations in blood flow may play a critical role in the development and progression of DME. Postoperative reduction in CRT, but not improvement in VA, appears to be related with the reduction in macular blood flow [50].

13.3.3 Unresponsive Cases

It is also known that some patients continue to have impaired visual outcomes and persistent DME despite adequate therapy with intravitreal anti-VEGFs and steroids [51]. In cases of patient's refractory to anti-VEGF therapy, intravitreal steroids represent an alternative. However, it has been demonstrated that anatomic improvements are not always accompanied by visual gains [52]. According to different studies, inadequate response to anti-VEGF agents may be defined as a reduction in CRT of less than 10–20%, or an improvement in BCVA of less than 5 letters, but also as a too frequent recurrence [39]. Studies have been performed in order to establish the role of PPV in the treatment of intractable DME. The results showed a reduction of DME with stabilization of the retinal anatomy maintained over a 1-year follow up. VA stabilized as well, but an improvement was noted only in those eyes presenting an ERM or a VMT preoperatively [51]. Due to its long lasting effect after a single procedure, PPV may be advised for cases resistant to anti-VEGF injections. It is also likely that some mechanisms in the genesis of the edema are not VEGF dependent. However, it is possible that the outcomes of vitrectomy in this type of patients are worse than expected, due to the difficulty in treating these eyes [43].

Even if it has been demonstrated that vitrectomy leads to stable anatomical improvements in cases of recalcitrant DME, there is a discrepancy between anatomical and functional results [8, 40]. In fact, 6 months and 1-year follow-ups after PPV show absent or only slight visual improvement [1, 19]. This finding suggests that factors other than macular thickness may influence the functional outcome [8].

An interesting study analyzed the effects of vitrectomy in eyes with non-tractional DME, unresponsive to non-surgical therapies including anti-VEGF injections. It showed that eyes with an enlarged foveal avascular zone (FAZ) did not show any anatomical or functional improvement, while recovery occurred in patients with a preserved FAZ, after a 6-months follow-up. This suggests that the reason for the recalcitrance of DME both to surgical and non-surgical therapies may be found in the extent of macular ischemia. Indeed, vitrectomy does not have any efficacy on the mechanisms of foveal thickening induced by macular ischemia, such as the necrosis of Müller cells [53]. This may give an explanation to the contrasting results of PPV for non-tractional edema, since in most studies the size of the FAZ is not evaluated postoperatively.

13.3.4 Special Situations

Anti-VEGF injections, which are the first line of treatment of DME, do not alleviate macular hypoxia and multiple injections for an extended timespan are usually needed [10]. Also, in some world areas anti-VEGFs may not be administered on a regular basis due to the cost and restrictions to their usage [32]. Therefore, surgery may be advised for those patients for whom intravitreal treatment is not feasible for multiple reasons [33, 43].

It needs to be kept in mind that, while benefit following anti-VEGF injections is quicker, visual and functional recovery following PPV is much slower. In fact, approximately 3–4 months are required for stabilization of macular edema, and the VA improvement occurs between 12 and 24 months postoperatively. On the other hand, the effects are more sustained than after intravitreal injections [43].

13.4 Surgical Technique

At present there is no consensus regarding the technique for pars plana vitrectomy for the treatment of DME [38]. In phakic patients, cataract surgery is performed at the same time as vitrectomy, if needed [42]. The studies on this topic describe progressively evolving techniques. In order to reduce surgical time and minimize the trauma to the eye, surgical techniques and instruments progressively improved.

Therefore, the diameter of the instruments progressively reduced, moving from 20 gauge vitrectomy to small gauge transconjunctival sutureless vitrectomy, i.e. 23-, 25-, and 27-gauge [10, 19]. Posterior segment visualization is also improving progressively, thanks to the introduction of wide-angle viewing systems [43]. Vitrectomy is performed with three pars plana sclerotomies, which are performed transconjunctivally with small gauge vitrectomy systems. The vitreous gel is completely removed. If PVD is not already present, it is usually induced using the vitrectomy probe with aspiration only. Triamcinolone acetonide can be used intraoperatively to visualize the vitreous during procedures such as posterior vitreous separation. Thanks to the improved visualization, it reduces the incidence of iatrogenic retinal breaks and retinal detachment. The most common complication is the elevation of the intraocular pressure due to residual triamcinolone in the eye [38, 42, 54]. The posterior hyaloid, which can be strongly attached, is removed as well as the peripheral vitreous, leaving only a small residual vitreous skirt [1, 16, 19, 26, 38, 41]. If a membrane is present on the retinal surface, it can be stained and subsequently removed, as it happens for the removal of idiopathic ERM [1, 26, 38, 41]. If the patient also presents a proliferative diabetic retinopathy, endophotocoagulation is performed as needed [26, 41]. Before the end of the operation, it is necessary to check the peripheral retina and perform laser or cryotherapy on retinal breaks if any [1, 38]. Suture of the sclerotomies may be performed according to the gauge of the vitrectomy. There is no conclusive evidence on the use of air tamponade [33]. Some authors also report the use of subconjunctival injection of 2 mg dexamethasone at the end of the operation [42, 55].

13.4.1 The Role of ILM Peeling

While there is consensus on ERM removal when present, a still debated issue regards the role of ILM peeling, since sufficient data on the topic is not yet available [33, 56]. The idea that ILM peeling may be effective in patients affected by DME derives from multiple observations. For instance, vitreous collagen covers the ILM, even in patients with a history of PVD or PPV. A layer of cortical vitreous remains at the vitreomacular interface, containing fibroblasts, astrocytes, and macrophages. Therefore, ILM peeling may lead to a more complete removal of inflammatory and tractional components from the retinal surface. It is important to evaluate the real utility of ILM peeling, since it also carries some risks, such as retinal breaks, dissociated optic nerve fiber layer, damage to Müller cells [31]. Multiple studies evaluating the role of vitrectomy on different types of DME do not often provide a comparison between PPV with and without ILM peeling [31, 51]. ILM peeling may afford improved structural but not functional outcomes over vitrectomy alone [28]. The first studies on the subject showed a faster resolution of DME and a lower recurrence rate when performing ILM peeling during vitrectomy. The advocated mechanism was the release of all the traction forces on the retinal surface and the removal of the scaffold used by astrocytes for proliferation on the retinal surface [57]. The greater structural improvement after ILM peeling may result from the additional removal of residual vitreous cortex after PVD [58]. However, it has also been found that the acceleration of DME resolution was not associated with final VA and rate of DME resolution [59]. A study with a long-term follow-up of patients undergoing PPV with and without ILM peeling showed a significant progressive VA improvement until 1 year postoperatively. VA remained stable during the next 4 years and started to slightly decline afterwards, even if no significant complications occurred. More than half the eyes had a visual improvement of at least two lines at the final visit, compared to the preoperative assessment. All the eyes included in the study presented a diffuse DME without tractions. At 6 months and 1 year follow-up PPV with ILM peeling showed better VA results than PPV alone. However, at 5 years there was no significant difference in visual outcomes [55]. This study, as well as others, concluded that ILM peeling did not seem to affect the visual outcomes of the patients [47, 55, 58]. The literature shows no significant difference between patient groups undergoing vitrectomy with or without ILM peeling, in terms of either visual acuity or CRT [56]. In cases of diffuse non-tractional DME, there is evidence that PPV leads to a sustained visual improvement, regardless of ILM peeling [34]. Indeed, it appears that in cases of diffuse DME both the anatomical and the visual outcomes are not different whether ILM is peeled or not [60]. Multiple studies have not shown a statistically significant difference regarding VA and CRT outcomes following PPV with or without ILM peeling for the treatment of non-tractional DME, with a follow-up between 12 and 80 months [61]. However, the studies show heterogeneous results. Indeed, there are also reports sustaining that ILM peeling provides greater VA improvement when compared to PPV alone [62]. Some studies report good results when performing PPV with ILM peeling in cases refractory to other treatments [19]. When comparing multiple studies on the subject, the main issue is the absence of randomized clinical trials. At this point of our knowledge, it is likely that the most suitable surgical strategy should be tailored on every single patient, also considering the ILM anatomy [56, 61]. Another problem affecting interpretation of studies on the role of ILM peeling is the heterogeneity of systemic factors that contribute to VA outcomes, such as HbA1c and duration of diabetes [31].

It must also be noted that, before the introduction of modern products for ILM staining, indocyanine green (ICG) was used. It was usually injected under balanced salt solution and immediately washed to reduce the incidence of side effects [42]. This agent has been associated with retinal toxicity and could therefore have had a negative effect on treatment outcomes [28]. As an example, a study showed that ILM staining with triamcinolone acetonide led to better visual results when compared to non-peeling or ICG staining. However, there was no difference in CRT reduction among the three groups [63]. Nowadays, the mostly used vital dyes contain trypan blue and brilliant blue G (triphenylmethane). They are injected under balanced salt solution, usually with closed infusion, and they are washed away after 2 min [19, 42]. In diabetic patients, the ILM may be more difficult to remove since it is usually strongly adherent and it is easier to break than in non-diabetic patients. Therefore, its staining is even more important [42].

13.4.1.1 Present Knowledge on ILM Peeling

The current knowledge on the role of ILM and on the consequences of its peeling is more detailed than it was in the past decades. ILM peeling is a traumatic procedure that can cause retinal damage, especially in pathologically impaired retinas. The diabetic ILM appears thicker than a normal ILM due to the proliferation of cell populations such as neutrophils, macrophages, lymphocytes, fibroblast-like cells. Moreover, Müller cells and ILM astrocytes in the presence of epiretinal gliosis are associated with an overexpression of the intermediate filament glial fibrillary acid protein (GFAP), which acts as a bridge between Müller cells and ILM, increasing their adhesion. Therefore, ILM peeling in diabetic eyes may lead to further damage to Müller cells, with structural collapse of the retina and damage of the outer retinal layers. The postoperative visual outcome appears to be worse when vitrectomy with ILM peeling is performed in presence of intraretinal cysts higher than 390 μm. The subfoveal atrophy may be responsible of the significant reduction in central retinal thickness in these eyes, in which the height of the cysts decreases but BCVA worsens. Therefore, vitrectomy with ILM peeling in these patients is not recommended [8]. However, a recent study showed that severe disruption of the external limiting membrane may be responsible of many cases of postoperative macular atrophy, which were previously considered caused by ILM peeling. This same study did not show any association between PPV with ILM peeling and macular atrophy during a 2-year follow up [64]. Moreover, while in eyes with idiopathic ERM ILM peeling reduces ERM recurrence, in diabetic eyes there is no evidence of a similar benefit [45].

13.4.2 Combined Treatments

The beneficial effects of vitrectomy may improve using combined treatments [8, 10, 35]. It has been reported that intraoperative usage of triamcinolone acetonide may be associated to a less significant breakdown of the blood–ocular barrier than when performing PPV alone [10]. A study showed that the association of PPV with ILM peeling, intravitreal injection of triamcinolone acetonide, peripheral, and grid/focal laser photocoagulation for the treatment of non-tractional unresponsive DME leads to functional and anatomical recovery, starting at 3 weeks postoperatively and persisting at a 3-year follow-up [65]. In eyes with non-tractional DME, PPV can also be combined with focal laser and 0.7 mg dexamethasone intravitreal implant, with an improvement of VA and CRT, persistent at 1-year follow-up [66]. However, also on this subject there is a relevant lack of consensus.

Indeed, other studies claim that there is no significant association between steroid injections at the end of PPV and improved visual outcomes [47]. It was observed that, in cases of diffuse DME without tractions, either ILM peeling

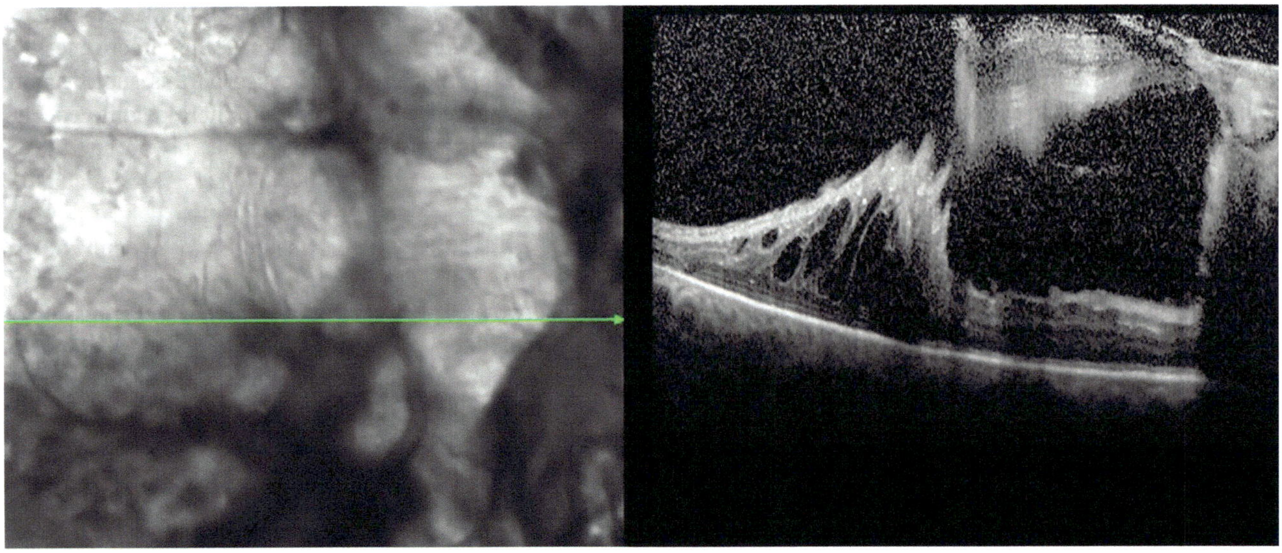

Fig. 13.2 SD-OCT horizontal line of the right eye. The complete alteration of the macular structure is evident as well as the traction exerted by the preretinal fibrosis

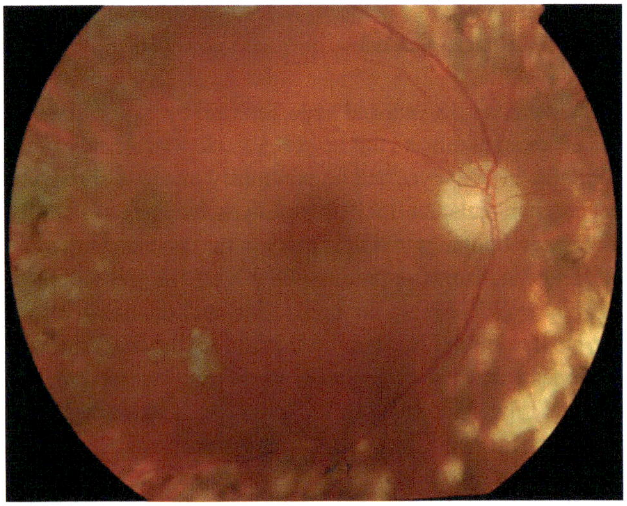

Fig. 13.3 Color photography of the right eye 12 months after surgery. Neither preretinal fibrosis nor neovascularization are present

20/100. Surgery was therefore planned. One week before vitrectomy, an intravitreal injection of anti-VEGF was performed in order to help with the dissection of the fibrosis and to reduce the risk of intraoperative bleeding. He subsequently underwent 27-gauge PPV in his right eye, with dissection and complete removal of the preretinal fibrosis. The PRP was also completed intraoperatively. After the operation, he did not receive further treatment but he underwent regular examinations. Twelve months after vitrectomy was performed, neither preretinal fibrosis nor DME were evident, and the foveal profile returned to normal, without any signs of traction (Figs. 13.3 and 13.4). The VA improved to 20/50, 12 months postoperatively.

It is interesting to observe how the foveal architecture may postoperatively return to normal even if severely disrupted by the traction exerted by a preretinal membrane. The preoperative injection of anti-VEGF may improve surgical out- comes without increasing retinal traction.

13.6.2 Clinical Case 2

This patient is a 61-year-old male, with a 15 years history of type II diabetes. His most recent Hba1c was 7.3%. He was pseudophakic in both eyes and he had a bilateral PDR, for which he underwent PRP in both eyes. When he was firstly evaluated, his VA in the right eye was 20/100. He presented DME and a thickened posterior hyaloid strongly attached to the retina in the macular region. The CRT measured with SS-OCT was 580 μm and a complete alteration of the macular profile was evident (Figs. 13.5, 13.6 and 13.7). He underwent 27-gauge vitrectomy with removal of the posterior hyaloid. Six months postoperatively, DME was no more present and the CRT reduced to 210 μm, with an improvement of the macular profile. The VA improved to 20/63 (Figs. 13.8, 13.9 and 13.10).

This case underlines how, in selected cases of DME with a relevant tractional component, vitrectomy with removal of the thickened and taut posterior hyaloid and relaxation of the tractions, can be considered the treatment of choice with no need of performing intravitreal injections first.

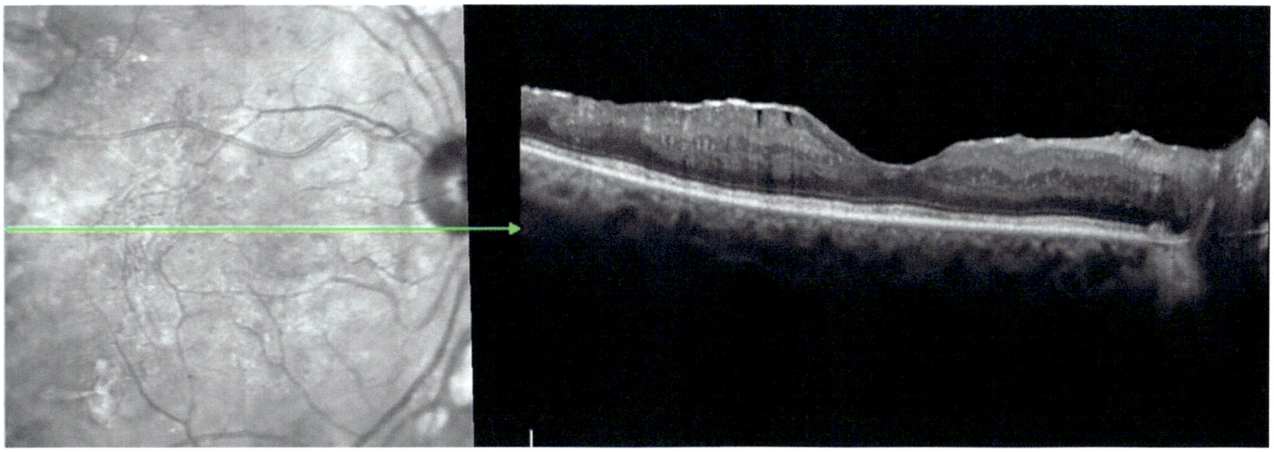

Fig. 13.4 SD-OCT horizontal line of the right eye 12 months postoperatively. The restoration of the normal macular morphology is evident, with restoration of the normal foveal depression

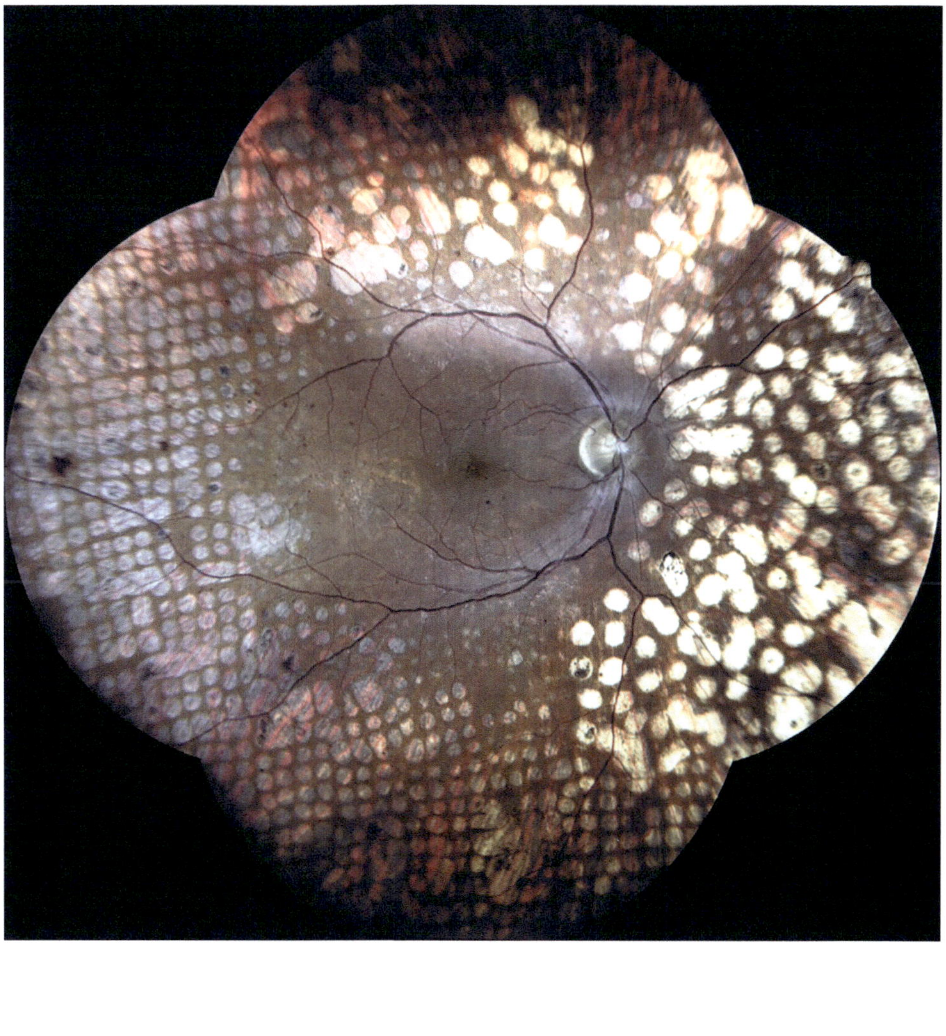

Fig. 13.5 Color fundus photography of the right eye of the patient

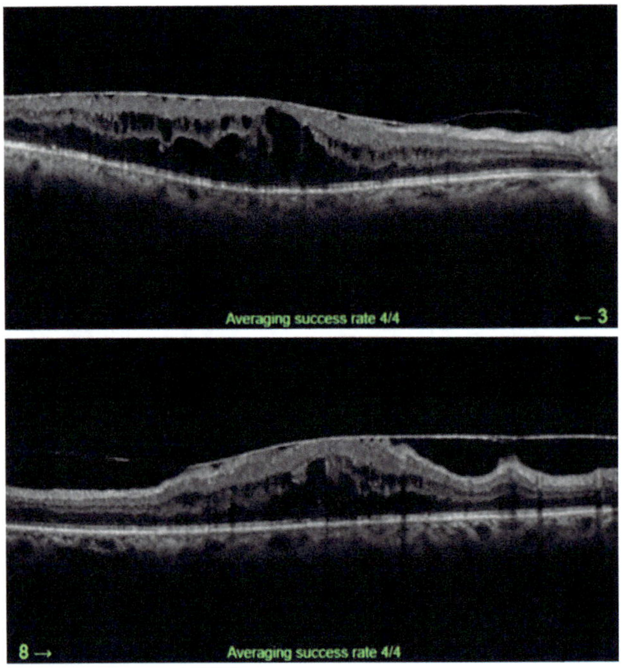

Fig. 13.6 Macular horizontal and vertical lines of the right eye, taken with a SS-OCT. DME and thickened and taut posterior hyaloid are evident

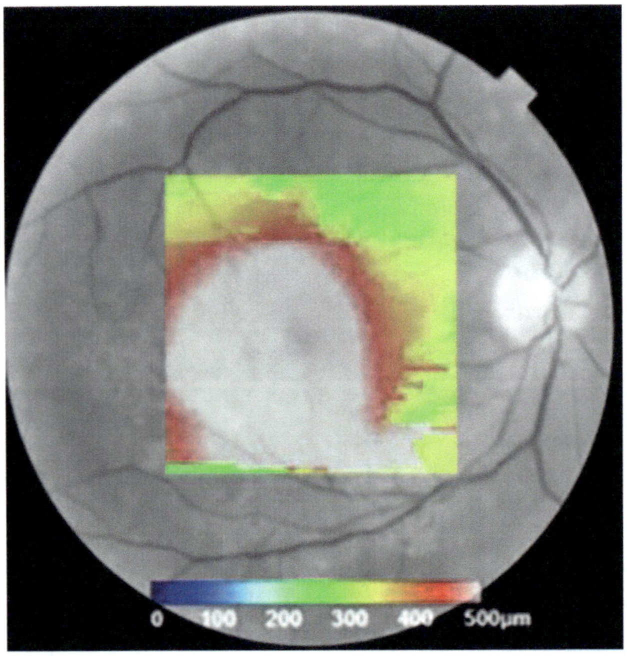

Fig. 13.7 SS-OCT map showing severely increased retinal thickness in the macular region

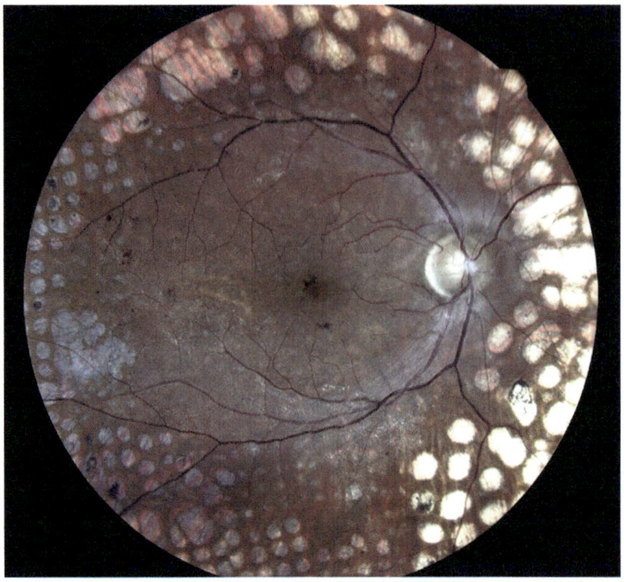

Fig. 13.8 Color fundus photography of the posterior pole of the right eye, 6 months postoperatively

13.6.3 Clinical Case 3

This patient is a 71-year-old man, affected by type 2 diabetes. He already under- went cataract surgery in the past, as well as PRP for a PDR. He was referred for a DME unresponsive to dexamethasone intravitreal implant performed on both eyes 2 months earlier. His VA was 20/50 on both the right and the left eye. Both eyes had an ERM with increased CRT and DME. Remarkably, the retinal profile on the left eye also showed a pseudo-hole appearance (Figs. 13.11, 13.12, 13.13 and 13.14). One month after the visit, 25-gauge PPV was performed on the left eye, with ERM removal and ILM peeling after staining with a combination of trypan blue and brilliant blue G. An intravitreal injection of anti-VEGF was also performed at the end of the operation. One month postoperatively, the macular profile improved, with resolution of the pseudo-hole and of the retinal wrinkling and improvement of the DME as well. VA was stable at 20/50 (Fig. 13.15). At the same time, also the right eye was evaluated. VA had decreased to 20/100 and the anatomical situation was stable. The patient decided to undergo surgery on the right eye 2 months later. The surgeon was the same, as well as the surgical technique. The only difference was that no intravitreal injection was performed at the end of the operation. One month later, the VA on the right eye improved

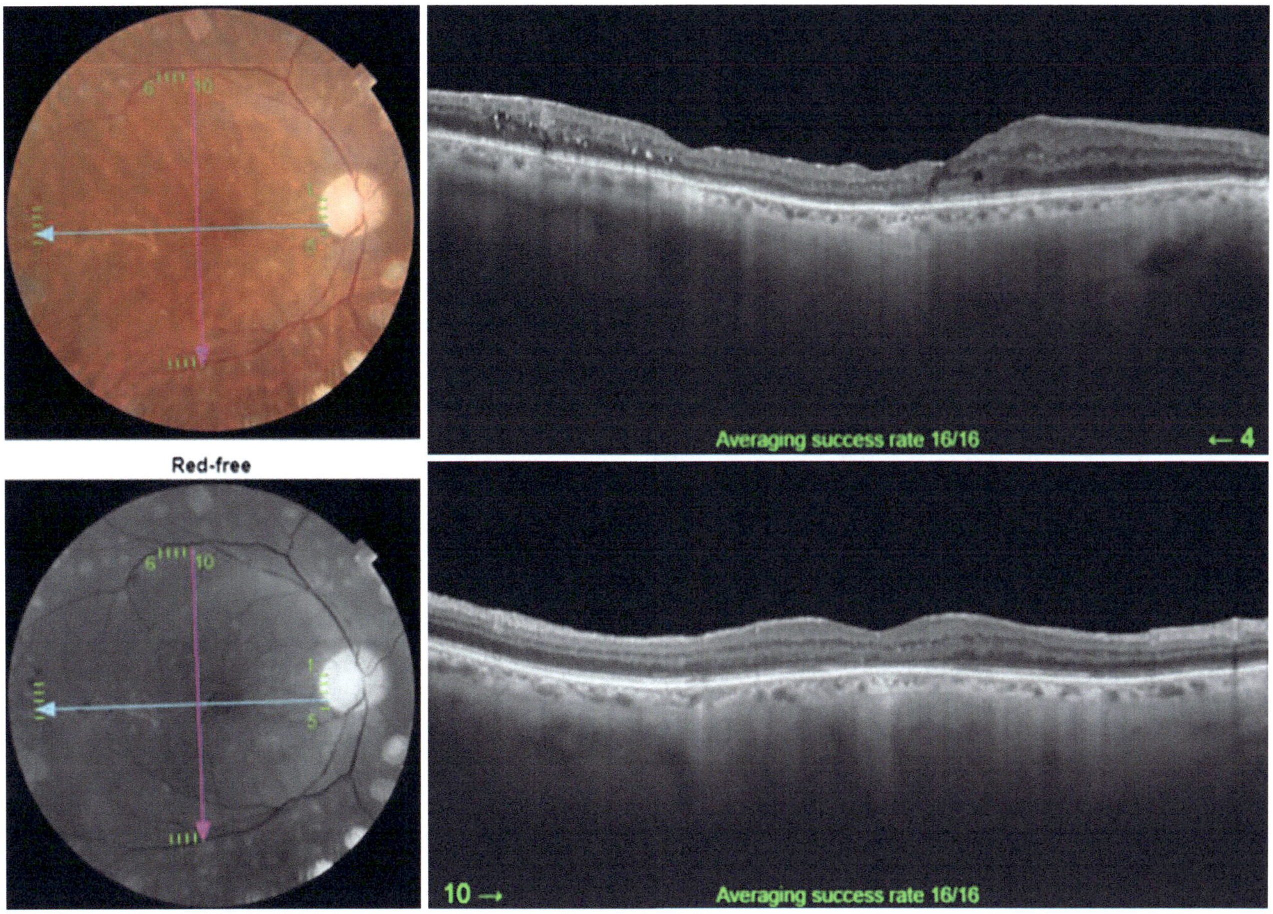

Fig. 13.9 Horizontal and vertical line centered on the macula, taken with SS-OCT, 6 months after vitrectomy

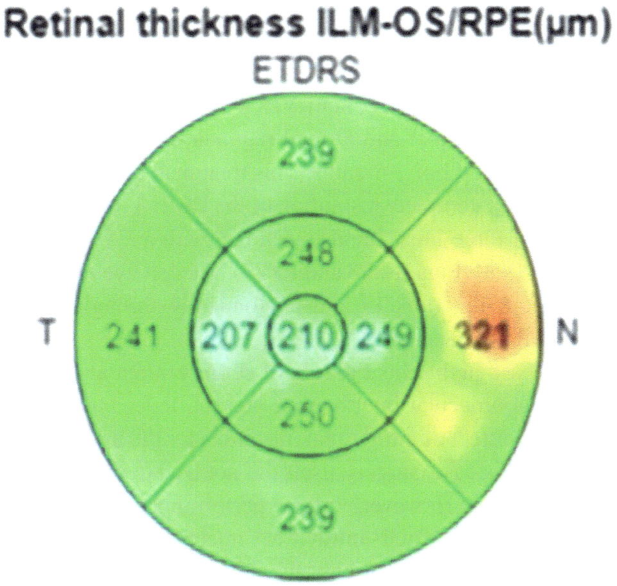

Fig. 13.10 Macular thickness cube obtained with SS-OCT, which shows the normalization of the CRT 6 months after surgery

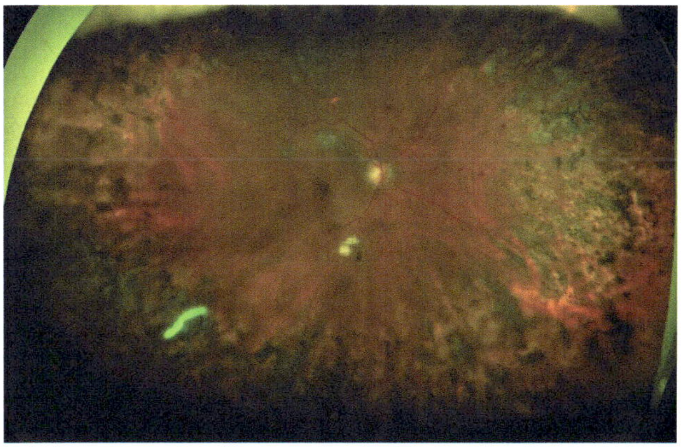

Fig. 13.11 Color fundus photography of the right eye at baseline. The dexamethasone implant is still visible in the inferotemporal sector of vitreous chamber

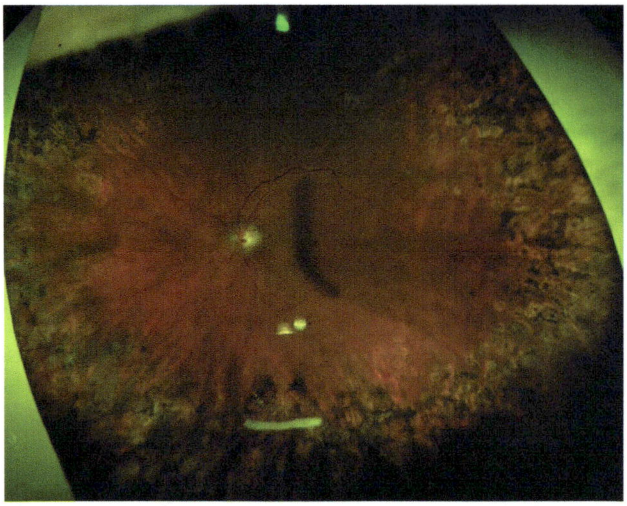

Fig. 13.12 Color fundus photography of the left eye at baseline. The visualization of the macular area is impaired by the shadow of the dexamethasone implant still present in the vitreous chamber

to 20/50, and an improvement was noted also from an anatomical point of view. The foveal anatomy improved and the DME reduced. A marked reduction in CRT was noted (Figs. 13.16 and 13.17) The left eye, which was at the fourth postoperative month, was also evaluated on the same day. No further treatments were performed after surgery. The VA was stable and a further anatomical improvement was remarked, in absence of further treatment after surgery. The foveal profile improved and the CRT reduced. No significant DME was present (Figs. 13.18 and 13.19).

This case presents a particular interest since it highlights that intravitreal injections are not always mandatory during surgery. Indeed, the macular anatomy of the right eye improved even in absence of injections performed at the end of surgery. It must also be noted that the postoperative improvement may be progressive and slow over time, as seen in the left eye of this patient, without the need of performing further medical or surgical treatment. Surgery appears to be effective also on those potentially associated anomalies, such as the pseudo-hole in this case.

Another remark concerns the difference between different imaging modalities. Indeed, while the alterations of the macular profile and the ERM are well evident on the SD-OCT images and appear to be severe, the macular appearance at the fundus photography does not reflect this grade of severity. Moreover, while the postoperative improvement is relevant in both eyes by evaluating the OCT images, the fundus photographs show a less relevant difference compared to baseline. This highlights the importance of multimodal imaging when studying these macular alterations, since the clinical observation alone may not be sufficient in certain cases.

13.6.4 Clinical Case 4

This is a 72-year-old woman, affected by type 2 diabetes since she was 39 years old. She had been on insulin therapy for 18 years. She was regularly followed in the retina service of the hospital for a severe NPDR, treated with PRP. She underwent uneventful bilateral cataract surgery. On the right eye she had a visual acuity of 20/50 and she presented a VMT and a DME, for which she was treated with an intravitreal implant of dexamethasone (Fig. 13.20). On the left eye the VA was 20/25 and she presented an almost normal foveal profile, with a very mild noncentral macular edema, therefore no treatment was performed (Figs. 13.21 and 13.22). Two months after the dexamethasone implant, the VA remained stable on the right eye and only a mild reduction in CRT was noted (Fig. 13.23). Five months after the intravitreal implant the DME persisted, and both ERM and VMT were noted (Fig. 13.24). There was a mild visual loss with a VA of 20/60. The patient, however, was not willing to undergo surgery, therefore 3 monthly injections of anti-VEGF were performed. One month after the third injection, VA was further reduced to 20/100 and there was no anatomical improvement (Figs. 13.25 and 13.26). The patient decided to undergo surgery. One month after, a 25-gauge PPV was performed on the right eye in order to release the vitreomacular traction and remove the ERM. The posterior hyaloid was completely detached during surgery, the ERM was removed and the ILM was peeled after staining with trypan blue and brilliant blue G. A complete fluid-air exchange was realized. An intravitreal injection of anti-VEGF was performed at the end of the surgery. One month postoperatively the VA was stable. As it concerns the macular anatomy, the DME persisted even if the ERM was no longer present and the VMT was released (Fig. 13.27). Therefore, anti-VEGF injections were performed with a Treat and Extend regimen, with a maximum injection interval of 2 months. This treatment eventually led to the almost complete resolution of the DME 3 months after the last of three intravitreal injections, with a VA improvement to 20/50 (Figs. 13.28 and 13.29). The left eye remained stable both functionally and anatomically throughout the entire follow-up period.

This case highlights the role of surgery when alterations of the vitreomacular interface are present. Indeed, they may impair the effect of intravitreal injections for the treatment of DME. In this case, surgery itself did not lead to a significant improvement. However, after performing surgery the response to anti-VEGF intravitreal injections changed dramatically. Moreover, not only the injections led to a greater anatomical and functional improvement, but also the interval between the injections was longer than it was before surgery.

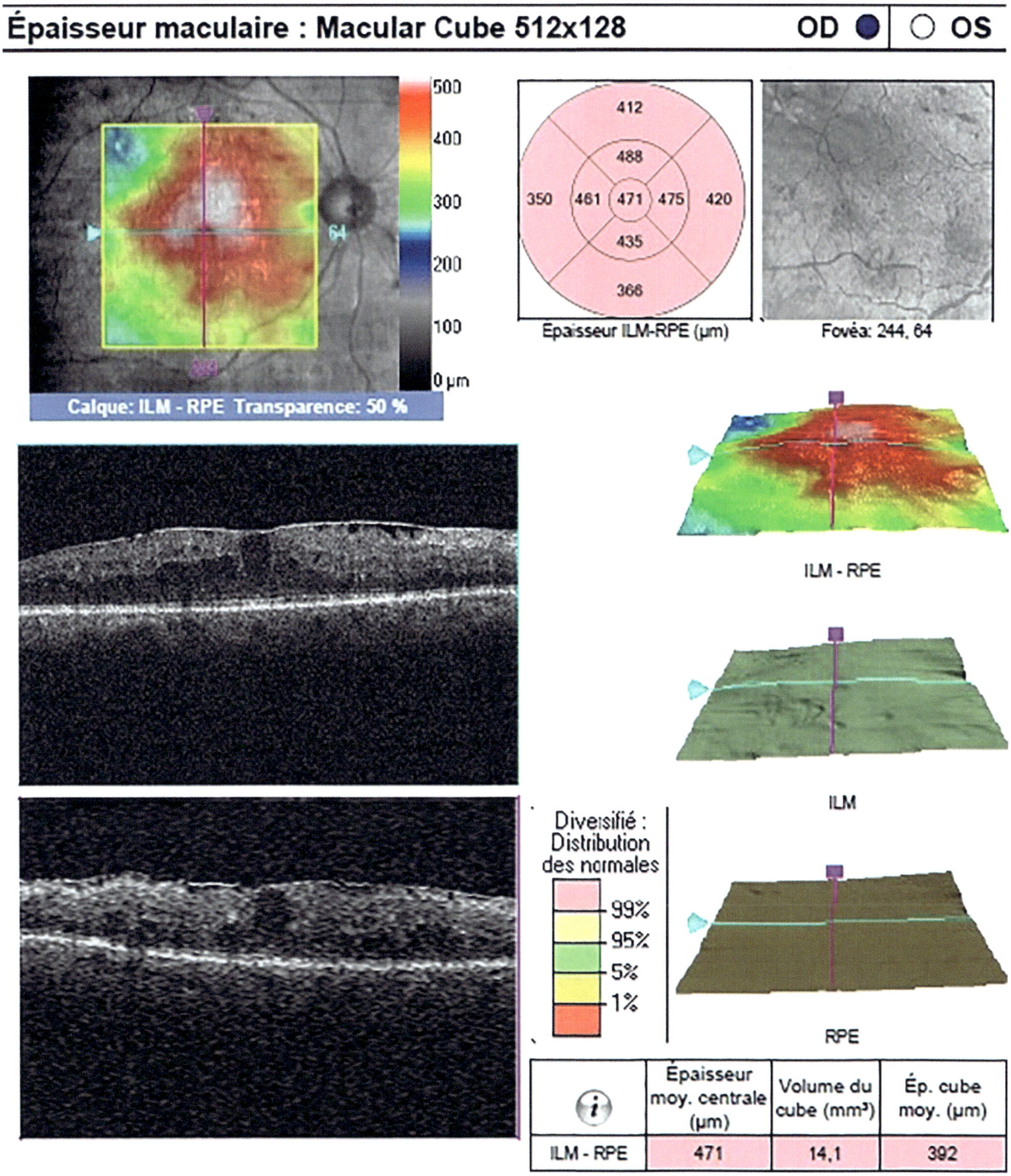

Fig. 13.13 SD-OCT macular cube of the right eye at baseline

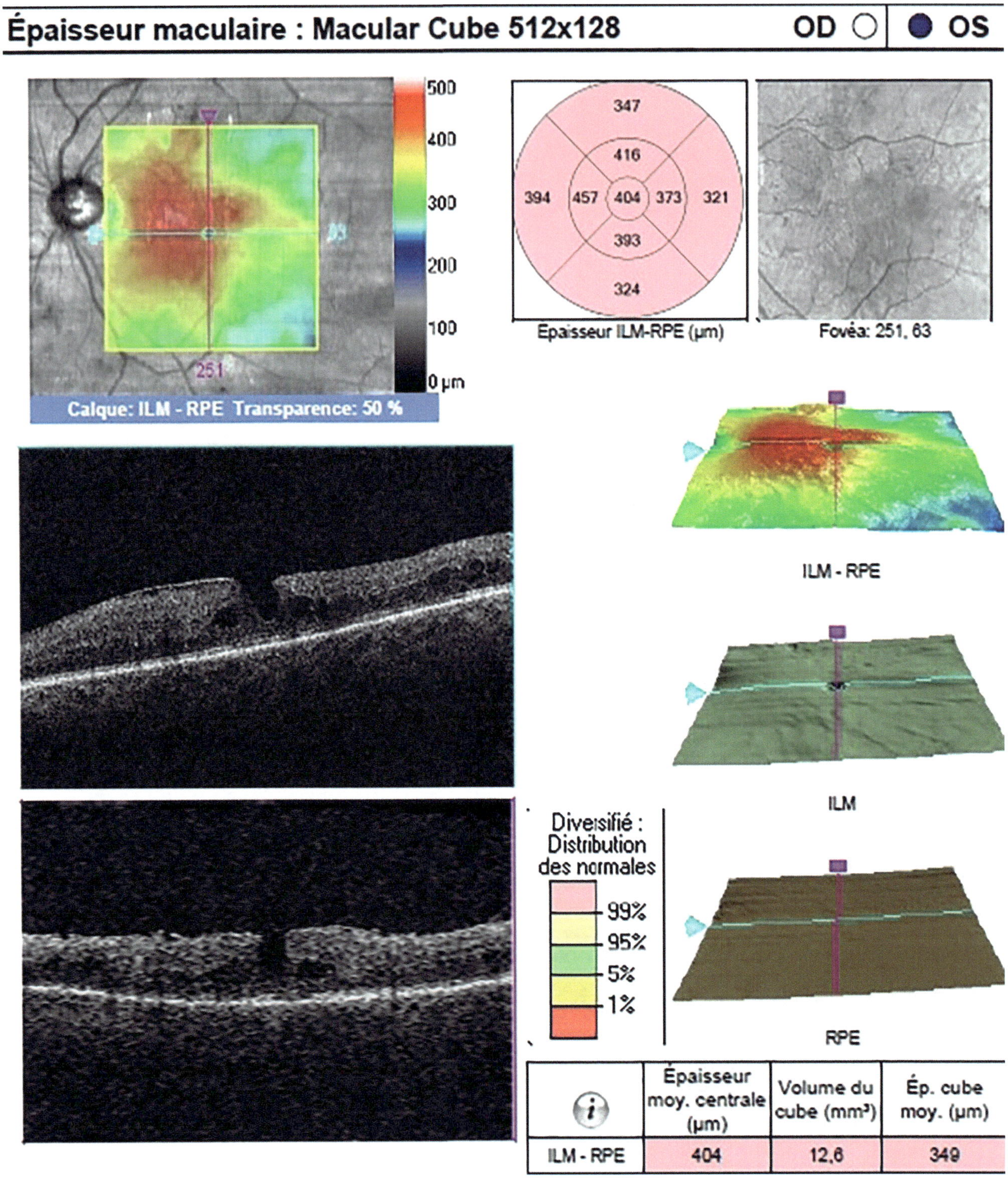

Fig. 13.14 SD-OCT macular cube of the left eye at baseline

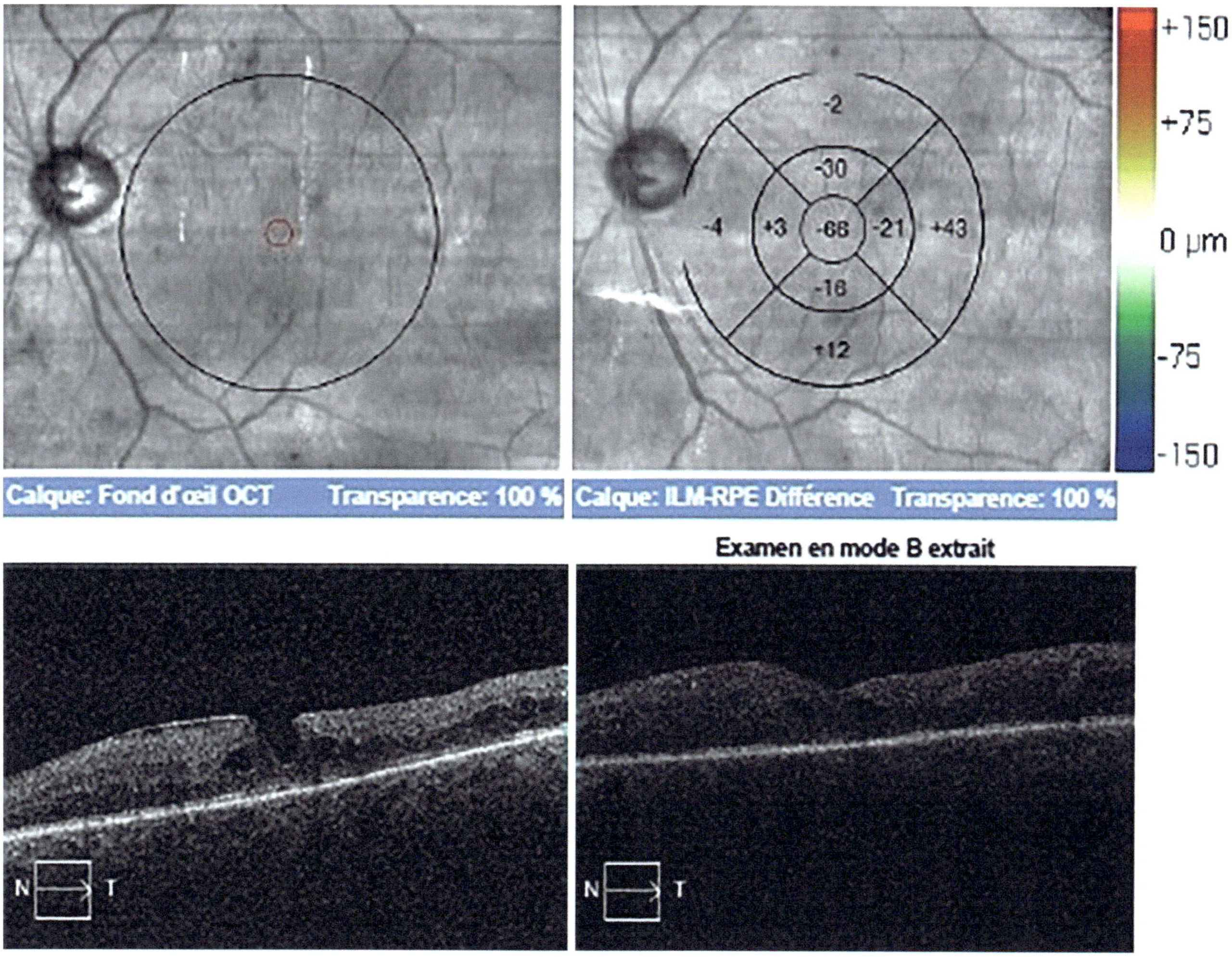

Fig. 13.15 Left eye: comparison between the macular cube at baseline (on the left) and 1 month after surgery (on the right)

13.6.5 Clinical Case 5

This patient is a 54-year-old woman, with an history of type 2 diabetes and an HbA1c of 8.8%. She had a PDR treated with partial PRP in both eyes. She was regularly followed in the hospital for a bilateral DME treated with multiple bilateral injections of anti-VEGF. She was pseudophakic in both eyes. The right eye did not present any major anomalies apart of the DME, which responded well to anti-VEGF (Figs. 13.30 and 13.31). On the opposite, during her follow-up, the development of a thick VMT on the left eye was noted, and she was addressed to surgery. VA was 20/20 on the right eye and 20/50 on the left eye (Figs. 13.32 and 13.33). A 25-gauge PPV was performed, detaching the thickened posterior hyaloid from the retina. Triamcinolone acetonide was used intraoperatively to improve vitreal visualization. ILM peeling was realized after staining with trypan blue and brilliant blue G. PPR was completed intraoperatively, and anti-VEGF injection was performed at the end of surgery. One month postoperatively, VA raised to 20/30 and the macular profile improved dramatically, with a restoration of the foveal depression and a relevant reduction of the DME (Fig. 13.34). The patient was subsequently treated with intravitreal injections of anti-VEGF and steroids. After 2 years from the intervention, the VA was preserved, and from an anatomical point of view the DME responded well to the intravitreal treatment (Figs. 13.35 and 13.36).

In this case, the prolonged benefits obtained performing surgery in eyes with DME and concomitant VMT and/or ERM are well evident, as well as the optimal postoperative response to intravitreal injections. Moreover, also in this case a discrepancy between the severity of the vitreomacular interface alterations observed at color fundus photography and at OCT is noted. Once again, this remarks the importance of a multimodal imaging approach in these patients.

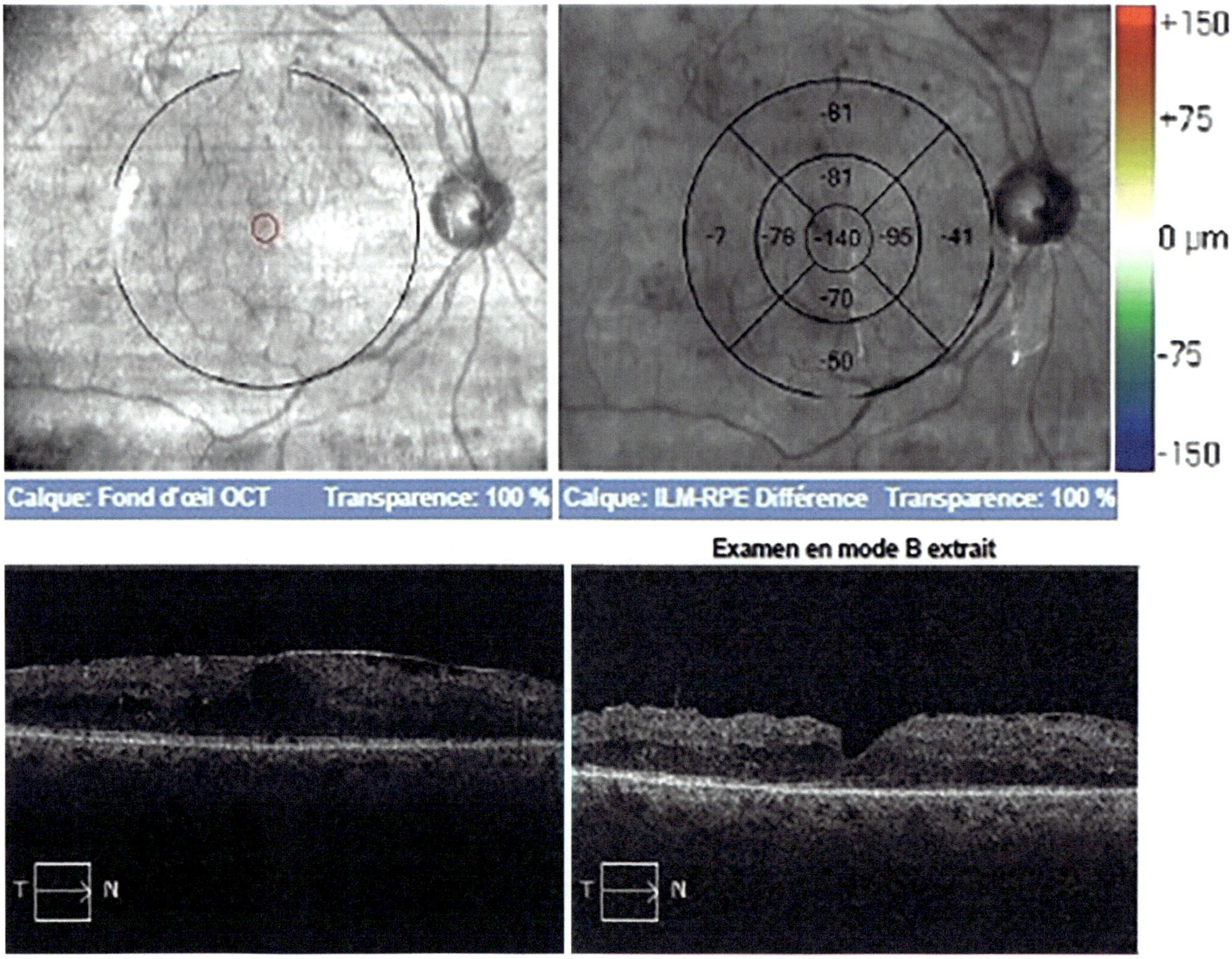

Fig. 13.16 Right eye: comparison between the macular cube 2 months preoperatively (on the left) and 1 month after surgery (on the right)

Fig. 13.17 Color fundus photography of the right eye 1 month after the operation

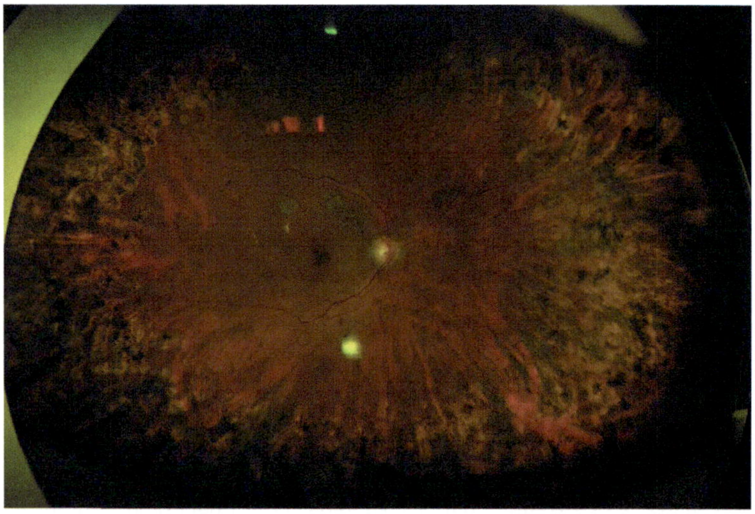

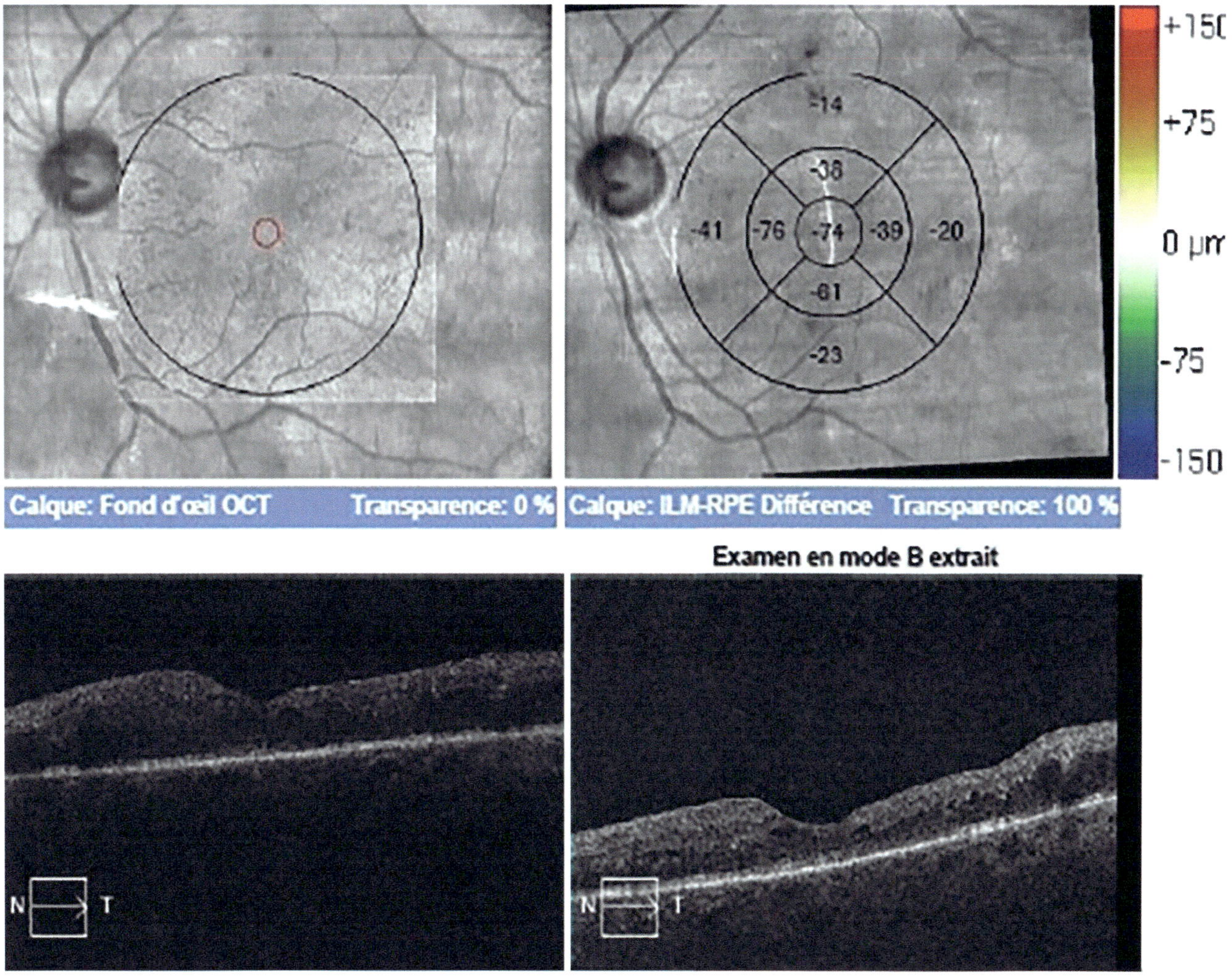

Fig. 13.18 Left eye: comparison between the macular cube 1 month (on the left) and 4 months (on the right) after surgery

Fig. 13.19 Color fundus photography of the left eye 4 months after the operation

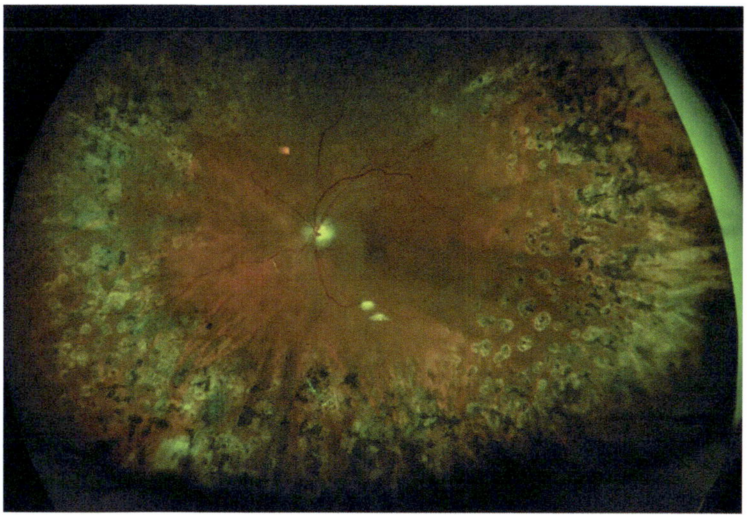

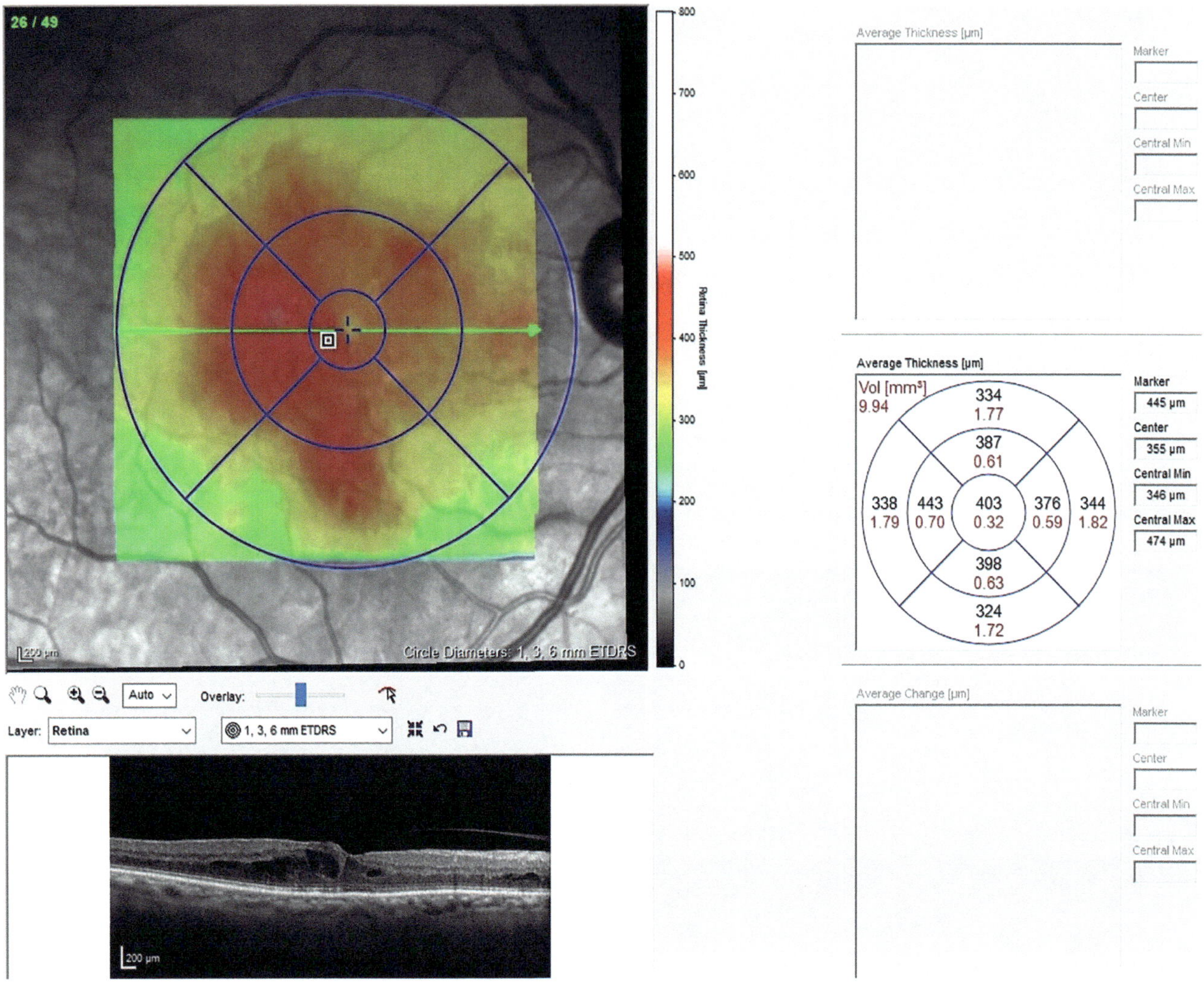

Fig. 13.20 SD-OCT macular map of the right eye at baseline

Fig. 13.21 Color fundus photography of the left eye at baseline

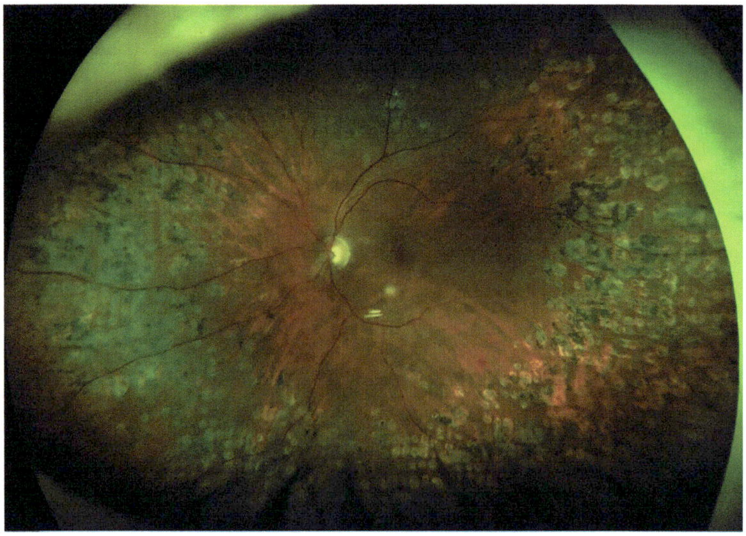

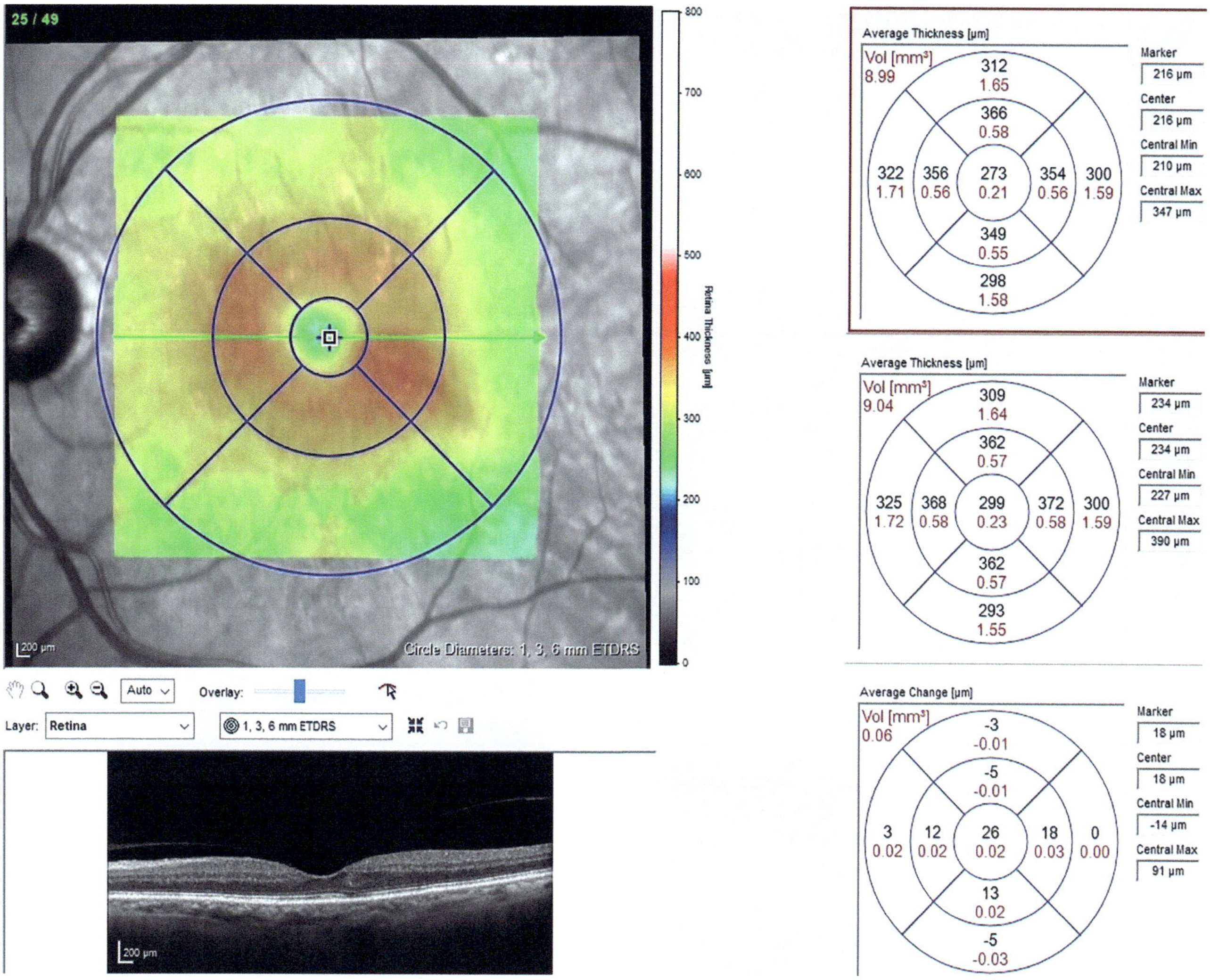

Fig. 13.22 SD-OCT macular map of the left eye at baseline. The thickness comparison on the right side of the image show that the macular thickness was stable over time, compared to the previous examinations

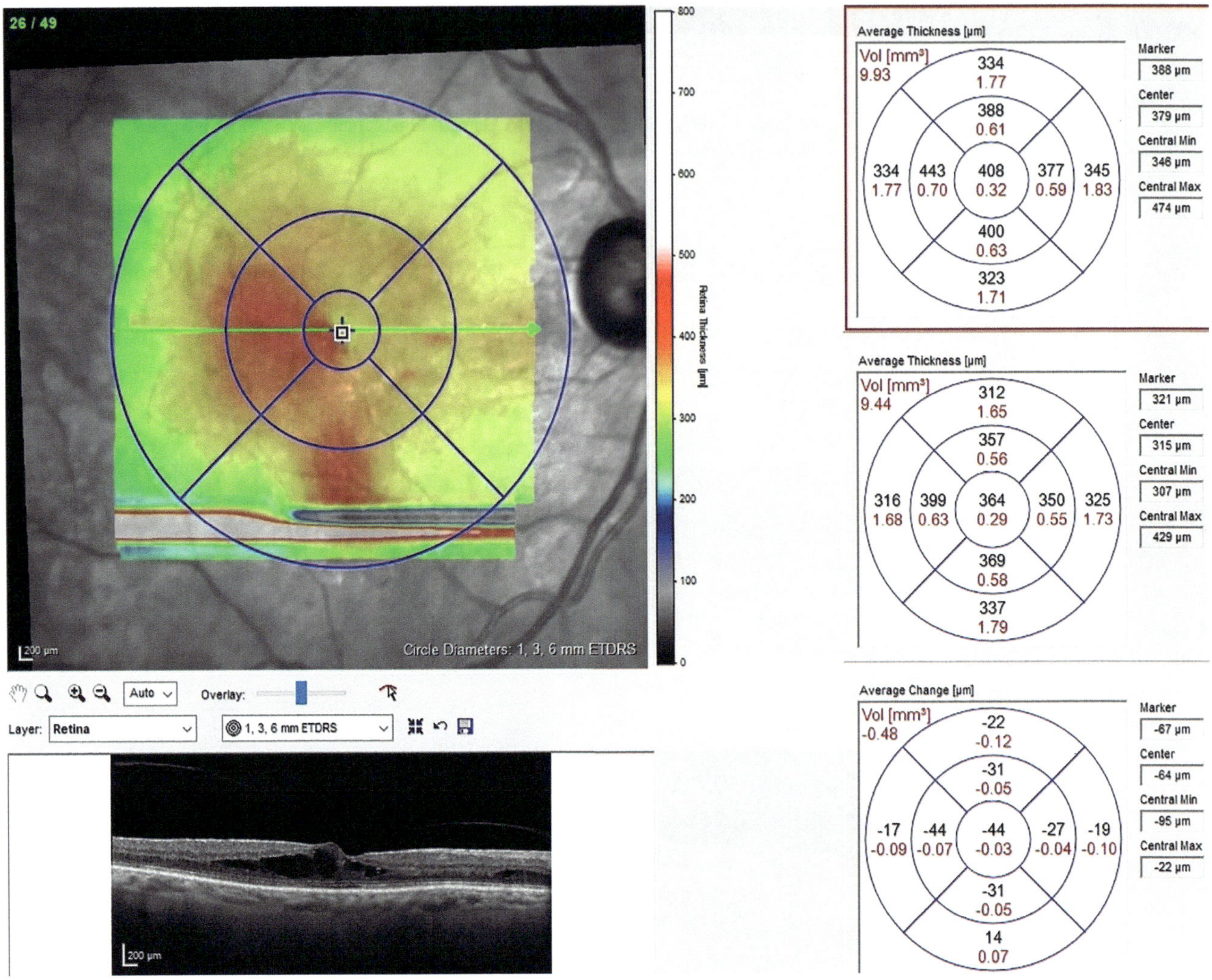

Fig. 13.23 Macular map of the right eye 2 months after the intravitreal implant of dexamethasone. The macular thickness is compared with the exam performed at baseline (at the top right of the image)

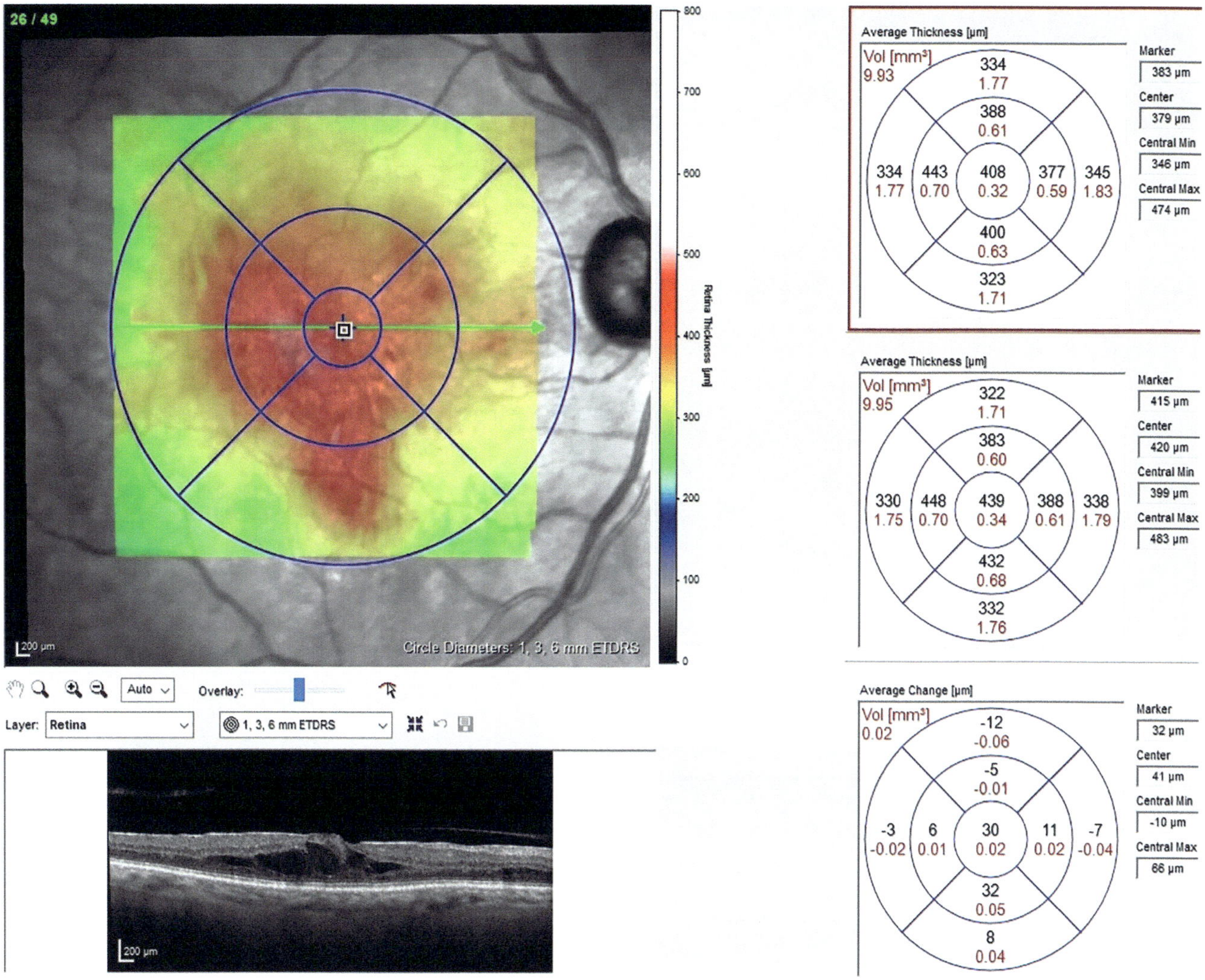

Fig. 13.24 Macular map of the right eye 5 months after the intravitreal implant of dexamethasone. The macular thickness is compared with the examination performed 2 months after the injection (on the top right of the image)

Fig. 13.25 Color fundus photography of the right eye preoperatively, 1 month after three intravitreal injections of anti-VEGF

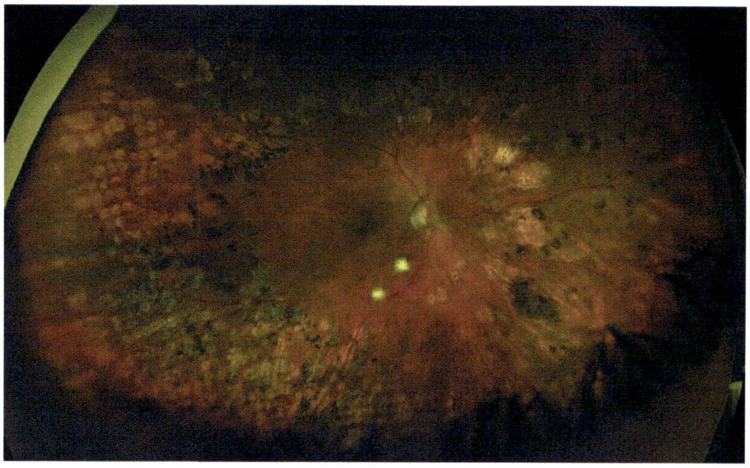

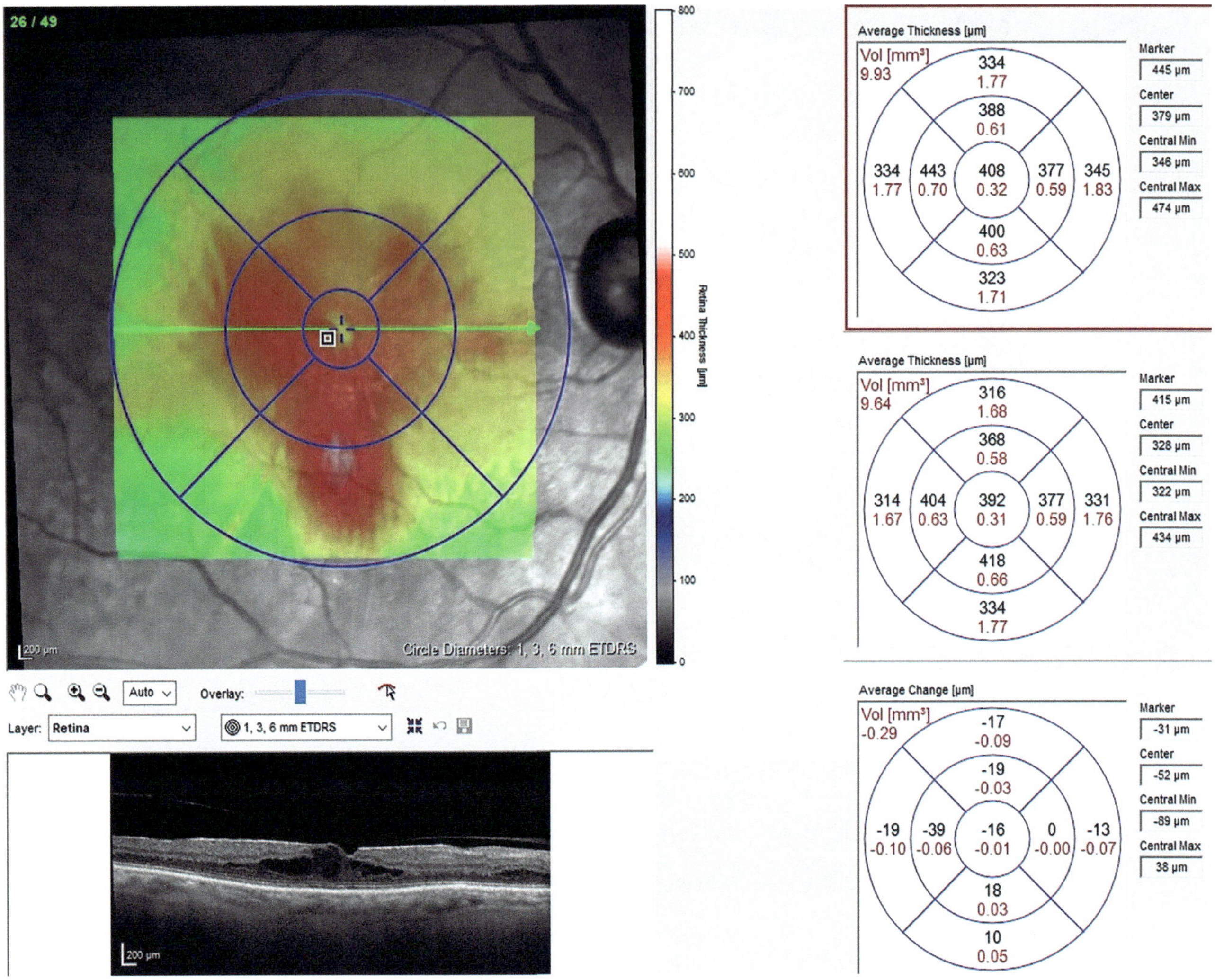

Fig. 13.26 Macular map of the right eye preoperatively, 1 month after 3 monthly injections of anti-VEGF. Comparison is made with the macular thickness before the injections (on the top right)

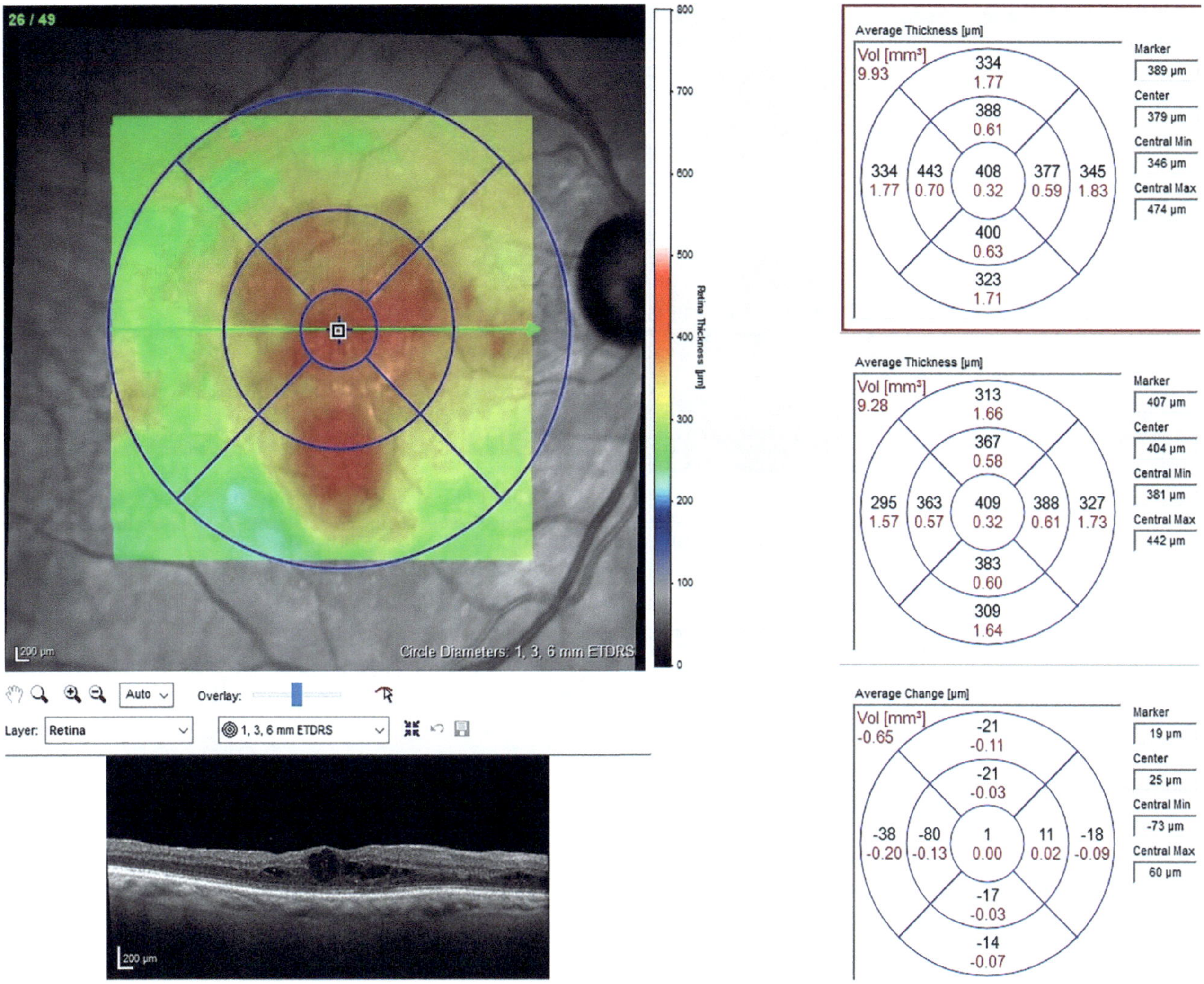

Fig. 13.27 Macular map of the right eye 1 month after vitrectomy. The macular thickness is compared to the exam performed 1 month before surgery (on the top right)

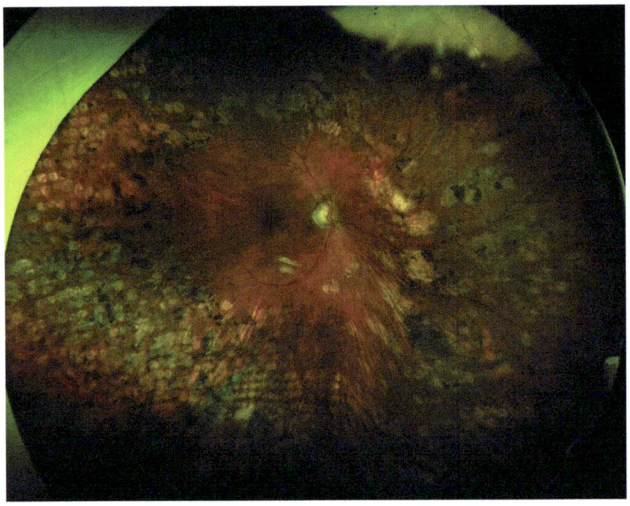

Fig. 13.28 Color fundus photography of the right eye performed at the last visit, 3 months after the last of three intravitreal injections of anti-VEGF

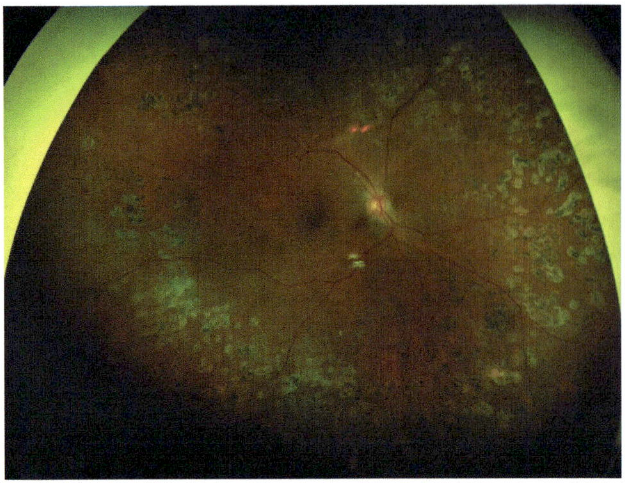

Fig. 13.30 Color fundus photography of the right eye while the patient was already undergoing therapy with anti-VEGF intravitreal injections

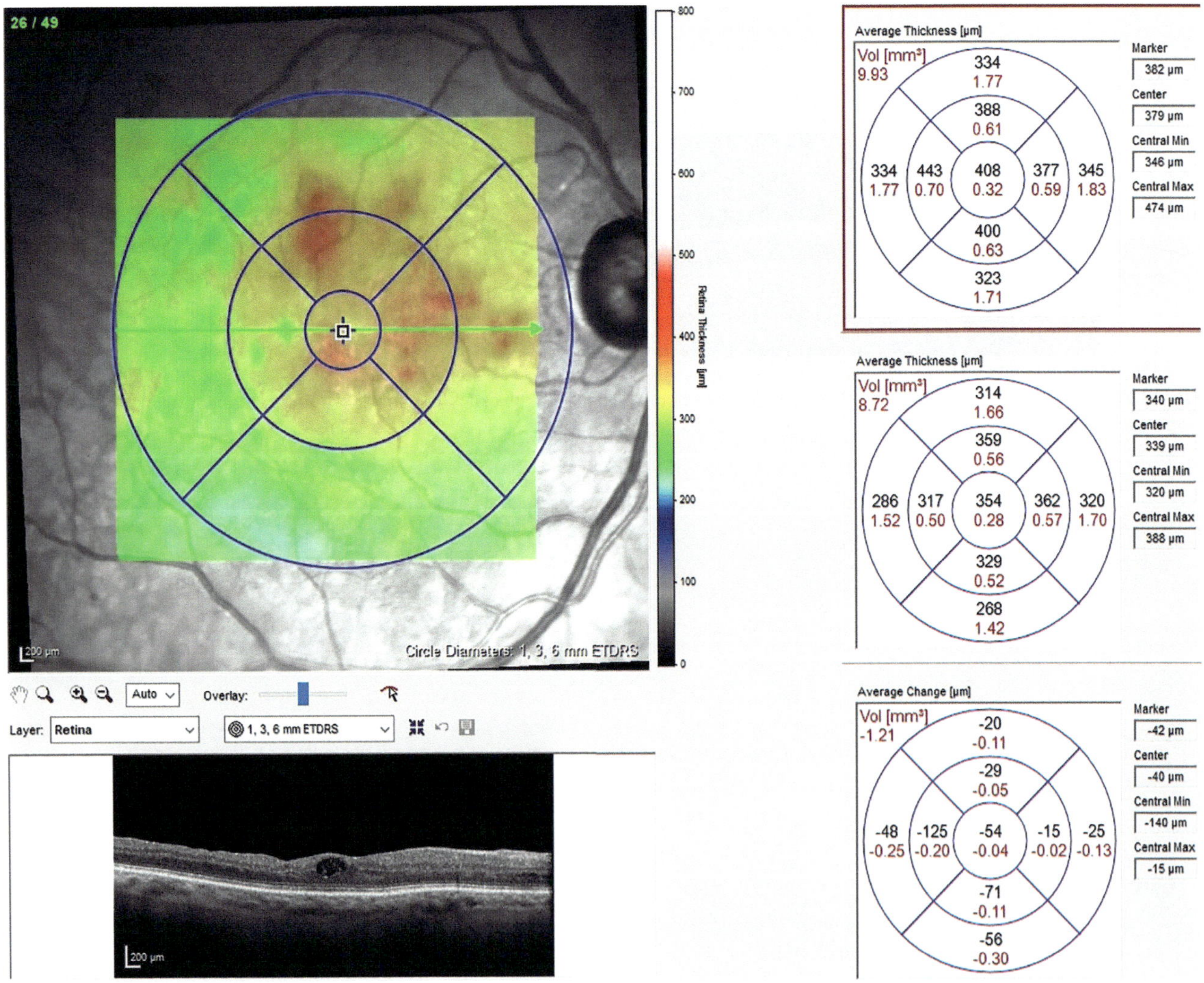

Fig. 13.29 Macular map of the right eye at the final visit of the patient, 3 months after three intravitreal injections of anti-VEGF. The macular thickness is compared to the exam performed 1 month postoperatively (on the top right)

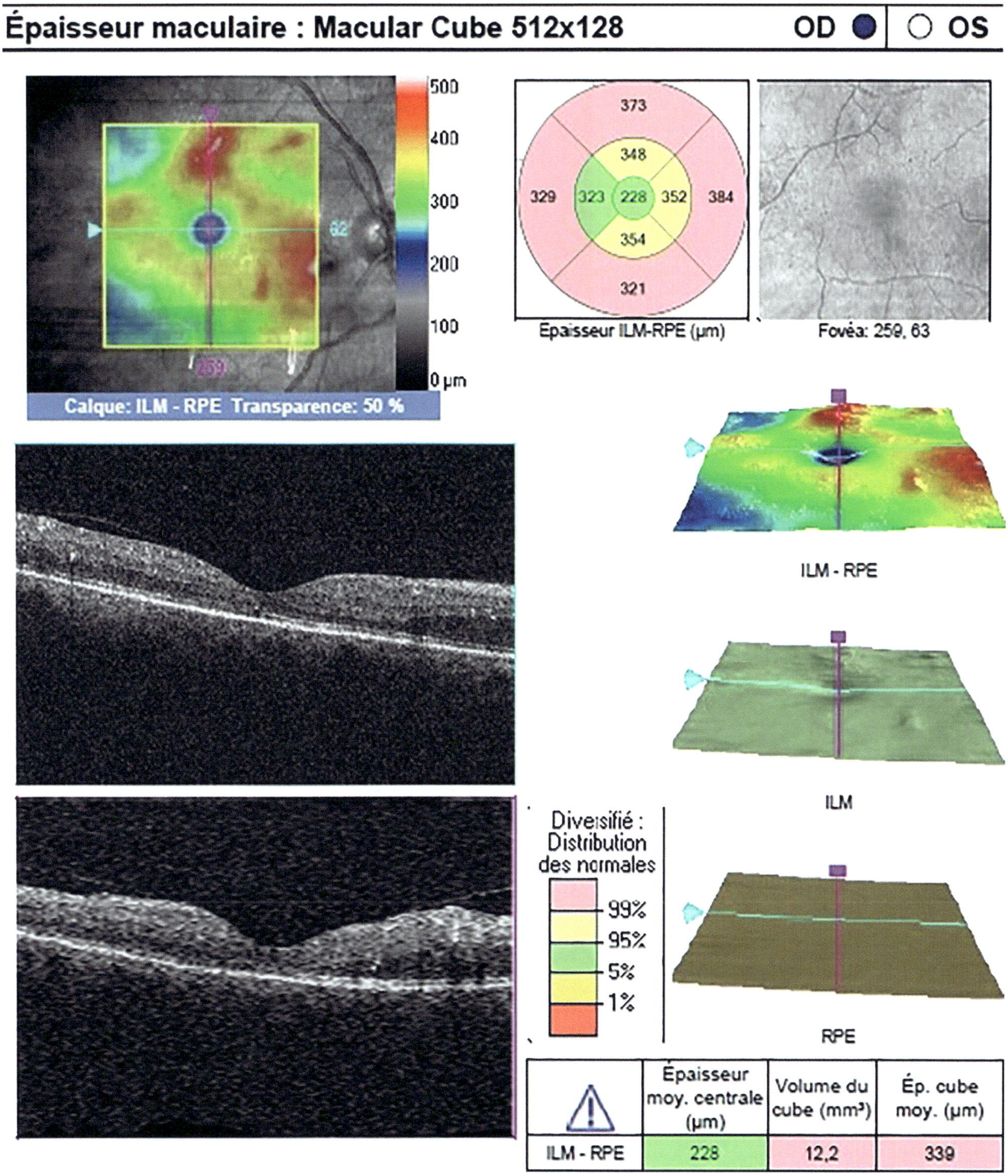

Fig. 13.31 SD-OCT macular cube of the right eye while the patient was already undergoing therapy with anti-VEGF intravitreal injections

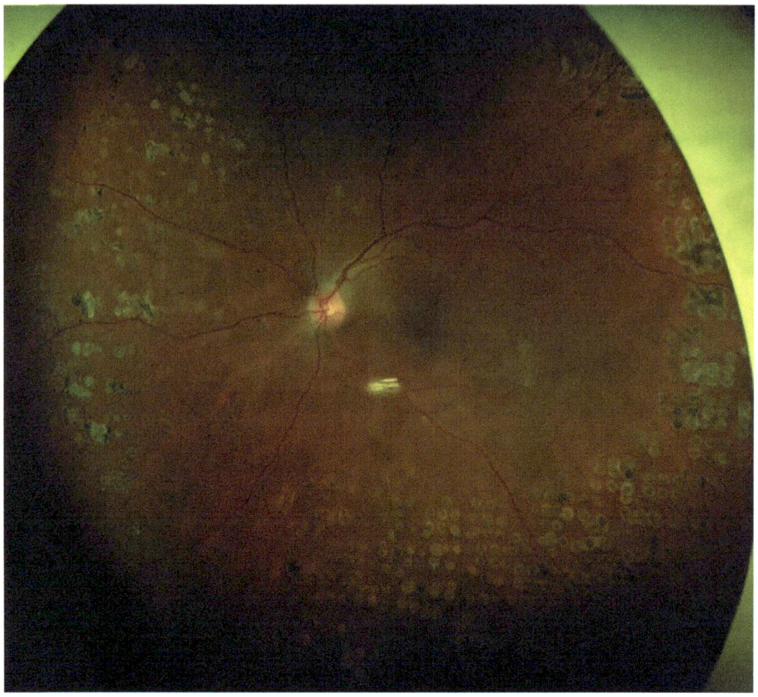

Fig. 13.32 Color fundus photography of the left eye before surgery

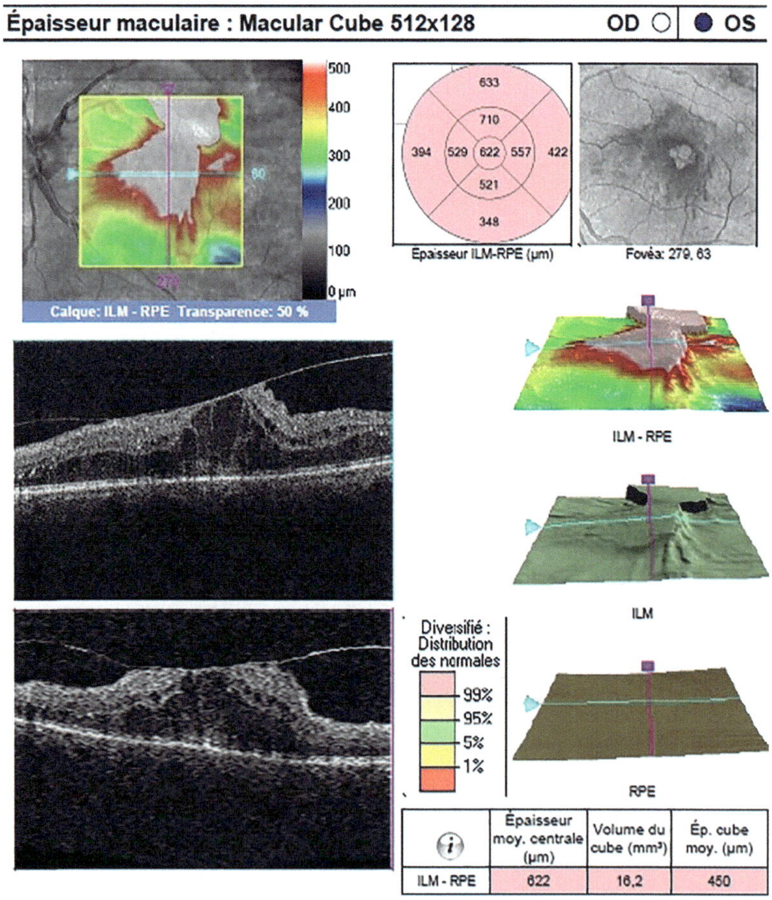

Fig. 13.33 Macular cube of the left eye before surgery

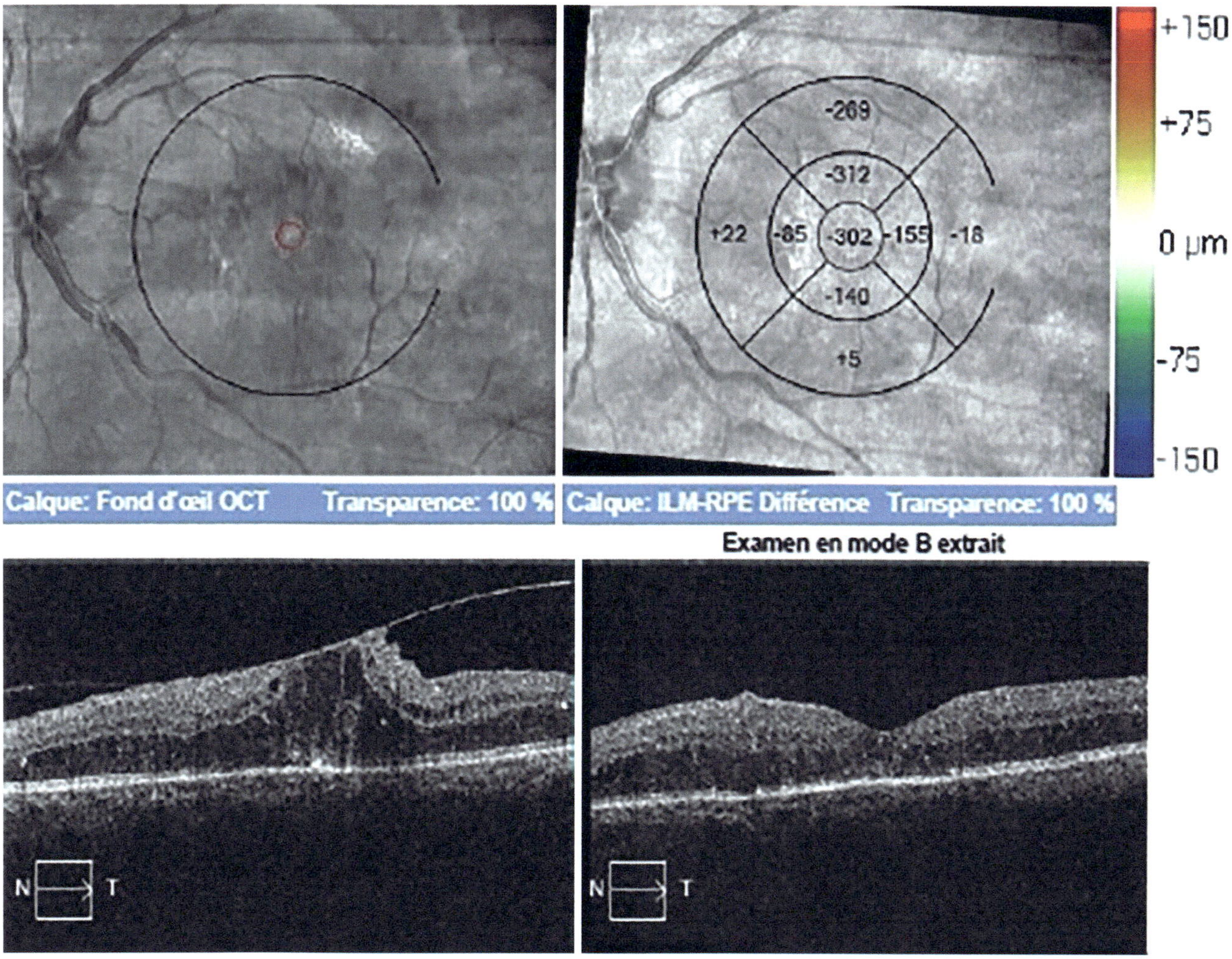

Fig. 13.34 Left eye: comparison between the macular cube before surgery (on the left) and 1 month after surgery (on the right)

Fig. 13.35 Color fundus photography of the left eye 2 years after surgery

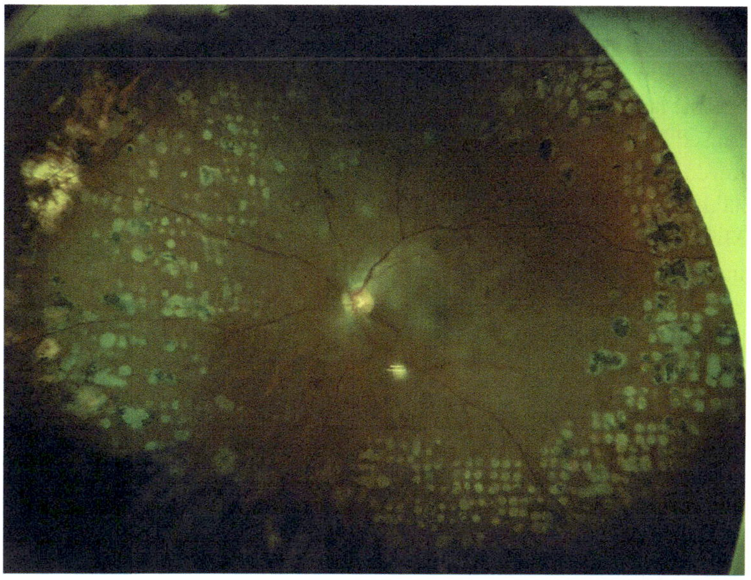

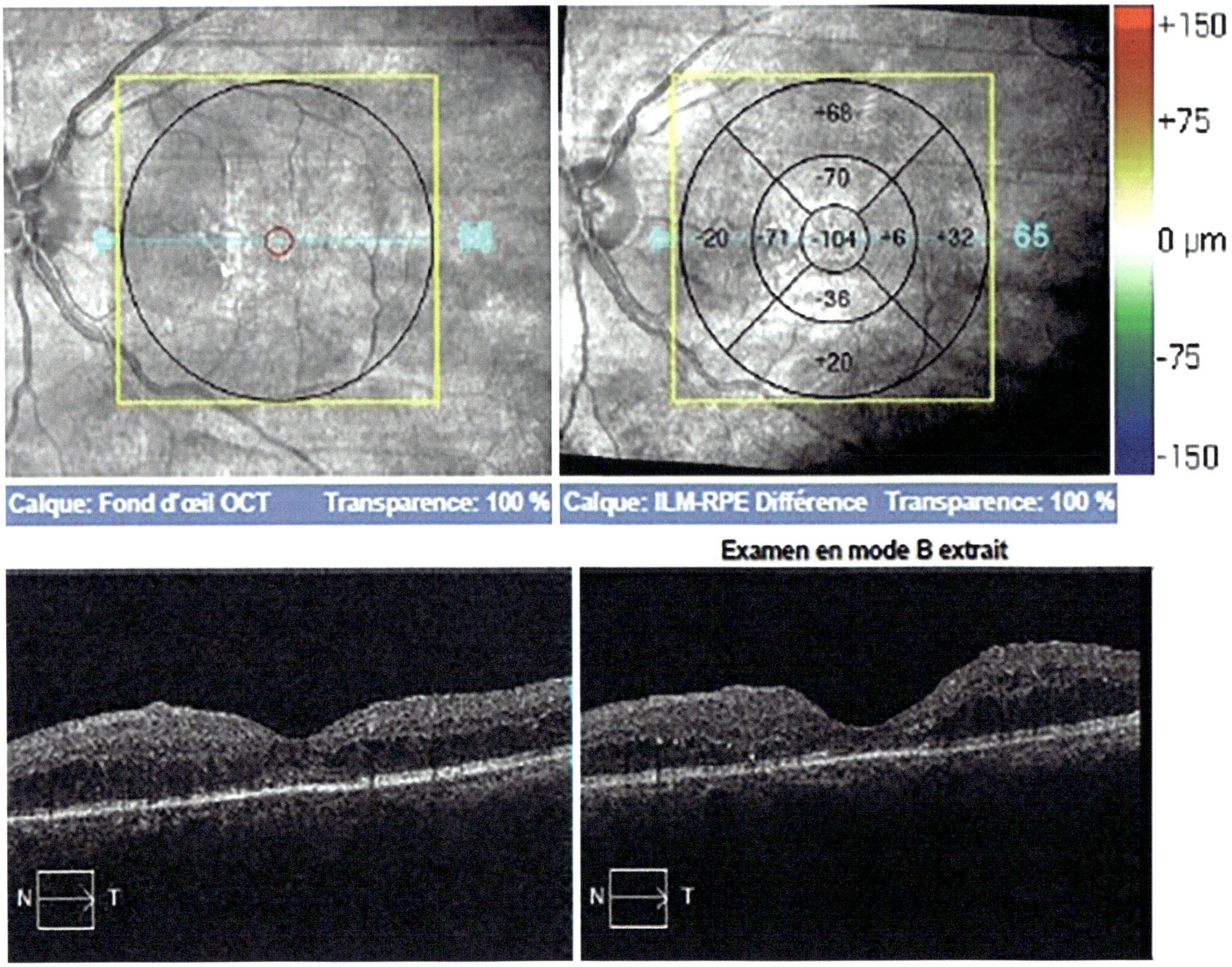

Fig. 13.36 Left eye: comparison between the macular cube realized 1 month (on the left) and 2 years (on the right) after surgery

References

1. Diabetic Retinopathy Clinical Research Network Writing Committee, Haller JA, Qin H, Apte RS, Beck RR, Bressler NM, et al. Vitrectomy outcomes in eyes with diabetic macular edema and vitreomacular traction. Ophthalmology. 2010;117(6):1087–1093.e3.
2. Sebag J, Buckingham B, Charles MA, Reiser K. Biochemical abnormalities in vitreous of humans with proliferative diabetic retinopathy. Arch Ophthalmol. 1992;110(10):1472–6.
3. Nasrallah FP, Jalkh AE, Van Coppenolle F, Kado M, Trempe CL, McMeel JW, et al. The role of the vitreous in diabetic macular edema. Ophthalmology. 1988;95(10):1335–9.
4. Hikichi T, Fujio N, Akiba J, Azuma Y, Takahashi M, Yoshida A. Association between the short-term natural history of diabetic macular edema and the vitreomacular relationship in type II diabetes mellitus. Ophthalmology. 1997;104(3):473–8.
5. Sebag J, Balazs EA. Pathogenesis of cystoid macular edema: an anatomic consideration of vitreoretinal adhesions. Surv Ophthalmol. 1984;28(Suppl):493–8.
6. Lopes de Faria JM, Jalkh AE, Trempe CL, McMeel JW. Diabetic macular edema: risk factors and concomitants. Acta Ophthalmol Scand. 1999;77(2):170–5.
7. Gaucher D, Tadayoni R, Erginay A, Haouchine B, Gaudric A, Massin P. Optical coherence tomography assessment of the vitreoretinal relationship in diabetic macular edema. Am J Ophthalmol. 2005;139(5):807–13.
8. Romano MR, Allegrini D, Della Guardia C, Schiemer S, Baronissi I, Ferrara M, et al. Vitreous and intraretinal macular changes in diabetic macular edema with and without tractional components. Graefes Arch Clin Exp Ophthalmol. 2019;257(1):1–8.
9. Mansour SE, Browning DJ, Wong K, Flynn HW, Bhavsar AR. The evolving treatment of diabetic retinopathy. Clin Ophthalmol. 2020;14:653–78.
10. Golan S, Loewenstein A. Surgical treatment for macular edema. Semin Ophthalmol. 2014;29(4):242–56.
11. Tsotridou E, Loukovitis E, Zapsalis K, Pentara I, Asteriadis S, Tranos P, et al. A re- view of last decade developments on epiretinal membrane pathogenesis. Med Hypothesis Discov Innov Ophthalmol. 2020;9(2):91–110.
12. Kang YK, Park HS, Park DH, Shin JP. Incidence and treatment outcomes of secondary epiretinal membrane following intravitreal injection for diabetic macular edema. Sci Rep. 2020;10(1):528.
13. Yamaguchi Y, Otani T, Kishi S. Resolution of diabetic cystoid macular edema associated with spontaneous vitreofoveal separation. Am J Ophthalmol. 2003;135(1):116–8.

14. Kaiser PK, Riemann CD, Sears JE, Lewis H. Macular traction detachment and diabetic macular edema associated with posterior hyaloidal traction. Am J Ophthalmol. 2001;131(1):44–9.
15. Lewis H, Abrams GW, Blumenkranz MS, Campo RV. Vitrectomy for diabetic macular traction and edema associated with posterior hyaloidal traction. Ophthalmology. 1992;99(5):753–9.
16. Tachi N, Ogino N. Vitrectomy for diffuse macular edema in cases of diabetic retinopathy. Am J Ophthalmol. 1996;122(2):258–60.
17. Browning DJ, Stewart MW, Lee C. Diabetic macular edema: evidence-based management. Indian J Ophthalmol. 2018;66(12):1736–50.
18. Stolba U, Binder S, Gruber D, Krebs I, Aggermann T, Neumaier B. Vitrectomy for persistent diffuse diabetic macular edema. Am J Ophthalmol. 2005;140(2):295–301.
19. Navarrete-Sanchis J, Zarco-Bosquets J, Tomas-Torrent JM, Diago T, Ortega- EL. Long-term effectiveness of vitrectomy in diabetic cystoid macular edema. Graefes Arch Clin Exp Ophthalmol. 2015;253(5):713–9.
20. Harbour JW, Smiddy WE, Flynn HW, Rubsamen PE. Vitrectomy for diabetic macular edema associated with a thickened and taut posterior hyaloid membrane. Am J Ophthalmol. 1996;121(4):405–13.
21. Grigorian R, Bhagat N, Lanzetta P, Tutela A, Zarbin M. Pars plana vitrectomy for refractory diabetic macular edema. Semin Ophthalmol. 2003;18(3):116–20.
22. La Heij EC, Hendrikse F, Kessels AG, Derhaag PJ. Vitrectomy results in diabetic macular oedema without evident vitreomacular traction. Graefes Arch Clin Exp Ophthalmol. 2001;239(4):264–70.
23. Massin P, Duguid G, Erginay A, Haouchine B, Gaudric A. Optical coherence tomography for evaluating diabetic macular edema before and after vitrectomy. Am J Ophthalmol. 2003;135(2):169–77.
24. Figueroa MS, Contreras I, Noval S. Surgical and anatomical outcomes of pars plana vitrectomy for diffuse nontractional diabetic macular edema. Retina. 2008;28(3):420–6.
25. Ikeda T, Sato K, Katano T, Hayashi Y. Improved visual acuity following pars plana vitrectomy for diabetic cystoid macular edema and detached posterior hyaloid. Retina. 2000;20(2):220–2.
26. Sato Y, Lee Z, Shimada H. Vitrectomy for diabetic cystoid macular edema. Jpn J Ophthalmol. 2002;46(3):315–22.
27. Terasaki H, Kojima T, Niwa H, Piao C-H, Ueno S, Kondo M, et al. Changes in focal macular electroretinograms and foveal thickness after vitrectomy for diabetic macular edema. Invest Ophthalmol Vis Sci. 2003;44(10):4465–72.
28. Simunovic MP, Hunyor AP, Ho I-V. Vitrectomy for diabetic macular edema: a systematic review and meta-analysis. Can J Ophthalmol. 2014;49(2):188–95.
29. Jackson TL, Nicod E, Angelis A, Grimaccia F, Pringle E, Kanavos P. Pars plana vitrectomy for diabetic macular edema: a systematic review, meta-analysis, and synthesis of safety literature. Retina. 2017;37(5):886–95.
30. Schmidt-Erfurth U, Garcia-Arumi J, Bandello F, Berg K, Chakravarthy U, Gerendas BS, et al. Guidelines for the management of diabetic macular edema by the European Society of Retina Specialists (EURETINA). Ophthalmologica. 2017;237(4):185–222.
31. Bae JH, Al-Khersan H, Yannuzzi NA, Hasanreisoglu M, Androudi S, Albini TA, et al. Surgical therapy for macular edema: what we have learned through the decades. Ocul Immunol Inflamm. 2019;27(8):1242–50.
32. Michalewska Z, Stewart MW, Landers MB, Bednarski M, Adelman RA, Nawrocki J. Vitrectomy in the management of diabetic macular edema in treatment-naïve patients. Can J Ophthalmol. 2018;53(4):402–7.
33. Berrocal MH, Acaba LA, Chenworth ML. Surgical innovations in the treatment of diabetic macular edema and diabetic retinopathy. Curr Diab Rep. 2019;19(10):106.
34. Kumagai K, Hangai M, Ogino N, Larson E. Effect of internal limiting membrane peeling on long-term visual outcomes for diabetic macular edema. Retina. 2015;35(7):1422–8.
35. Gundogan FC, Yolcu U, Akay F, Ilhan A, Ozge G, Uzun S. Diabetic macular edema. Pak J Med Sci. 2016;32(2):505–10.
36. Adelman R, Parnes A, Michalewska Z, Parolini B, Boscher C, Ducournau D. Strategy for the management of diabetic macular edema: the European vitreo-retinal society macular edema study. Biomed Res Int. 2015;2015:352487.
37. Hagenau F, Vogt D, Ziada J, Guenther SR, Haritoglou C, Wolf A, et al. Vitrectomy for diabetic macular edema: optical coherence tomography criteria and pathology of the vitreomacular interface. Am J Ophthalmol. 2019;200:34–46.
38. Yoshida S, Murakami T, Nozaki M, Suzuma K, Baba T, Hirano T, et al. Review of clinical studies and recommendation for a therapeutic flow chart for diabetic macular edema. Graefes Arch Clin Exp Ophthalmol. 2021;259(4):815–36.
39. AlQahtani AS, Hazzazi MA, Waheeb SA, Semidey VA, Semidey VA, Elgendy HK, et al. Saudi Arabia guidelines for diabetic macular edema: a consensus of the Saudi Retina Group. Saudi Med J. 2021;42(2):131–45.
40. Lin H-C, Yang C-M, Chen S-N, Hsieh Y-T. Vitrectomy with internal limiting membrane peeling versus nonsurgical treatment for diabetic macular edema with massive hard exudates. PLoS One. 2020;15(7):e0236867.
41. Pessoa B, Dias DA, Baptista P, Coelho C, Beirão JNM, Meireles A. Vitrectomy out- comes in eyes with tractional diabetic macular edema. Ophthalmic Res. 2019;61(2):94–9.
42. Patelli F, Radice P, Giacomotti E. Diabetic macular edema. Dev Ophthalmol. 2014;54:164–73.
43. Terasaki H, Ogura Y, Kitano S, Sakamoto T, Murata T, Hirakata A, et al. Management of diabetic macular edema in Japan: a review and expert opinion. Jpn J Ophthalmol. 2018;62(1):1–23.
44. Flaxel CJ, Edwards AR, Aiello LP, Arrigg PG, Beck RW, Bressler NM, et al. Factors associated with visual acuity outcomes after vitrectomy for diabetic macular edema: diabetic retinopathy clinical research network. Retina. 2010;30(9):1488–95.
45. Ozturk M, Guven D, Kacar H, Karapapak M, Demir M. Functional and morphological results of epiretinal membrane surgery in idiopathic versus diabetic epiretinal membranes. Semin Ophthalmol. 2021;36(5–6):366–72.
46. Chhablani JK, Kim JS, Cheng L, Kozak I, Freeman W. External limiting membrane as a predictor of visual improvement in diabetic macular edema after pars plana vitrectomy. Graefes Arch Clin Exp Ophthalmol. 2012;250(10):1415–20.
47. Browning DJ, Lee C, Stewart MW, Landers MB. Vitrectomy for center-involved diabetic macular edema. Clin Ophthalmol. 2016;10:735–42.
48. Bonnin S, Sandali O, Bonnel S, Monin C, El Sanharawi M. Vitrectomy with internal limiting membrane peeling for tractional and nontractional diabetic macular edema: long-term results of a comparative study. Retina. 2015;35(5):921–8.
49. Nguyen QD, Shah SM, Van Anden E, Sung JU, Vitale S, Campochiaro PA. Supplemental oxygen improves diabetic macular edema: a pilot study. Invest Ophthalmol Vis Sci. 2004;45(2):617–24.
50. Park JH, Woo SJ, Ha YJ, Yu HG. Effect of vitrectomy on macular microcirculation in patients with diffuse diabetic macular edema. Graefes Arch Clin Exp Ophthalmol. 2009;247(8):1009–17.
51. Mukai R, Matsumoto H, Akiyama H. Surgical outcomes of vitrectomy for intractable diabetic macular edema. Graefes Arch Clin Exp Ophthalmol. 2021;259(2):363–8.
52. Maturi RK, Glassman AR, Liu D, Beck RW, Bhavsar AR, Bressler NM, et al. Effect of adding dexamethasone to continued ranibizumab treatment in patients with persistent diabetic macular edema: a DRCR network phase 2 randomized clinical trial. JAMA Ophthalmol. 2018;136(1):29–38.

53. Kim J, Kang SW, Shin DH, Kim SJ, Cho GE. Macular ischemia and outcome of vitrectomy for diabetic macular edema. Jpn J Ophthalmol. 2015;59(5):295–304.
54. Yamakiri K, Sakamoto T, Noda Y, Nakahara M, Ogino N, Kubota T, et al. Reduced incidence of intraoperative complications in a multicenter controlled clinical trial of triamcinolone in vitrectomy. Ophthalmology. 2007;114(2):289–96.
55. Kumagai K, Furukawa M, Ogino N, Larson E, Iwaki M, Tachi N. Long-term follow-up of vitrectomy for diffuse nontractional diabetic macular edema. Retina. 2009;29(4):464–72.
56. Nakajima T, Roggia MF, Noda Y, Ueta T. Effect of internal limiting membrane peeling during vitrectomy for diabetic macular edema: systematic review and meta- analysis. Retina. 2015;35(9):1719–25.
57. Gandorfer A, Messmer EM, Ulbig MW, Kampik A. Resolution of diabetic macular edema after surgical removal of the posterior hyaloid and the inner limiting membrane. Retina. 2000;20(2):126–33.
58. Bahadir M, Ertan A, Mertoğlu O. Visual acuity comparison of vitrectomy with and without internal limiting membrane removal in the treatment of diabetic macular edema. Int Ophthalmol. 2005;26(1–2):3–8.
59. Christoforidis JB, D'Amico DJ. Surgical and other treatments of diabetic macular edema: an update. Int Ophthalmol Clin. 2004;44(1):139–60.
60. Yamamoto T, Hitani K, Sato Y, Yamashita H, Takeuchi S. Vitrectomy for diabetic macular edema with and without internal limiting membrane removal. Ophthalmologica. 2005;219(4):206–13.
61. Rinaldi M, dell'Omo R, Morescalchi F, Semeraro F, Gambicorti E, Cacciatore F, et al. ILM peeling in nontractional diabetic macular edema: review and metanalysis. Int Ophthalmol. 2018;38(6):2709–14.
62. Stefaniotou M, Aspiotis M, Kalogeropoulos C, Christodoulou A, Psylla M, Ioachim E, et al. Vitrectomy results for diffuse diabetic macular edema with and without inner limiting membrane removal. Eur J Ophthalmol. 2004;14(2):137–43.
63. Yamakoshi T, Kachi S, Sugita J, Asami T, Ishikawa K, Ito Y, et al. Triamcinolone- assisted removal of internal limiting membrane enhances the effect of vitrectomy for diabetic macular edema. Ophthalmic Res. 2009;41(4):203–9.
64. Ivastinovic D, Haas A, Weger M, Seidel G, Mayer-Xanthaki C, Lindner E, et al. Vitrectomy for diabetic macular edema and the relevance of external limiting mem- brane. BMC Ophthalmol. 2021;21(1):334.
65. Kim YT, Kang SW, Kim SJ, Kim SM, Chung SE. Combination of vitrectomy, IVTA, and laser photocoagulation for diabetic macular edema unresponsive to prior treatments; 3-year results. Graefes Arch Clin Exp Ophthalmol. 2012;250(5):679–84.
66. Boyer DS, Faber D, Gupta S, Patel SS, Tabandeh H, Li X-Y, et al. Dexamethasone intravitreal implant for treatment of diabetic macular edema in vitrectomized patients. Retina. 2011;31(5):915–23.
67. Lee DH, Kim YJ, Yoon YH. Minimally invasive microincision vitrectomy surgery with an intraoperative dexamethasone implant for refractory diabetic macular edema. Ophthalmologica. 2016;235(3):150–6.
68. Kim KT, Jang JW, Kang SW, Chae JB, Cho K, Bae K. Vitrectomy combined with intraoperative dexamethasone implant for the management of refractory diabetic macular edema. Korean J Ophthalmol. 2019;33(3):249–58.
69. Hwang S, Kang SW, Kim KT, Noh H, Kim SJ. Three-year outcomes of vitrectomy combined with intraoperative dexamethasone implantation for non-tractional refractory diabetic macular edema. Sci Rep. 2021;11(1):1292.
70. Watanabe A, Tsuzuki A, Arai K, Gekka T, Kohzaki K, Tsuneoka H. Efficacy of intravitreal triamcinolone acetonide for diabetic macular edema after vitrectomy. J Ocul Pharmacol Ther. 2016;32(1):38–43.
71. Uji A, Murakami T, Suzuma K, Yoshitake S, Arichika S, Ghashut R, et al. Influence of vitrectomy surgery on the integrity of outer retinal layers in diabetic macular edema. Retina. 2018;38(1):163–72.
72. Ichiyama Y, Sawada O, Mori T, Fujikawa M, Kawamura H, Ohji M. The effectiveness of vitrectomy for diffuse diabetic macular edema may depend on its preoperative optical coherence tomography pattern. Graefes Arch Clin Exp Ophthalmol. 2016;254(8):1545–51.
73. Pendergast SD. Vitrectomy for diabetic macular edema associated with a taut premacular posterior hyaloid. Curr Opin Ophthalmol. 1998;9(3):71–5.
74. Yang CM. Surgical treatment for severe diabetic macular edema with massive hard exudates. Retina. 2000;20(2):121–5.
75. Otani T, Kishi S. Tomographic assessment of vitreous surgery for diabetic macular edema. Am J Ophthalmol. 2000;129(4):487–94.
76. Amoaku WM, Ghanchi F, Bailey C, Banerjee S, Banerjee S, Downey L, et al. Diabetic retinopathy and diabetic macular oedema pathways and management: UK Consensus Working Group. Eye (Lond). 2020;34(Suppl 1):1–51.

Management of DME: One Minute Preceptor

14

Practical Management Approach for DME

Rachel S. Mogil and Sophie J. Bakri

14.1 Introduction

When a patient presents to clinic for a diabetic eye exam, a history is first obtained. Risk factors for diabetic retinopathy include duration of disease, presence of hypertension, elevated hemoglobin A1c (HbA1c) levels, and male gender [1]. The following data is collected: years since diagnosis, presence or absence of insulin dependence, and medical history including renal disease, neuropathy, concomitant hypertension including most recent blood pressure reading, hyperlipidemia, and the most recent HbA1c. The trends in HbA1c values are then reviewed to ascertain glycemic control over the last few years.

History of any prior treatment for diabetic eye disease is obtained including laser photocoagulation, anti-vascular endothelial growth factor (anti-VEGF) or steroid treatment, or pars plana vitrectomy. If the patient has received prior intravitreal injections, information regarding the medications that were trialed, the interval at which they were used, and the date of the most recent injection is collected.

The patients are queried regarding any current visual symptoms such as floaters or blurry vision, and if they have noticed any recent or gradual visual changes over the last few months.

Clinical examination is then performed. This includes assessing best-corrected visual acuity, intraocular pressure, pupillary responses, extraocular motility, and confrontational visual fields. Blood pressure readings may be obtained for those patients with hypertension with no available data.

During the anterior segment exam, it is important to assess the iris and/or angle for signs of neovascularization, especially in patients with elevated intraocular pressure. This may necessitate a gonioscopic evaluation, which is best performed prior to dilation. The lens is inspected for any signs of cataract frequently seen in diabetic patients, such as diabetic, cortical, or posterior subcapsular cataracts, which may contribute to poor vision.

Slit lamp biomicroscopy of the posterior pole is critical in the assessment of diabetic retinopathy. After assessing the vitreous for signs of hemorrhage, the nerve is then evaluated to ascertain the presence or absence of neovascularization of the disc (NVD). The vessels are inspected for signs of venous dilation or beading, intraretinal microvascular abnormalities, and neovascularization elsewhere (NVE). While noting the presence of new vessel growth is essential, it is also important to evaluate for the absence of capillaries, which can indicate ischemia in the setting of diabetic retinopathy.

Using a macular contact lens or a high-magnification noncontact lens (90D, 78D, or 66D), the macula is then assessed for the presence of microaneurysms (MAs), dot blot hemorrhages (DBHs), hard exudates, and cotton wool spots. The fovea is then examined to determine the presence of retinal thickening and intraretinal cysts, which can indicate macular edema.

A peripheral retinal examination is then performed at both the slit lamp and using indirect ophthalmoscopy.

Imaging is typically obtained as part of a patient's examination. Patients may undergo optical coherence tomography (OCT), especially if macular edema is suspected. Macular OCT confirms the presence and extent of retinal thickening and diabetic macular edema (DME). It also allows the assessment of retinal layers, the loss of which can help predict and explain visual prognosis in diabetic patients with chronic macular edema and poor vision. OCT is used to monitor DME in patients receiving treatment. Though, as previously documented, OCT findings do not always correlate with visual acuity [2, 3]. As such, visual acuity remains the key indicator of treatment success or failure.

Fluorescein angiography (FA) may also be obtained. FA confirms the presence of subtle NVD or NVE, MAs, and ischemic areas of retina with capillary non-perfusion. This helps guide the need for panretinal photocoagulation and focal laser treatment of DME. If the patient is unable to undergo FA, OCT angiography can be used. A non-invasive

R. S. Mogil · S. J. Bakri (✉)
Department of Ophthalmology, Mayo Clinic, Rochester, MN, USA
e-mail: bakri.sophie@mayo.edu

S. Saxena et al. (eds.), *Diabetic Macular Edema*, https://doi.org/10.1007/978-981-19-7307-9_14

imaging modality, OCT angiography can demonstrate macular vascular abnormalities such as retinal and choroidal neovascularization, ischemia, capillary non-perfusion, and MAs, but unlike FA, it cannot demonstrate leakage.

Color fundus photography is helpful in documenting abnormal findings such as NVD or NVE but is not routinely obtained on every patient.

For patients with DME and excellent vision (20/25 or better), they are offered the option of monitoring with close follow-up every 2–4 months with OCT and return precautions of worsening vision loss, as DRCR.net Protocol V found no difference in mean visual acuity after 2 years in eyes treated with aflibercept, focal laser with aflibercept, or observation with aflibercept [4]. As such, these patients can be observed until visual acuity is affected (20/30 or worse). All patients with DME are counseled to practice good blood pressure and blood glucose control, as well as continued management of any hyperlipidemia in the interim, as improvements in these values alone can reduce macular thickness [5].

Anti-VEGF treatment is selected based on the patient's best-corrected visual acuity. DRCR.net Protocol T demonstrated similar visual gains amongst patients with visual acuity of 20/40 or better receiving bevacizumab, ranibizumab, and aflibercept. For patients with visual acuity of 20/50 or worse, visual acuity gains were higher in those receiving aflibercept [6].

For patients with center-involving DME (CI-DME) and good vision (better than 20/40), treatment is initiated with a series of monthly bevacizumab, given its similar visual gains and cost effectivity, with a total of four injections. Patients are re-evaluated 4–5 weeks after the last injection with OCT.

For patients with CI-DME and vision of 20/50 or worse, a series of monthly aflibercept (given its documented superiority to bevacizumab or ranibizumab in DME eyes with worse baseline visual acuity) [6] is recommended with a total of four injections and evaluation 4–5 weeks after the last injection with OCT. While this is the preferred practice, the cost of aflibercept can be financially prohibitive. In those instances, patients are started on bevacizumab until financial support can be established.

For patients who have incomplete response (no improvement in or worsening of visual acuity or retinal thickness) to a series of bevacizumab on a tight 4-week interval, the patient may be switched to another anti-VEGF agent, for example aflibercept or ranibizumab, at the same interval for another series of four injections.

Monthly injections are continued until visual acuity and/or central retinal thickness improves with fluid resolution and becomes stable. If after one or two series of injections, the patient has reached stability, treatment is extended. Injection intervals are increased from 4- to 6-week intervals, and then to 8–10 week and 10–12-week intervals. At this time, stable patients are offered cessation of treatment with close monitoring.

For patients in which neither bevacizumab, aflibercept, or ranibizumab have shown effectiveness in providing any functional or anatomic benefit (after at least 3–6 injections or 4–6 months), intraocular corticosteroid treatment may be considered, such as with the dexamethasone intravitreal implant or fluocinolone acetonide insert. Both treatments have been demonstrated to reduce DME and improve visual acuity [7–10]. The effectiveness of the dexamethasone intravitreal implant usually decreases after approximately 3–6 months, at which time an additional treatment can be considered. The non-dissolving fluocinolone acetonide implant, which provides drug delivery for 36 months, can be considered in patients without prior steroid response with chronic macular edema [11]. Intraocular pressure is typically rechecked 4–6 weeks after intraocular corticosteroid injection and treatment success is re-evaluated with OCT at around 6–10 weeks. Corticosteroid treatments may be considered for patients who are unable to present for monthly injections. These treatments have a greater risk of elevated intraocular pressure and cataract progression than anti-VEGF therapy.

Focal and grid laser treatment, while once the standard of care for CI-DME in the pre-anti-VEGF era, is now used typically as an adjuvant. Focal laser can be utilized in patients with leaking MAs contributing to non-CI-DME [12]. A yellow or green laser is selected for focal treatment. The goal is to directly treat leaking MAs and grid areas of diffuse leakage and retinal thickening. Spots should be 1–2 burn widths of separation with a power of 50–100 mW and a duration of 0.05–0.1 s [12]. Laser spots should be applied no closer than 500 μm from the fovea and should have a light gray color. Subthreshold (modified ETDRS) grid laser treatment is preferred as it offers less thermal damage than typical grid treatment by using lighter burns that are less intense and more spaced out with a smaller spot size of 50 microns, without requiring treatment-induced change in MA color [13, 14]. Patients are re-evaluated 3–4 months after laser treatment and may need multiple treatment sessions to be successful.

Rarely, if patients are unable to maintain an injection schedule, are injection-averse, or are not appropriate candidates for focal laser or intraocular steroids, topical steroids, and non-steroidal anti-inflammatory drugs (NSAIDs) can be attempted. Treatment consists of topical prednisolone and topical ketorolac tromethamine four times daily, with reassessment in 1 month. There is little data on the effect of topical corticosteroids on DME, but previous studies have shown that topical difluprednate decreases retinal thickness and improves visual acuity in patients with persistent DME [15] and decreases retinal thickness in vitrectomized eyes with refractory DME [16] and eyes with diffuse DME [17]. Two other studies have shown that topical dexamethasone-cyclodextrin may reduce retinal thickness and improve visual acuity in eyes with DME, especially those that have been vitrectomized [18, 19]. Preliminary data show that topical NSAIDs may reduce central macular thickness in patients with DME [20, 21]. Furthermore, while an observational study found no visual or functional gain in combination therapy [22], a randomized clinical trial recently demonstrated that topical ketorolac in combination with intravitreal bevacizumab resulted in a greater reduction in mean central subfield thickness and improvement in visual acuity than bevacizumab alone [23].

Finally, surgical therapy may also be an option. Given that the altered vitreous in diabetic patients may be contributing to the development and maintenance of DME, pars plana vitrectomy can be considered in patients with diffuse DME unresponsive to laser or anti-VEGF treatment, especially in patients with associated vitreoretinal traction [24]. Vitrectomized eyes have been shown to produce less total anti-VEGF, making vitrectomy a viable option for patients with DME unresponsive to treatment, even in the absence of traction [12], although this is controversial. Traction due to an epiretinal membrane should be considered as a cause of persistent DME after an incomplete response has been shown to anti-VEGF or corticosteroid treatment. Epiretinal membrane removal has been shown to increase visual acuity in patients undergoing vitrectomy for DME [25].

14.2 Clinical Cases

Case #1

A 59-year-old Somali male with type 2 diabetes mellitus presents for a diabetic eye exam. He is taking metformin and glipizide and is being treated for hypertension and hyperlipidemia. He has a history of proliferative diabetic retinopathy for which he underwent panretinal photocoagulation of both eyes and reports a history of anti-VEGF injections 5 years prior to presentation. His HbA1c upon presentation was 7.6. Exam was notable for few MAs and panretinal photocoagulation in both eyes, but no NVD or NVE (Fig. 14.1). OCT showed intraretinal fluid of the left eye (Fig. 14.2), but given excellent visual acuity of 20/20 in both eyes, he elected to observe and follow-up in 3 months. Four months later he returned with subjective worsening vision and visual acuity of 20/40 in the right eye and 20/50 in the left eye. OCT showed new DME in the right eye and increased CI-DME in the left eye (Figs. 14.3 and 14.4). He was started on a series of four bevacizumab injections every 4–5 weeks in both eyes, though aflibercept was considered in the left eye given DRCR.net Protocol T but was initially cost prohibitive. Upon re-evaluation 4 months later, his vision was 20/60 in the right eye and 20/70 in the left eye, and his DME had worsened on

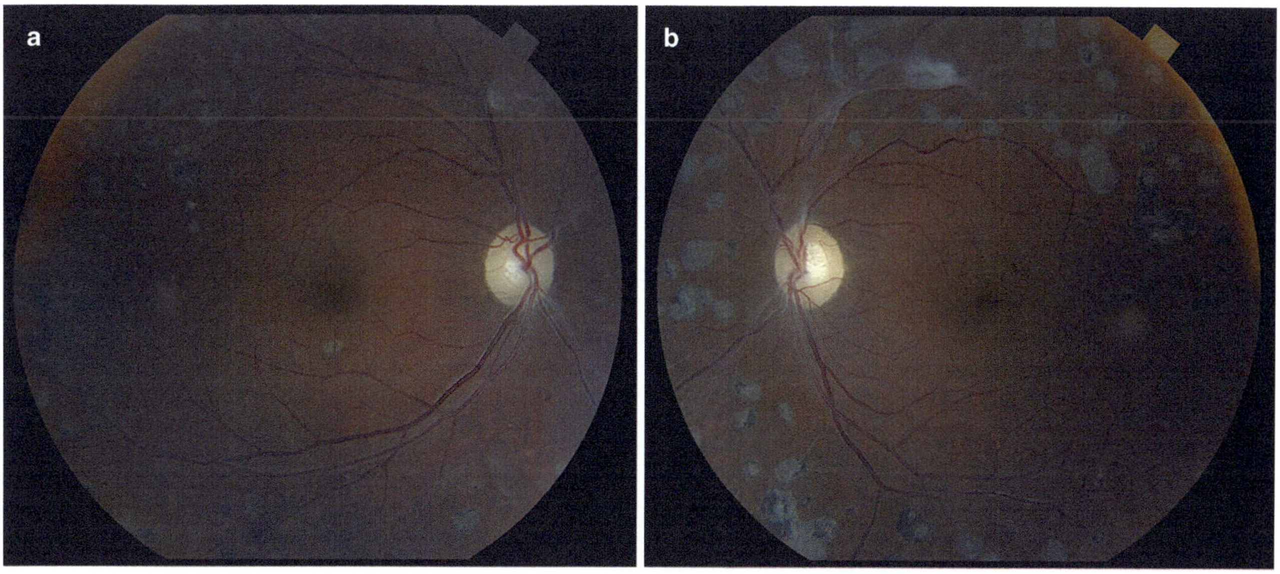

Fig. 14.1 Color fundus photo of the right (**a**) and left (**b**) eye notable for microaneurysms in both eyes, gliosis of the superior arcade (worse in the left eye), and prior panretinal photocoagulation of both eyes. There is no neovascularization of the disc or elsewhere in either eye

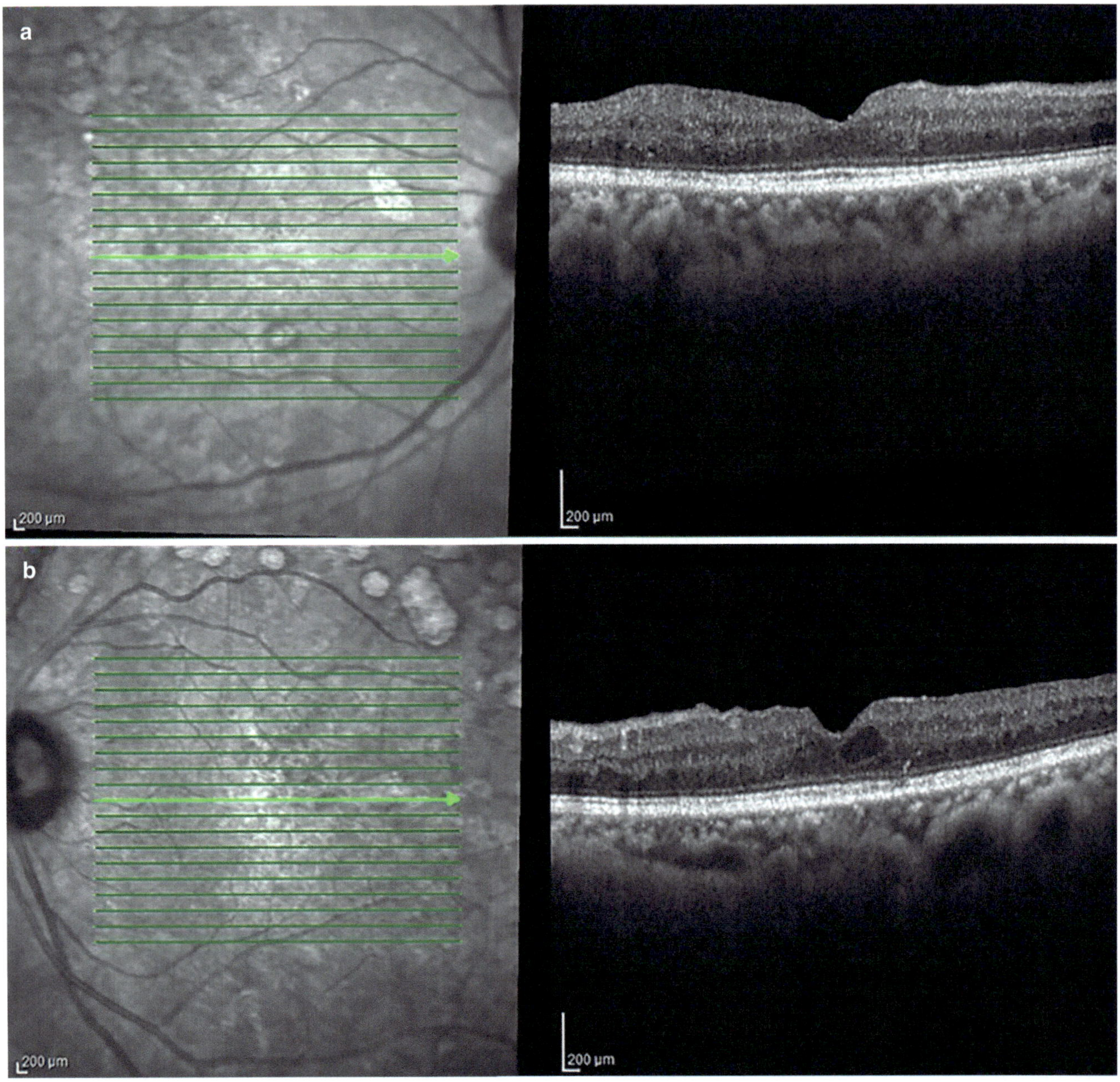

Fig. 14.2 Infrared (left image) and optical coherence tomography (right image) of the right (**a**) and left (**b**) eye showing intraretinal fluid of the left eye

OCT (Figs. 14.5 and 14.6). He was switched to a series of four aflibercept monthly in both eyes. At his most recent visit, his blood pressure was controlled and his HbA1c was 6.0. He will follow-up 4–5 weeks after his last injection.

Case #2

A 47-year-old Hispanic man with type 2 diabetes mellitus presents for his diabetic eye exam. He was diagnosed with diabetes 1 year prior to presentation and he currently takes metformin and glipizide. He is also being treated for hypertension and hyperlipidemia. His HbA1c at presentation was 7.2 (with a high of 9.6 in the last year). He has a history of amblyopia in the right eye. His best-corrected visual acuity was 20/30 and 20/20 in the right and left eyes, respectively. His exam was notable for DBHs, MAs, and few hard exudates in both eyes without NVD or NVE (Fig. 14.7). OCT showed CI-DME in the right eye and small intraretinal cysts in the left eye (Figs. 14.8 and 14.9). FA showed MAs and DME in the right eye worse than the left eye without NVD or NVE (Fig. 14.10). Given that he was asymptomatic and had good visual acuity, the patient elected to observe and return in 3 months. At his follow-up visit, his vision was stable by Snellen acuity, but he noted worsening distortion and blurry vision of the right eye. OCT showed worsening DME in that eye (Fig. 14.11). A trial of bevacizumab in the right eye was recommended (a series of three injections every 4–5 weeks).

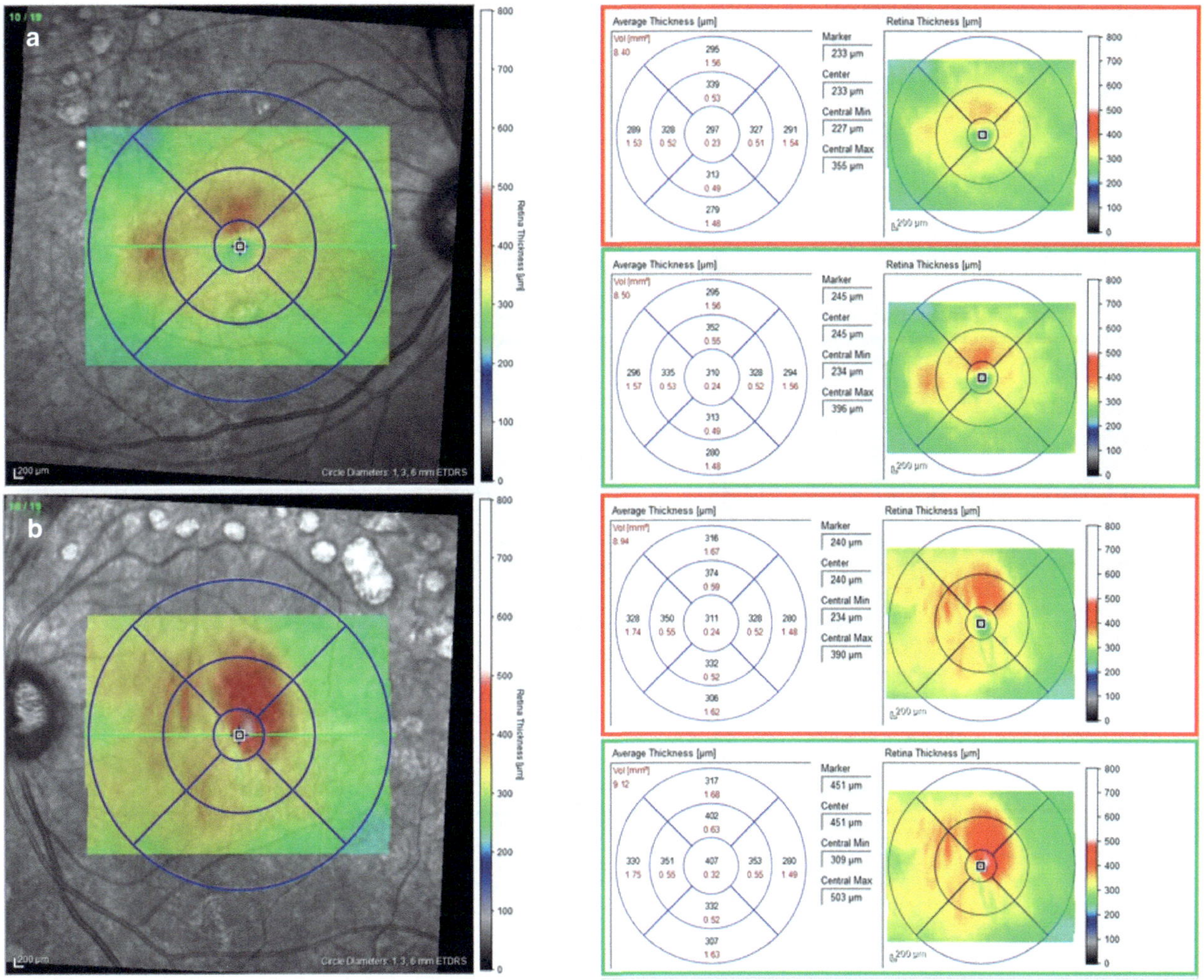

Fig. 14.3 Thickness maps of the right (**a**) and left (**b**) eye showing new thickening in both eyes. The red boxes indicate the maps from the examination 4 months prior. The green boxes indicate the maps from the current examination

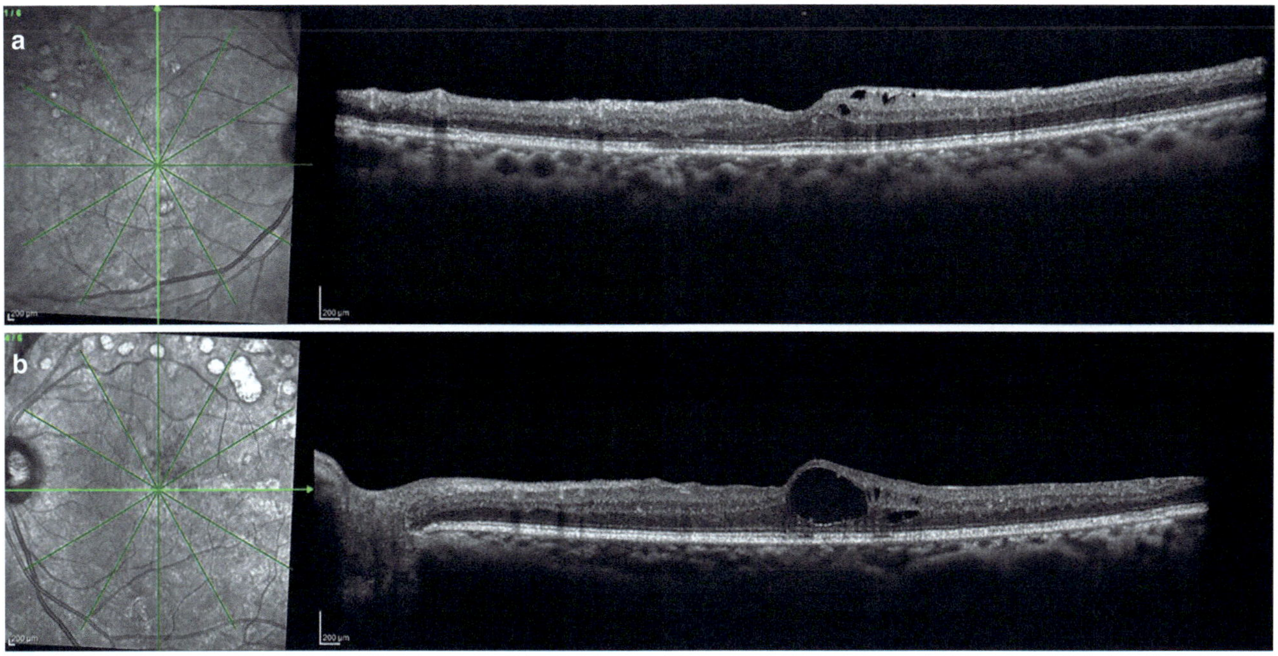

Fig. 14.4 Infrared (left image) and optical coherence tomography (right image) of the right (**a**) and left (**b**) eye showing new intraretinal fluid in the right eye and increased center-involving intraretinal fluid in the left eye

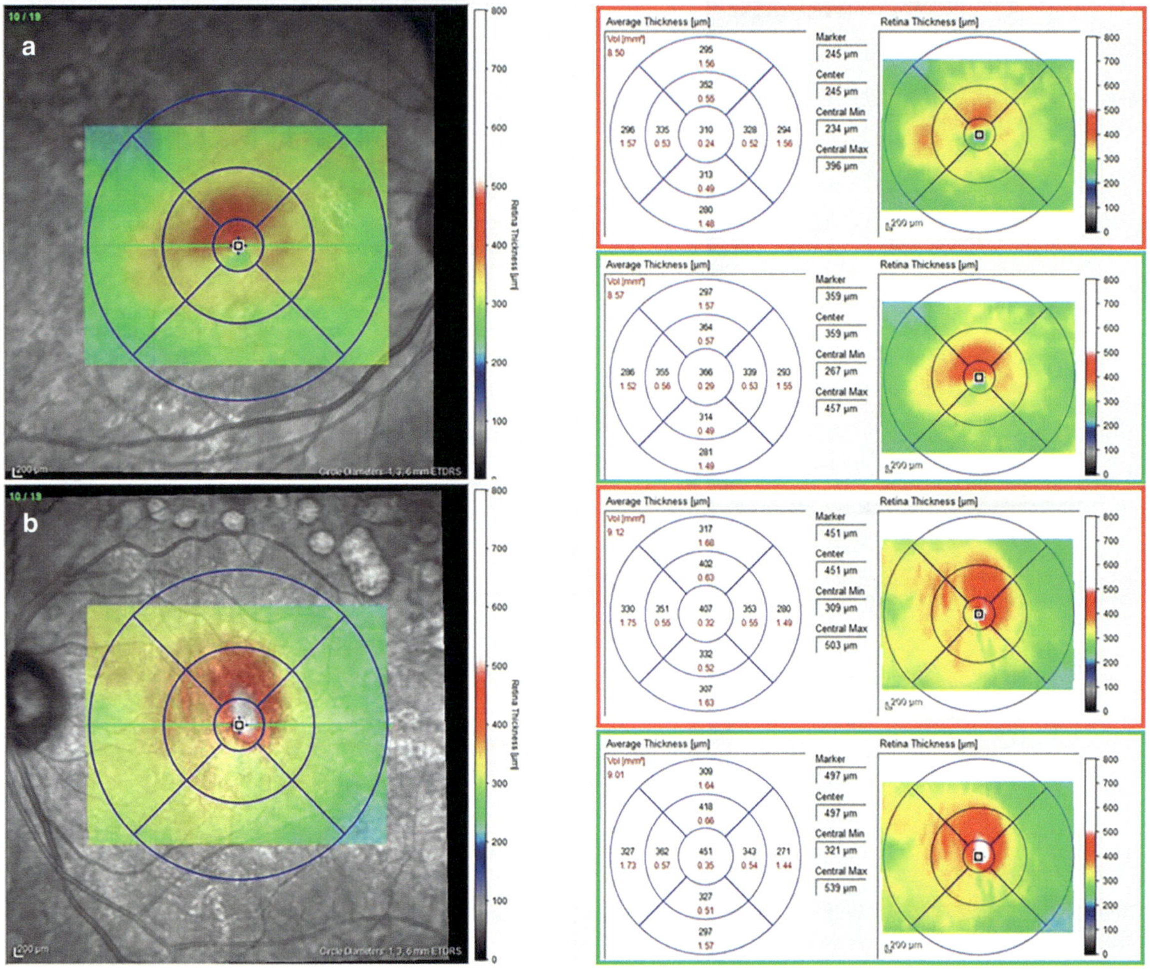

Fig. 14.5 Thickness maps of the right (**a**) and left (**b**) eye showing worsening thickening in both eyes after 4 months. The red boxes indicate the maps from the examination 4 months prior. The green boxes indicate the maps from the current examination

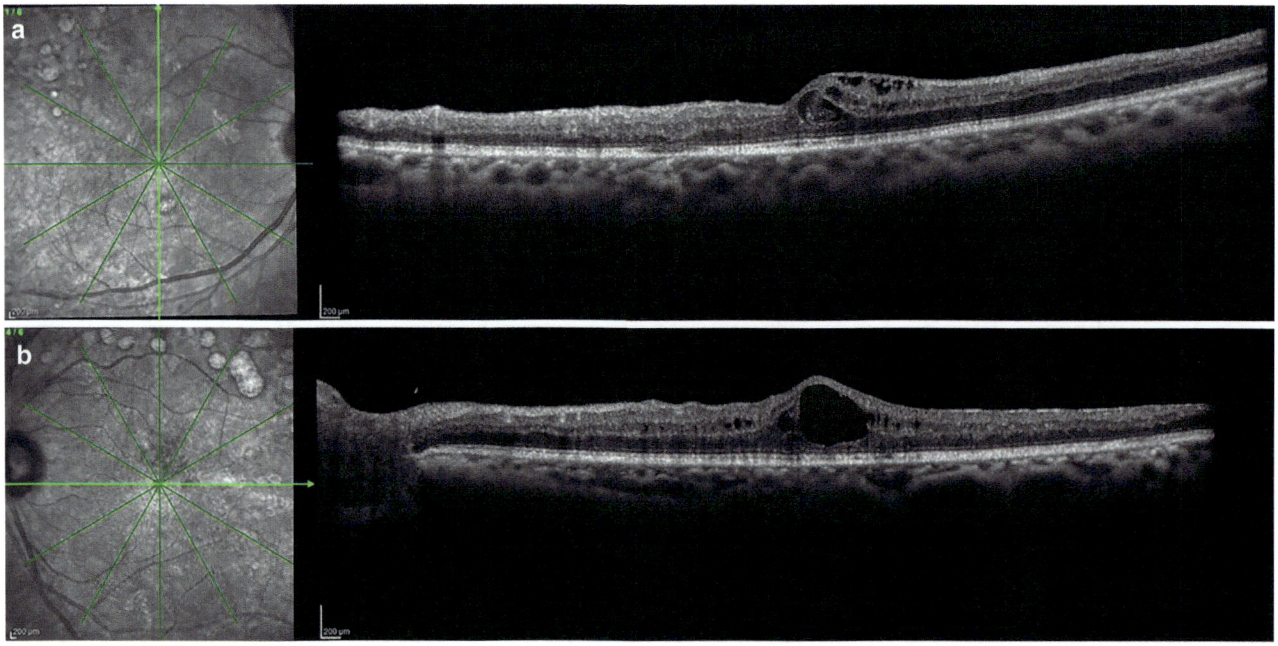

Fig. 14.6 Infrared (left image) and optical coherence tomography (right image) of the right (**a**) and left (**b**) eye showing increased intraretinal fluid in both eyes

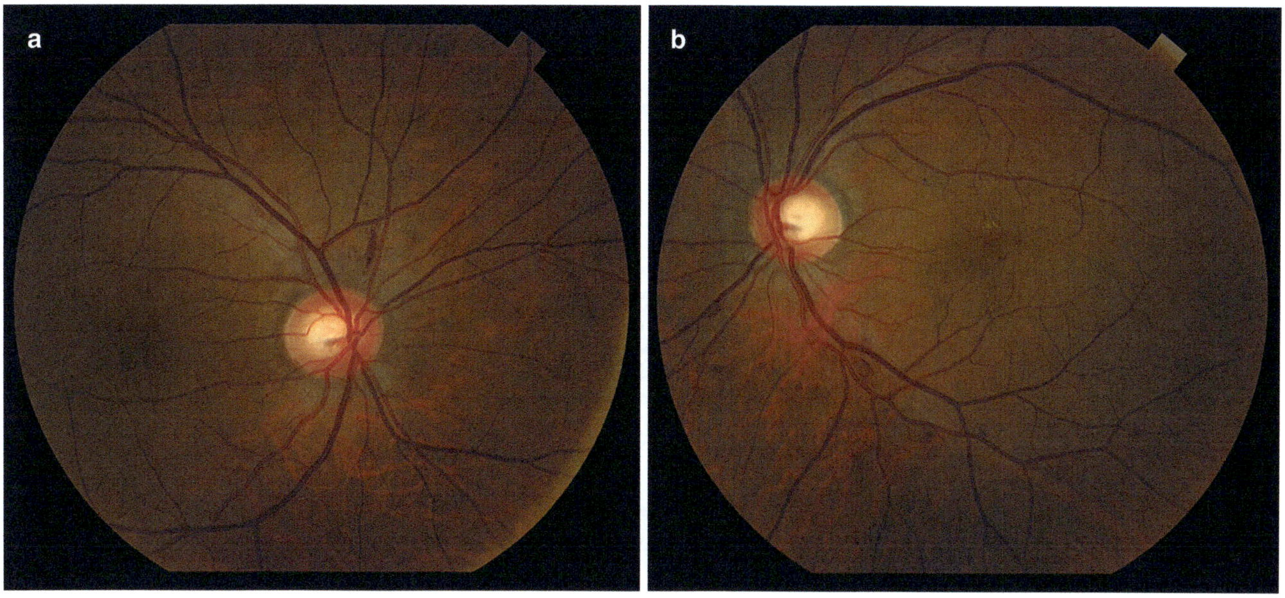

Fig. 14.7 Color fundus photos of the right (**a**) and left (**b**) eye showing dot blot hemorrhages, microaneurysms, and few hard exudates in both eyes without neovascularization

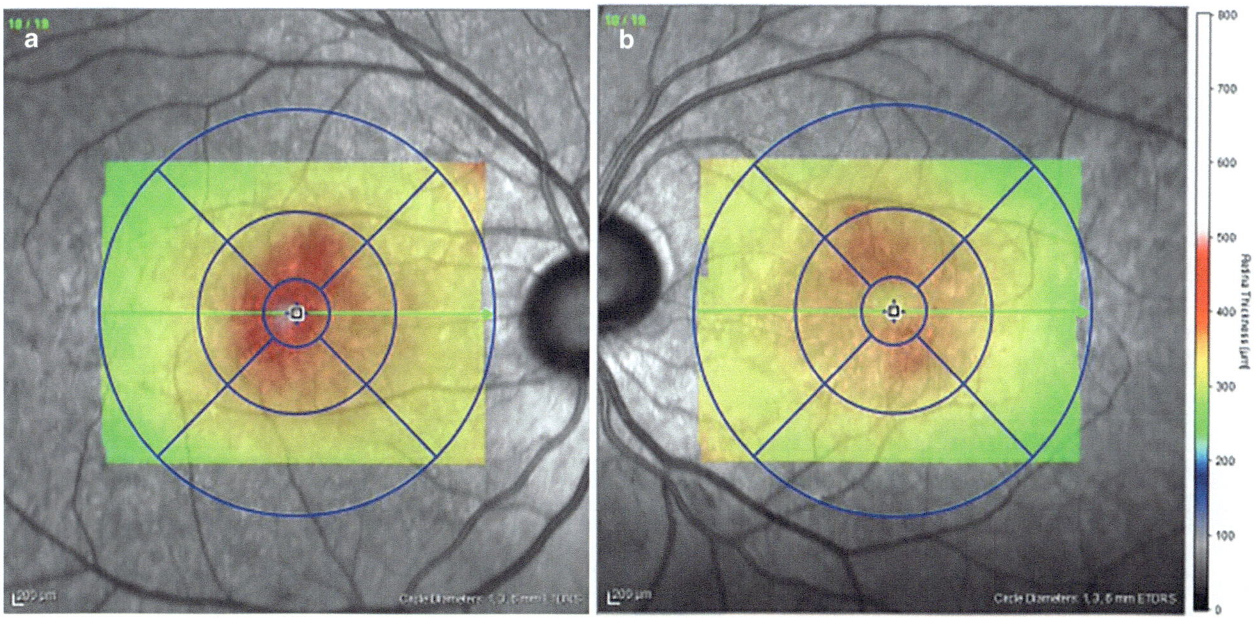

Fig. 14.8 Thickness maps of the right (**a**) and left (**b**) eye showing central thickening in the right eye greater than the left

Focal laser was considered, but his MAs were too close to the fovea to safely laser. He will follow-up 4–5 weeks after his last injection with OCT.

Case #3

A 79-year-old female with type 2 diabetes mellitus diagnosed 30 years ago, on insulin, who is also being treated for hypertension and hyperlipidemia presents as a referral for diabetic macular edema. She was diagnosed with DME in the left eye 2 years prior to presentation but had been observing given non-foveal location and good vision. Two months prior to presentation, the DME appeared worse and she was referred for evaluation. Her vision at presentation was 20/25 with correction in both eyes. Exam was notable for DBHs in the right eye, DBHs, MAs, hard exudates and intraretinal hemorrhages peripherally in the left eye, with mild arteriolar attenuation in both eyes (Fig. 14.12). OCT showed atrophy inferiorly in the right eye (in the context of prior inferior retinal detachment) and CI-DME with temporal exudates in the left eye (Fig. 14.13). FA showed scattered intraretinal leak-

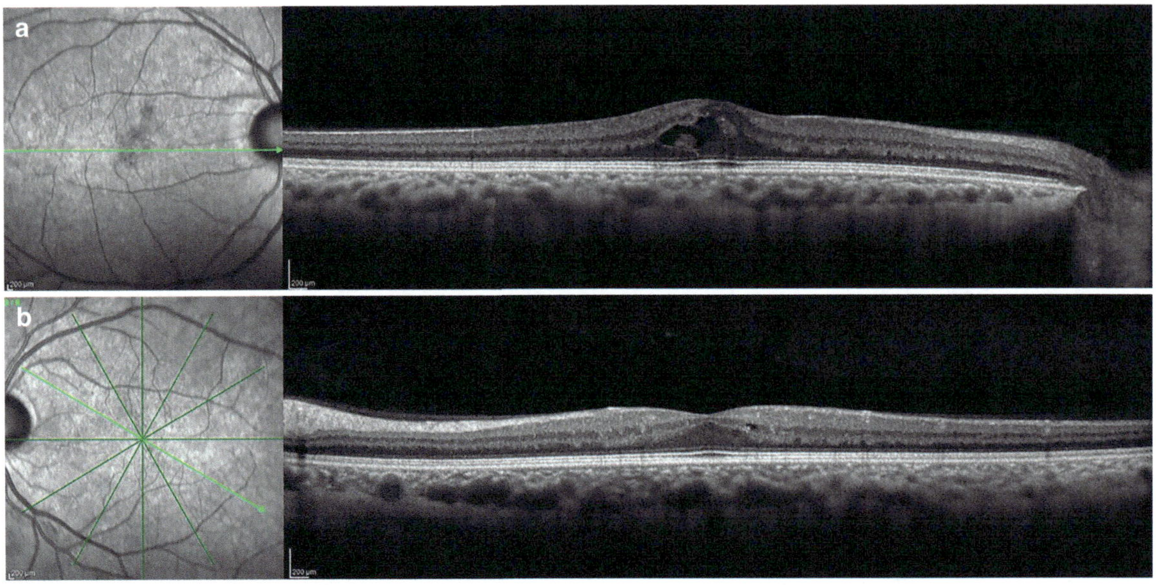

Fig. 14.9 Infrared (left image) and optical coherence tomography (right image) of the right (**a**) and left (**b**) eye showing intraretinal fluid worse in the right eye than left eye, with microaneurysms in the right eye

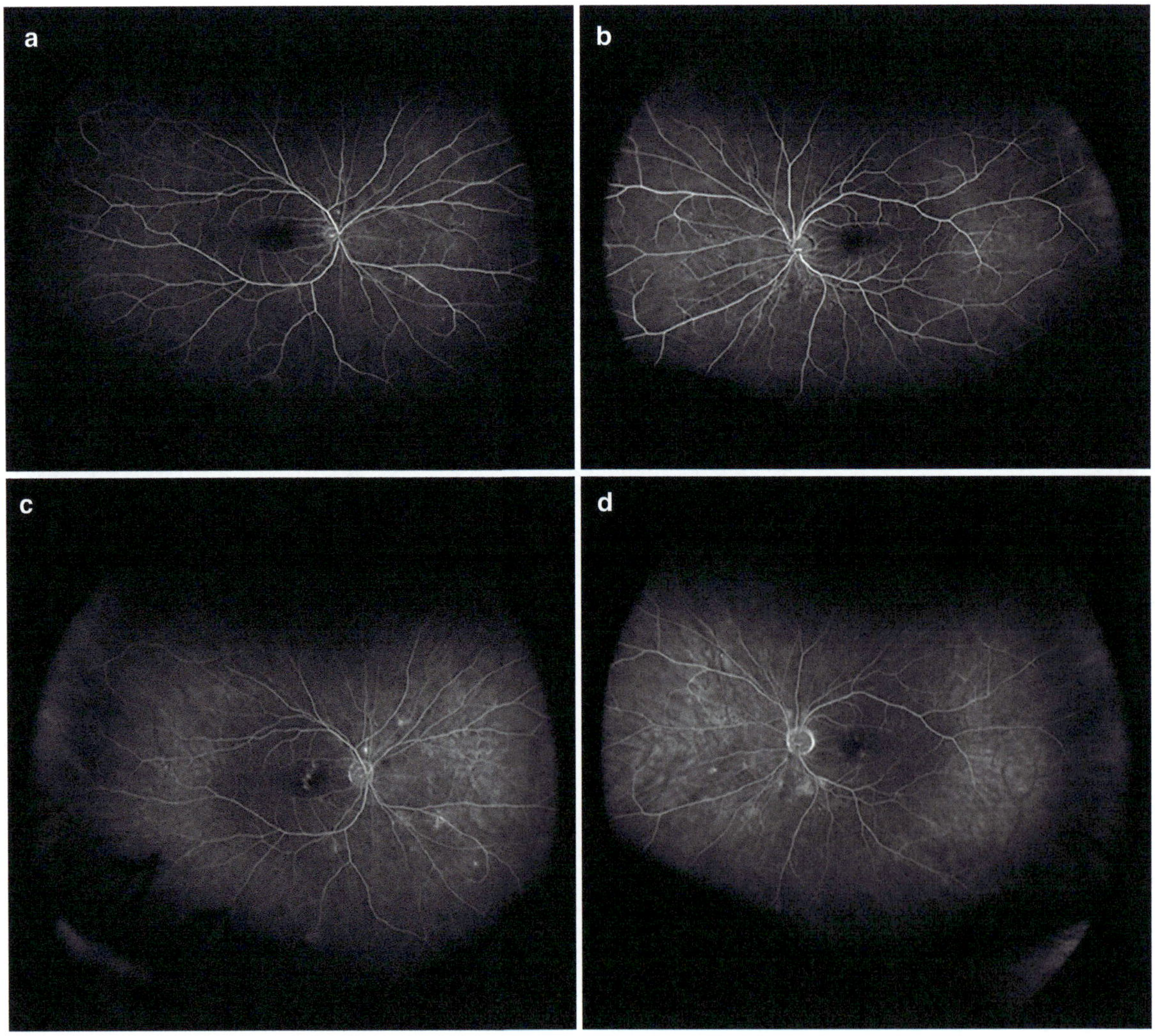

Fig. 14.10 Early fluorescein angiography images of the right (**a**) and left (**b**) eye and late images of the right (**c**) and left (**d**) eye showing microaneurysms and leakage around the fovea in the right eye worse than left eye. There is no neovascularization of the disc or elsewhere

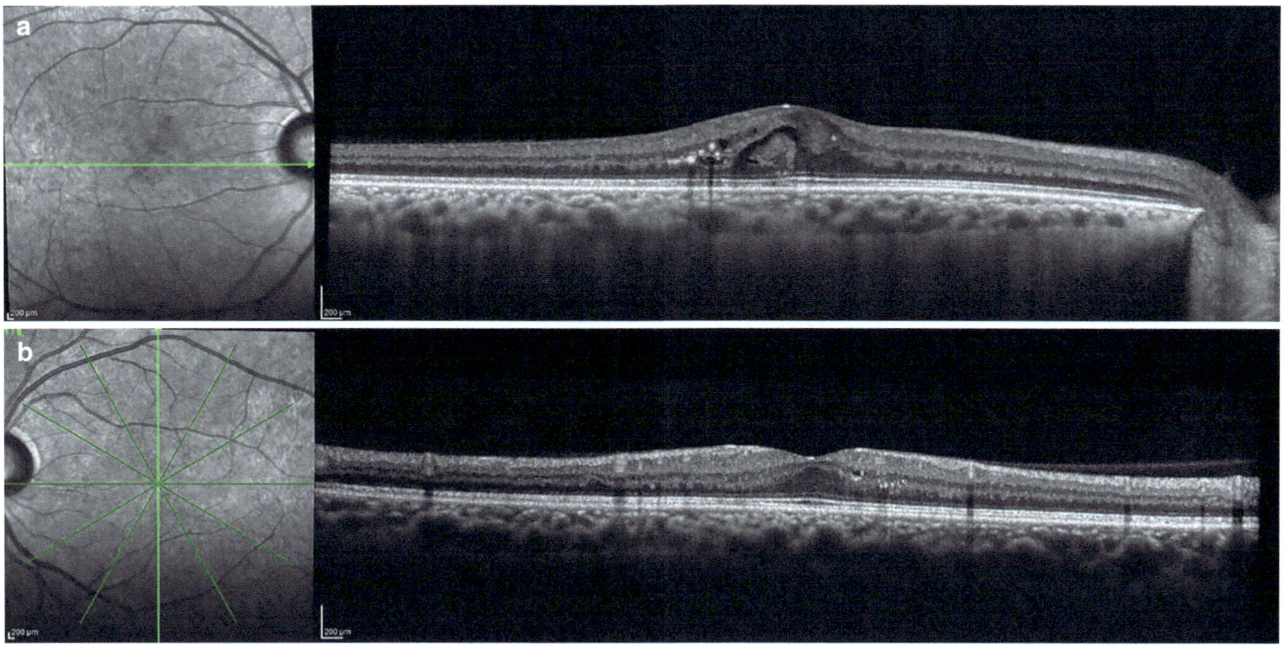

Fig. 14.11 Infrared (left image) and optical coherence tomography (right image) of the right (**a**) and left (**b**) eye showing intraretinal fluid, exudates and a microaneurysm of the right eye with trace intraretinal fluid and exudates of the left eye

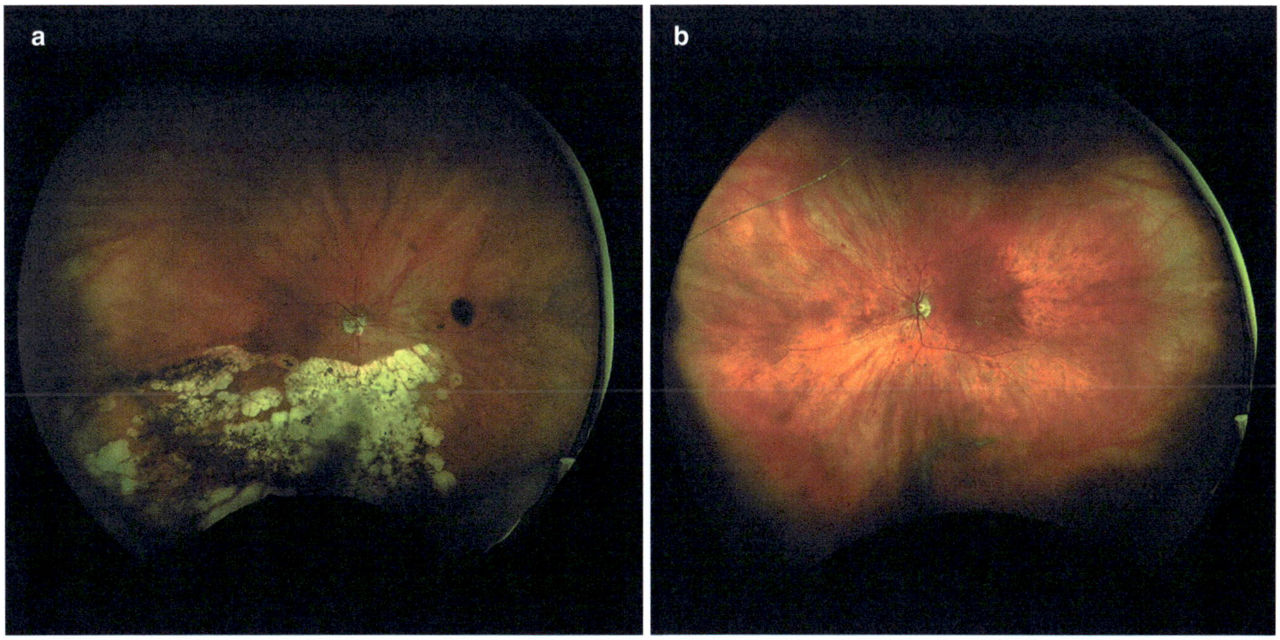

Fig. 14.12 Optos color fundus photos of the right (**a**) and left (**b**) eye showing dot blot hemorrhages in the right eye, dot blot hemorrhages, microaneurysms, hard exudates and intraretinal hemorrhages in the periphery of the left eye with mild arteriolar attenuation in both eyes. Of note, the patient had a history of a retinal detachment repaired by scleral buckling procedure, with inferior laser of the right eye

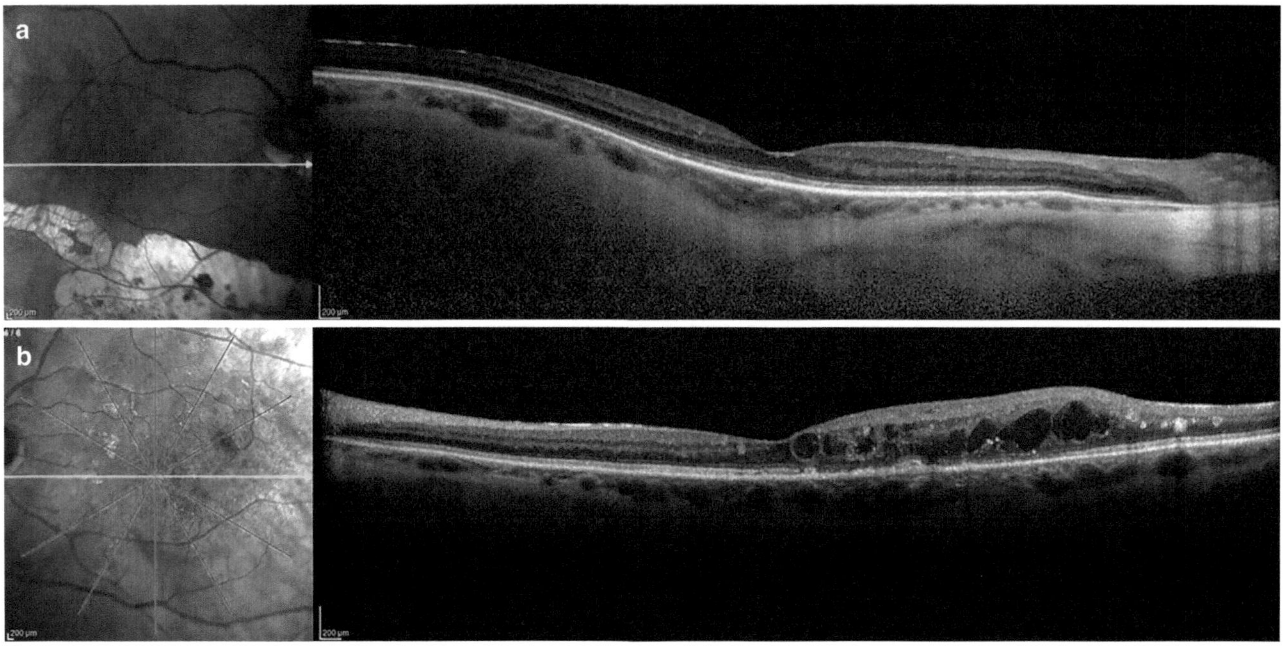

Fig. 14.13 Infrared (left image) and optical coherence tomography (right image) of the right (**a**) and left (**b**) eye showing atrophy inferiorly in the right eye and intraretinal fluid and hard exudates of the left eye

age in the left eye; there was no NVD or NVE in either eye (Fig. 14.14). She was started on a series of five bevacizumab injections every 4–5 weeks in the left eye. Upon follow-up, she was noted to have an incomplete response to bevacizumab (Figs. 14.15 and 14.16) and was switched to aflibercept for another series of five injections every 4–5 weeks. She had a better response to aflibercept (Figs. 14.17 and 14.18) and is undergoing another series of 5 injections at the same interval. She will follow-up 4–5 weeks after her last injection with OCT.

Case #4

A 67-year-old man with type 2 diabetes mellitus, hyperlipidemia, hypertension, and obstructive sleep apnea presents for diabetic evaluation. He has chronic DME for which he has received focal laser in both eyes. He also has a history of proliferative diabetic retinopathy status post panretinal photocoagulation of the right eye and is now quiescent. He has moderate non-proliferative diabetic retinopathy in the left eye. He has been receiving aflibercept monthly in the right eye after incomplete response to bevacizumab in the past, and aflibercept every 8–9 weeks in the left eye. Upon presentation his best-corrected visual acuity was 20/50 and 20/60 in the right and left eyes, respectively. His exam was notable for moderate non-proliferative diabetic retinopathy, focal laser scars (Fig. 14.19), MAs and DME in both eyes with panretinal photocoagulation in the right eye. OCT showed diffuse intraretinal fluid in both eyes, worse compared to 4 months prior (Figs. 14.20 and 14.21). Prior FA showed retinal vascular leakage of both eyes with no good focal laser targets (Fig. 14.22). Given worsening DME and large central cysts, a trial of triamcinolone acetonide 2 mg intravitreal injection was recommended in the right eye and his aflibercept interval was shorted back to every 4–6 weeks in the left eye. One month later, his best-corrected visual acuity was 20/40 in the right eye and 20/30 in the left eye. His intraocular pressure was normal in both eyes. OCT showed improvement in DME in both eyes (Fig. 14.23). As there was no steroid response, he underwent dexamethasone intravitreal implant of the right eye and continued aflibercept every 4–5 weeks in the left eye. He will follow-up in 12–15 weeks after he finishes his current aflibercept series in the left eye.

Case #5

A 75-year-old female with type 2 diabetes mellitus, stage 4 chronic kidney disease, hypertension, hypothyroidism, and coronary artery disease presents with moderate non-proliferative diabetic retinopathy with DME in both eyes. Her HbA1c is 7.9% and she is taking insulin. She underwent a series of bevacizumab injections every 4 weeks in both eyes with inadequate response and was switched to aflibercept at the same interval. Her vision uncorrected was 20/50 and 20/40 in the right and left eyes, respectively. Her exam was notable for moderate CI-DME and MAs as well as scattered hemorrhages in the periphery of both eyes. Prior FA

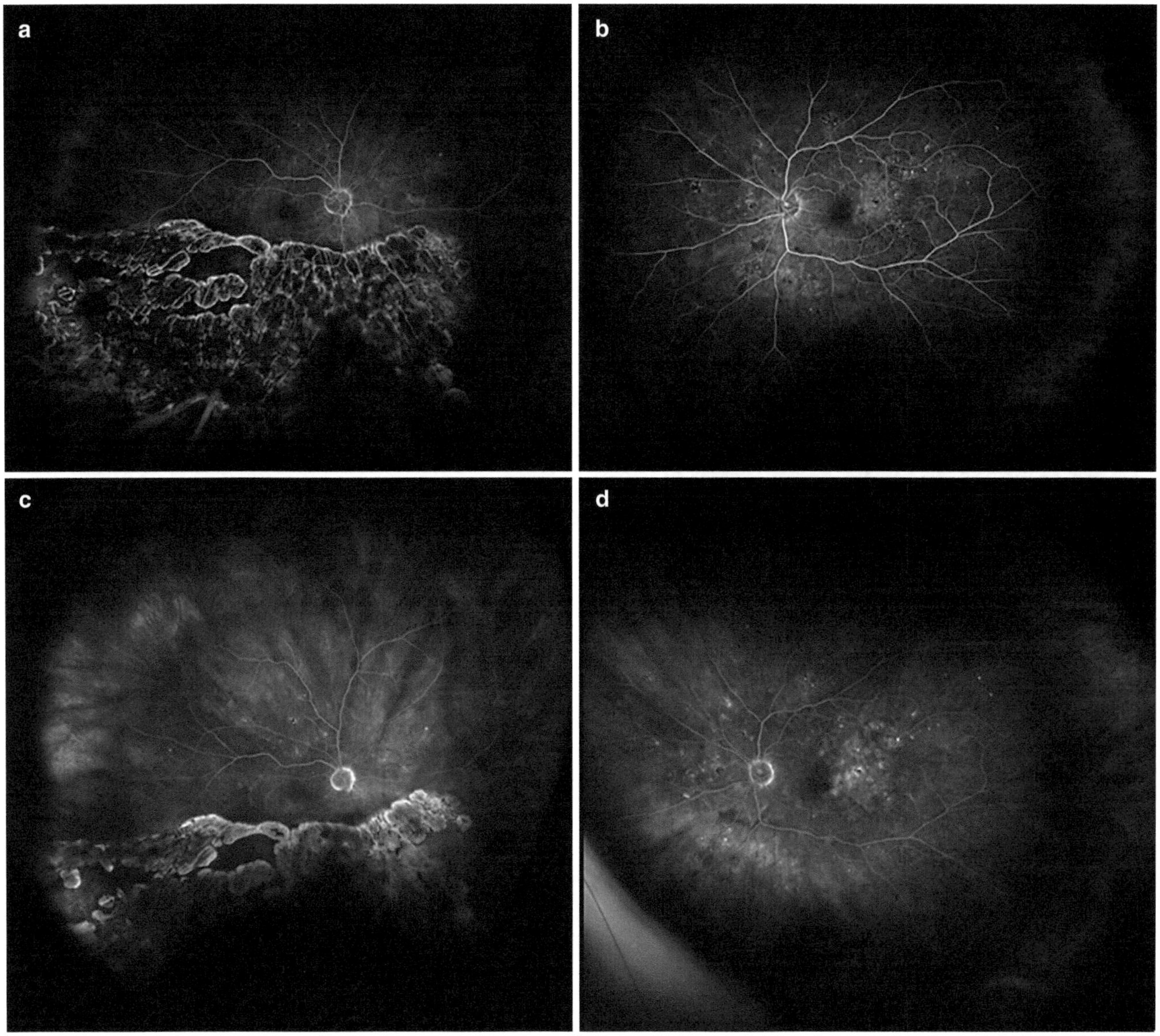

Fig. 14.14 Early fluorescein angiography images of the right (**a**) and left (**b**) eye and late images of the right (**c**) and left (**d**) eye showing scattered intraretinal leakage of the left eye. There is no neovascularization in either eye

showed many MAs with retinal vascular leakage and foveal leakage in both eyes but no NVD or NVE (Fig. 14.24). OCT was notable for increased intraretinal fluid compared to prior and trace subretinal fluid in the right eye, and stable intraretinal fluid in the left eye (Fig. 14.25). Given the worsening fluid in the right eye, and the incomplete response to bevacizumab and now aflibercept, she was trialed on intravitreal triamcinolone acetonide 2 mg in the right eye and continued on aflibercept in the left eye with a stricter interval of every 4 weeks. One month later, her vision was 20/60 and 20/30 uncorrected in the right and left eye respectively and her intraocular pressure was normal. Her OCT showed improvement in DME in both eyes (Figs. 14.26 and 14.27). As intravitreal triamcinolone acetonide was successful at reducing the intraretinal fluid, she was given the dexamethasone intravitreal implant in the right eye and continued on aflibercept in the left eye. She will follow-up 4–5 weeks after the last injection in the left eye with OCT. She will also get an OCT of both eyes prior to every injection visit to monitor for recurrence.

Case #6

A 71-year-old Somali female with type 2 diabetes mellitus on insulin (latest HbA1c was 9.5 with a high of 13 in the last 3 years) and hypertension presents for diabetic evaluation. She has been receiving aflibercept in both eyes for moderate non-proliferative diabetic retinopathy with DME (Fig. 14.28) for the last 4 years. She was initially treated with bevaci-

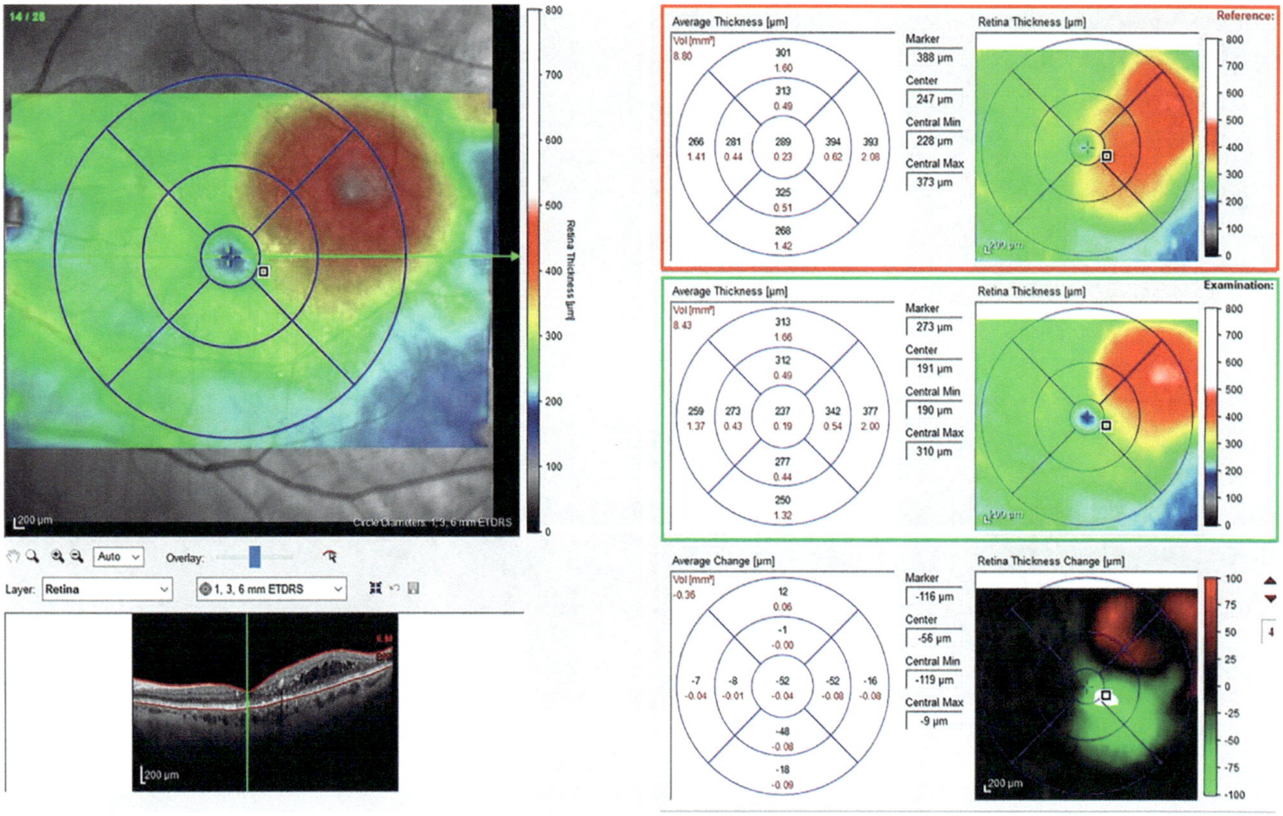

Fig. 14.15 Thickness map change report of the left eye showing persistent intraretinal fluid and retinal thickening despite treatment with bevacizumab for 5 months. The red box indicates the map from the examination 5 months prior. The green box indicates the map from the current examination

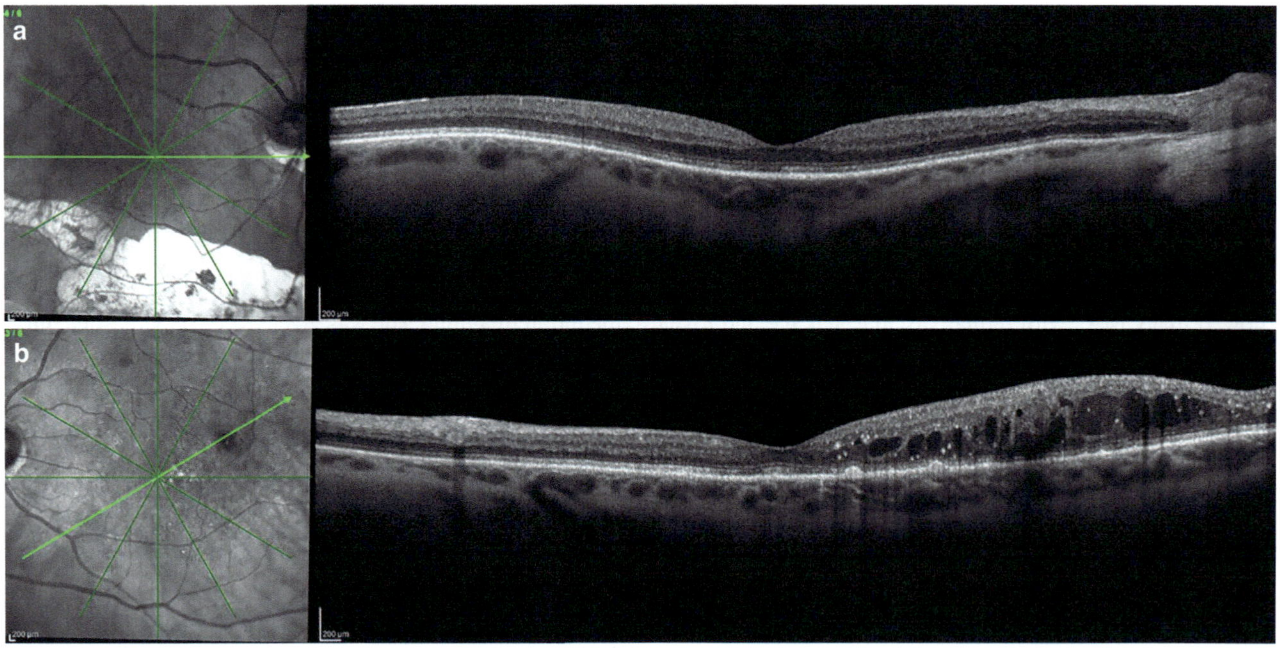

Fig. 14.16 Infrared (left image) and optical coherence tomography (right image) of the right (**a**) and left (**b**) eye showing incomplete response to bevacizumab with continued intraretinal fluid and hard exudates of the left eye

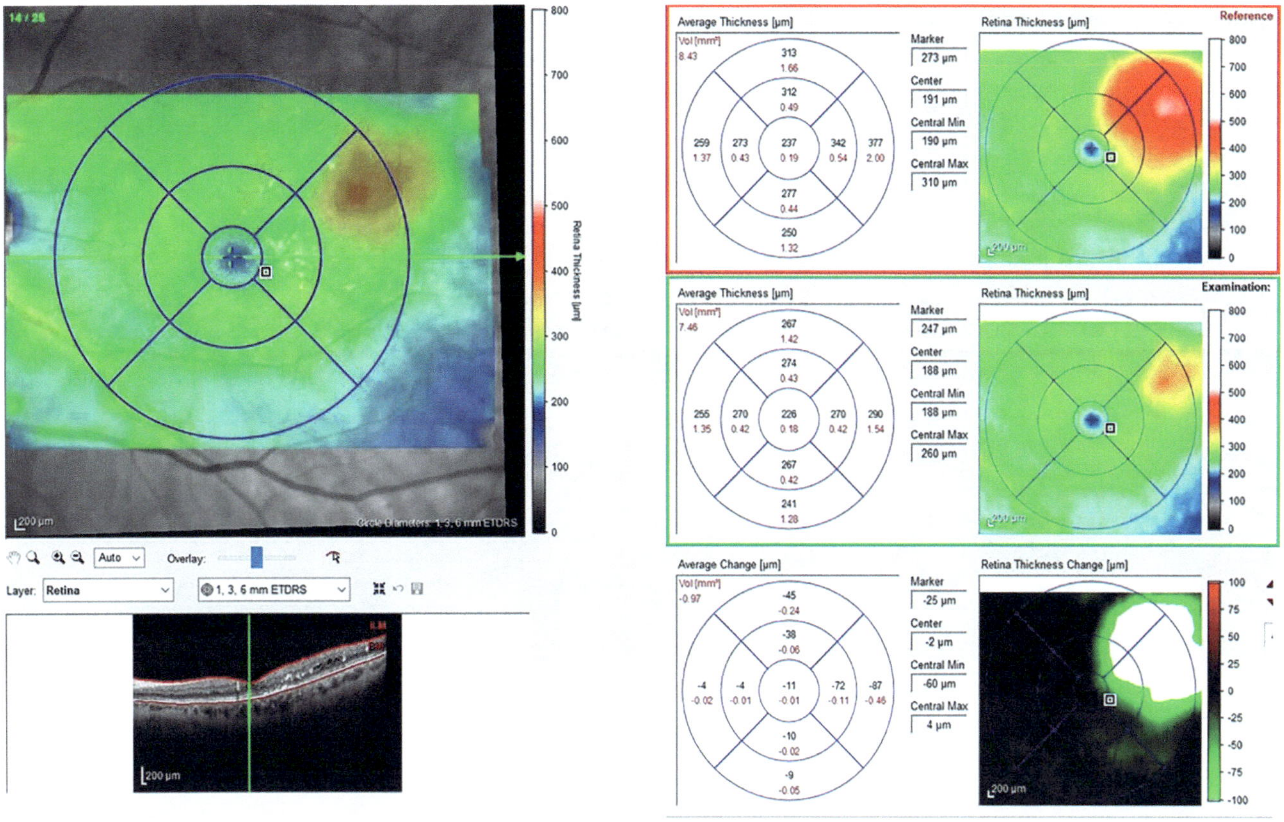

Fig. 14.17 Thickness map change report showing decreased thickness in the left eye after a series of aflibercept. The red box indicates the map from the examination 5 months prior. The green box indicates the map from the current examination

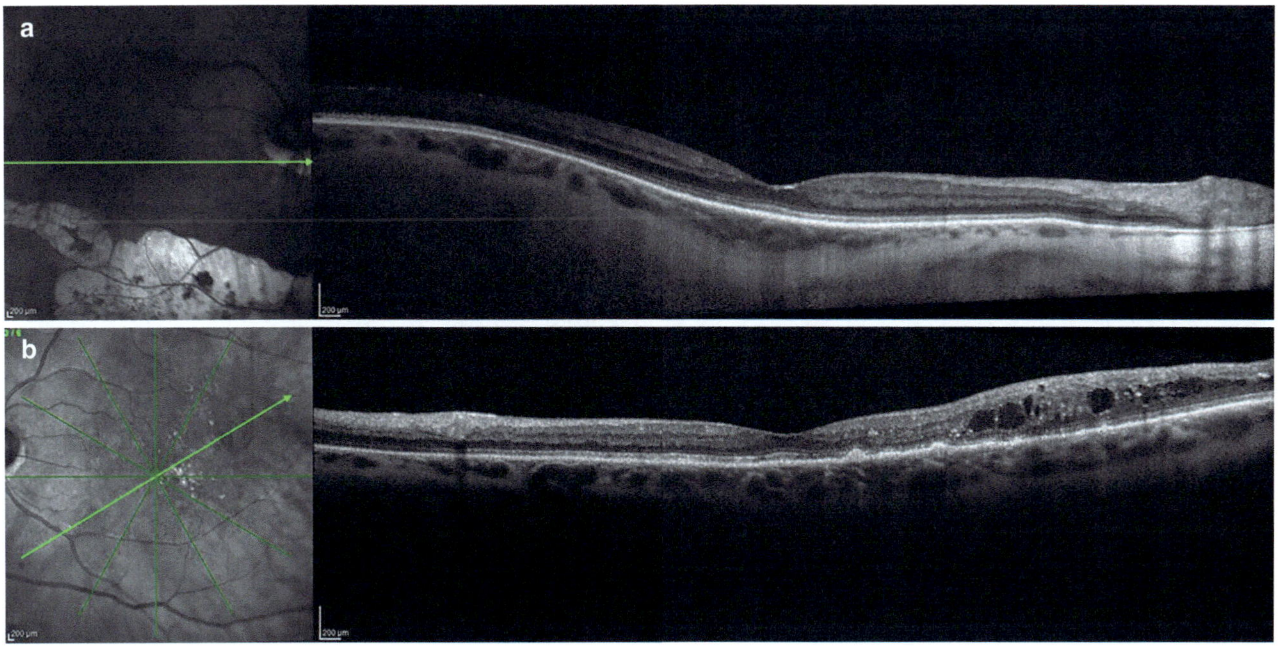

Fig. 14.18 Infrared (left image) and optical coherence tomography (right image) of the right (**a**) and left (**b**) eye showing better response to aflibercept with improved intraretinal fluid and exudates of the left eye

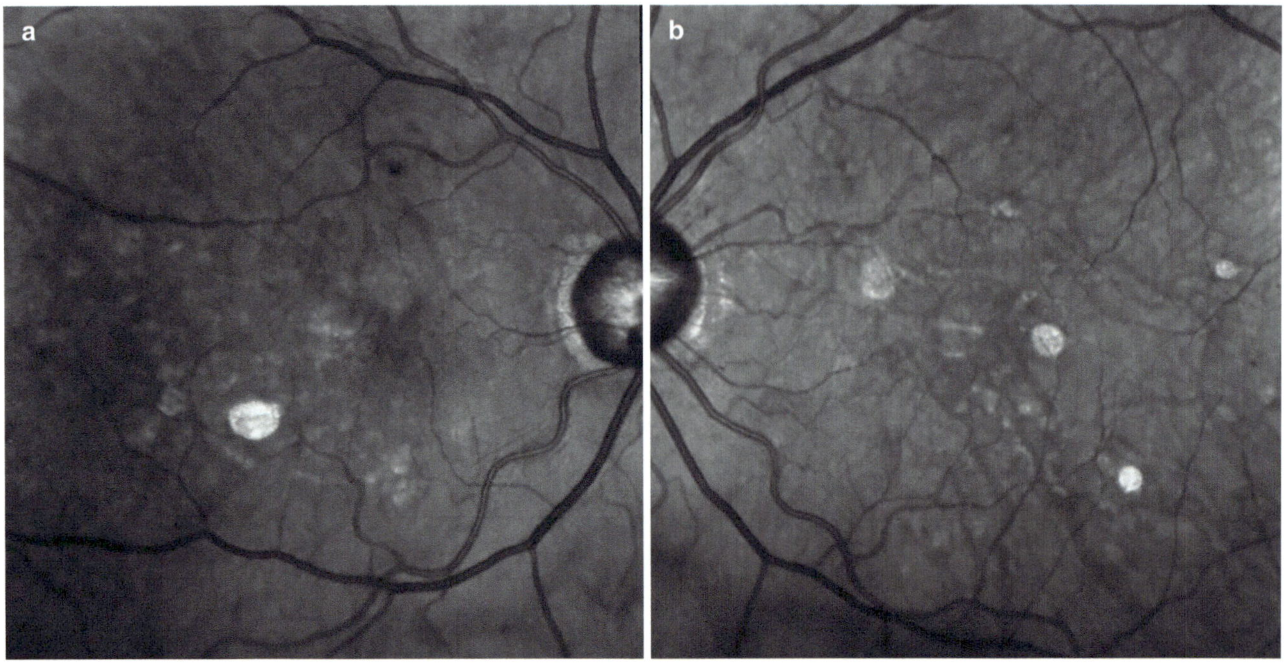

Fig. 14.19 Infrared photo of the right (**a**) and left (**b**) eye showing focal laser scars

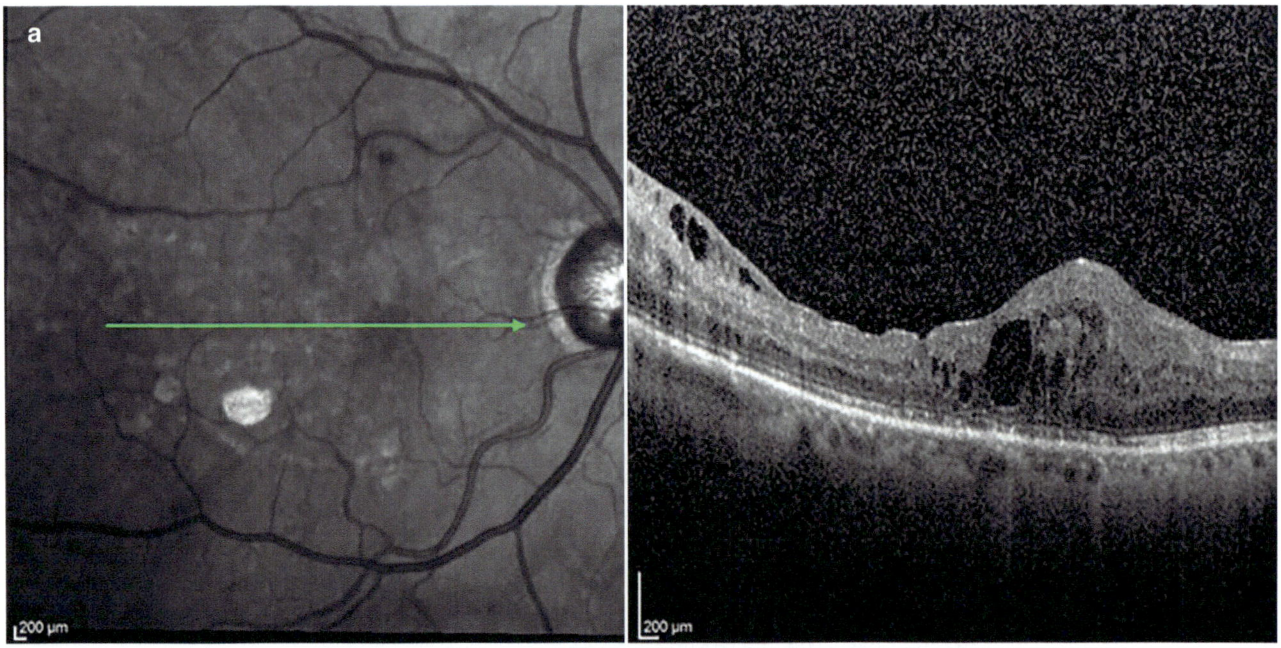

Fig. 14.20 Infrared (left image) and optical coherence tomography (right image) of the right (**a**) and left (**b**) eye showing intraretinal fluid worse in the right than left eye while undergoing a series of aflibercept in both eyes. The right eye also has a temporal epiretinal membrane

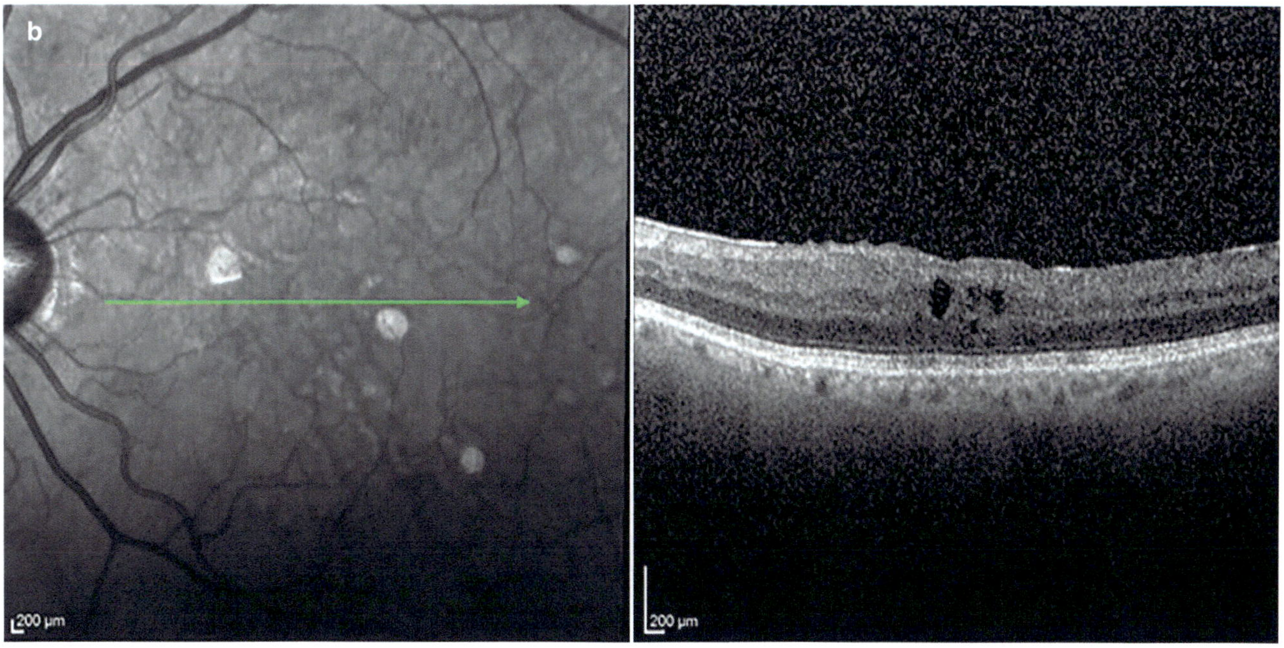

Fig.14.20 (continued)

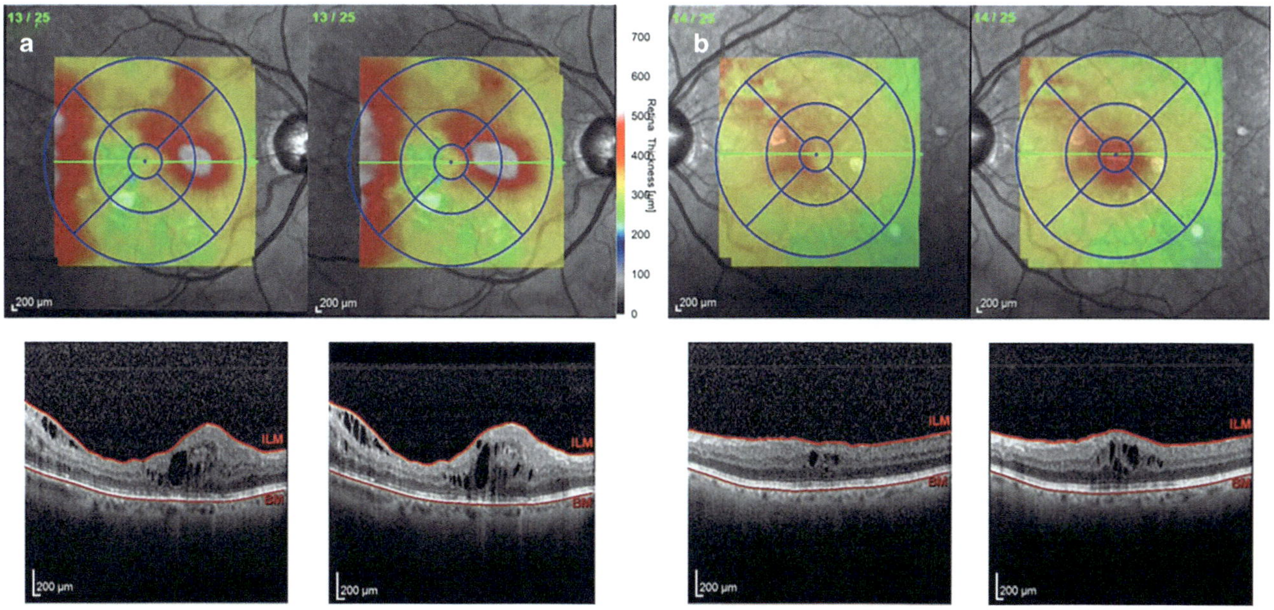

Fig. 14.21 Thickness map change report of the right (**a**) and left (**b**) eye showing worsening retinal thickening in both eyes. The image on the left of each panel indicates the study from 3 months prior. The image on the right of each panel indicates the study from the current evaluation

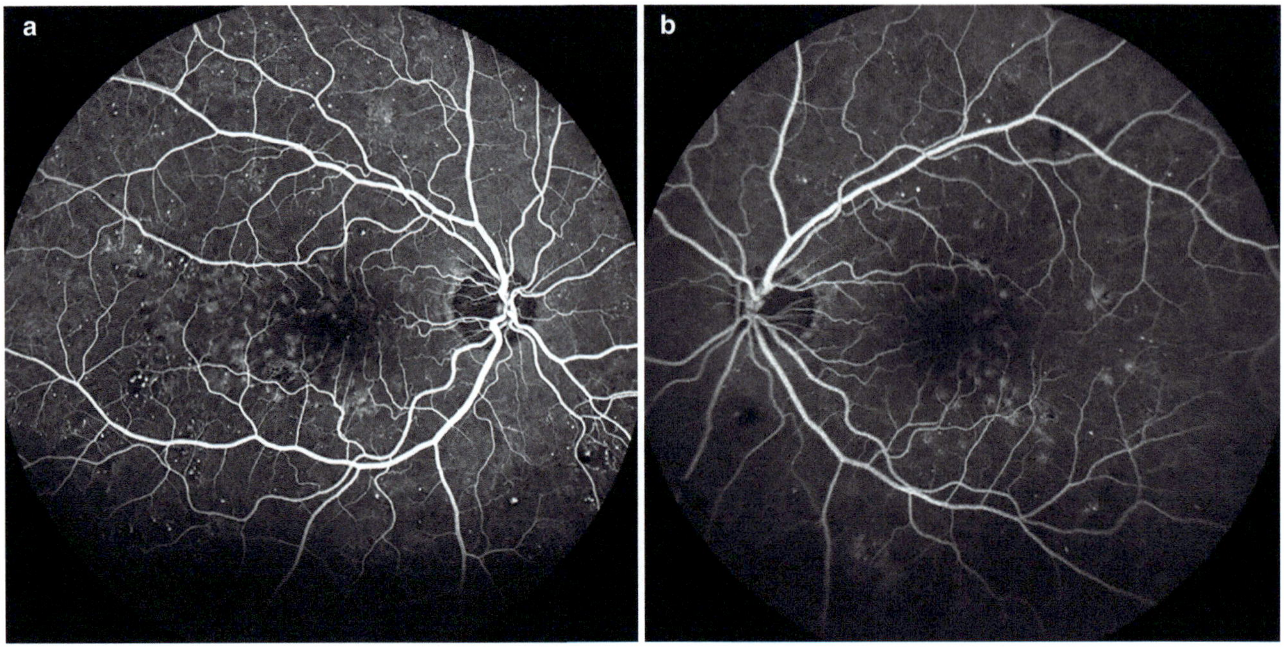

Fig. 14.22 Late fluorescein angiography images of the right (**a**) and left (**b**) eye showing retinal vascular leakage in both eyes without obvious microaneurysms contributing to macular edema. There are patchy areas of capillary drop-out in the right eye. There is no neovascularization in either eye

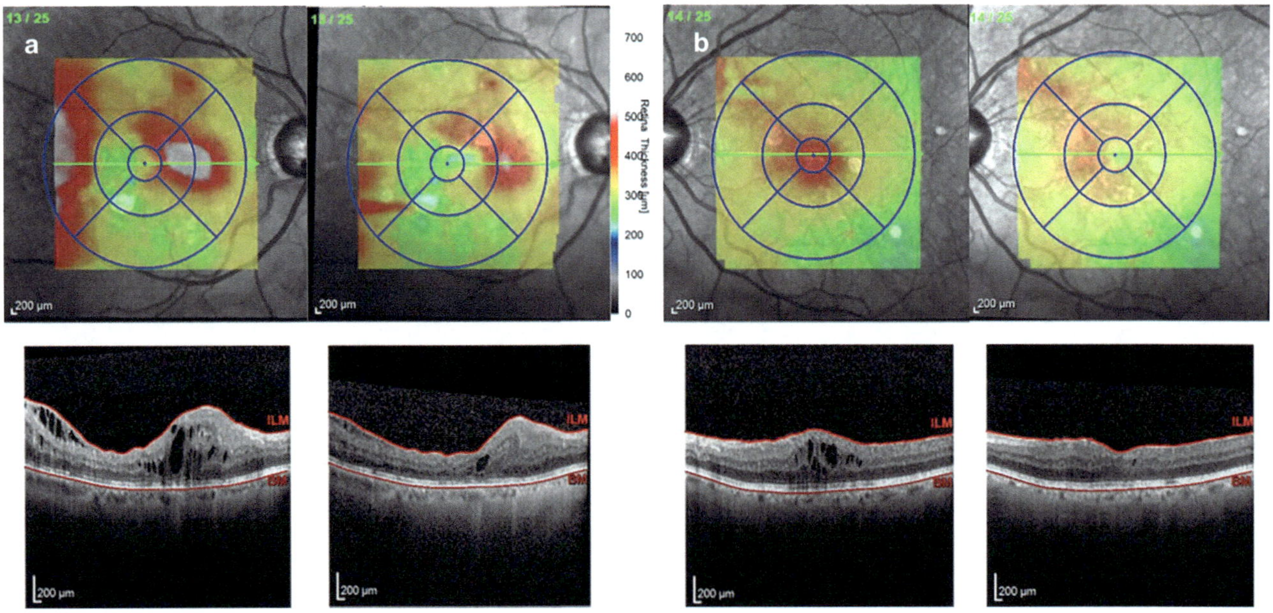

Fig. 14.23 Thickness map change report of the right (**a**) and left (**b**) eye showing improvement in retinal thickening in both eyes after intravitreal triamcinolone acetonide in the right eye and shortened aflibercept interval in the left eye. The image on the left of each panel indicates the study from 1 month prior. The image on the right of each panel indicates the study from the current evaluation

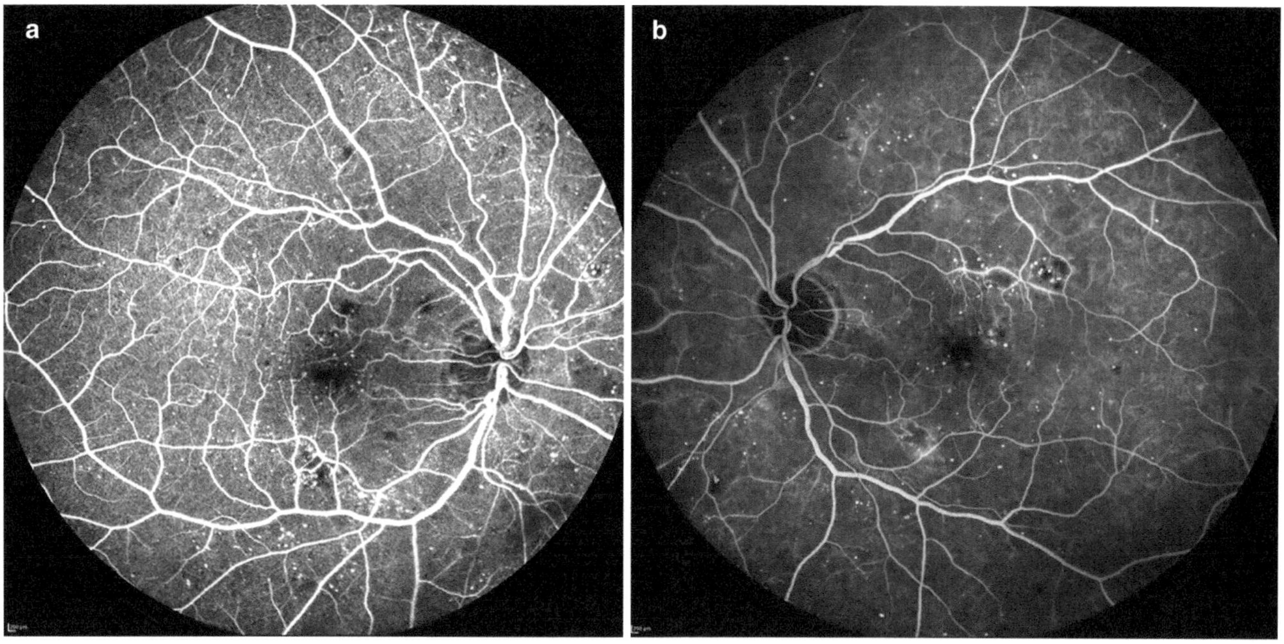

Fig. 14.24 Fluorescein angiography of the right (**a**) and left (**b**) eye showing microaneurysms and retinal vascular leakage in both eyes. The left eye image was captured later in the sequence. Subsequent images (not depicted) demonstrate foveal leakage in both eyes

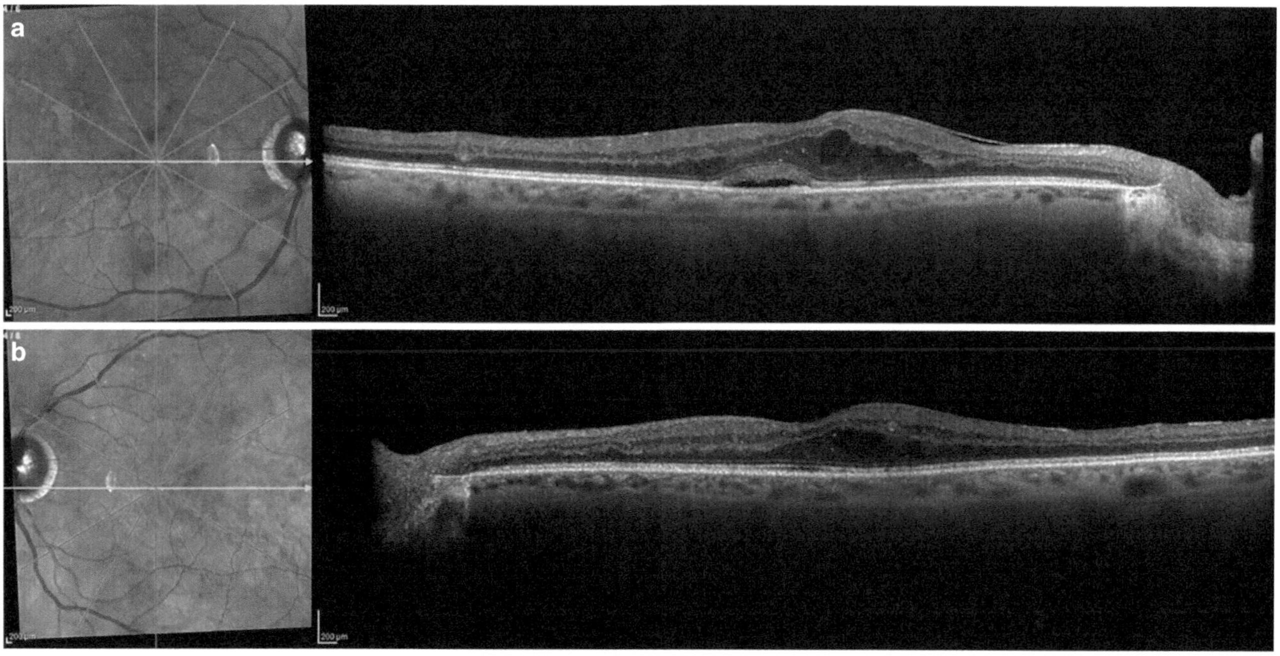

Fig. 14.25 Infrared (left image) and optical coherence tomography (right image) of the right (**a**) and left (**b**) eye showing worsening intraretinal fluid in the right eye with a pocket of subretinal fluid, and stable intraretinal fluid and thickening in the left eye

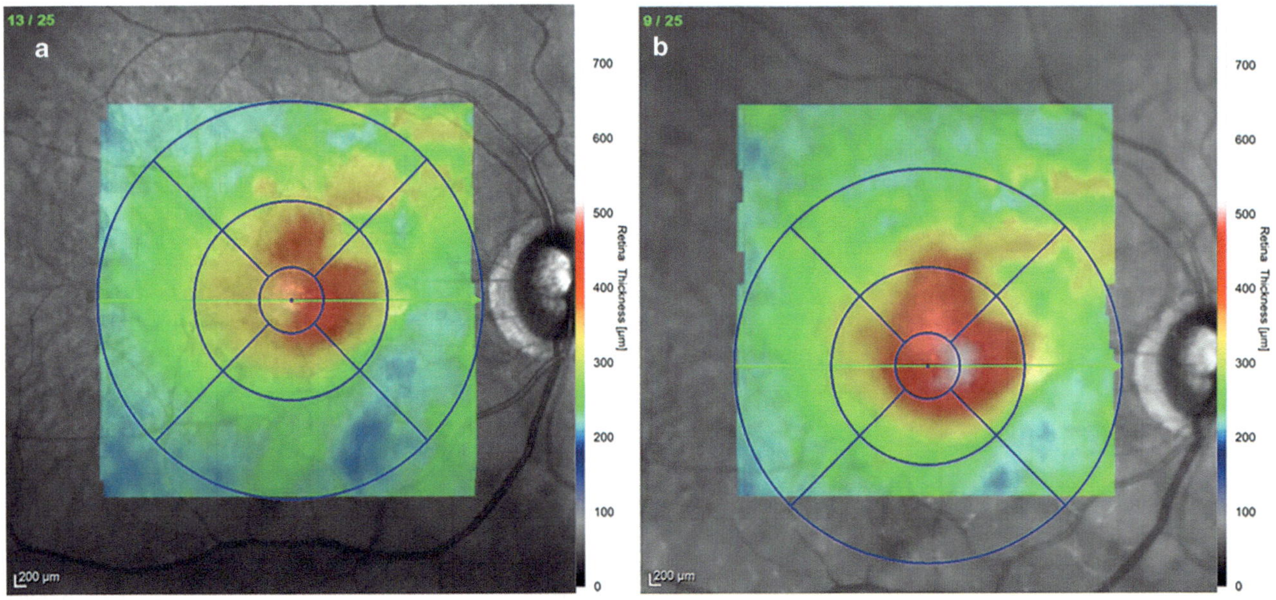

Fig. 14.26 Thickness map of the right eye after intravitreal triamcinolone acetonide (**a**) and 1 month prior (**b**) to injection showing improved retinal thickness with a decrease in intraretinal fluid and resolution of subretinal fluid (not shown)

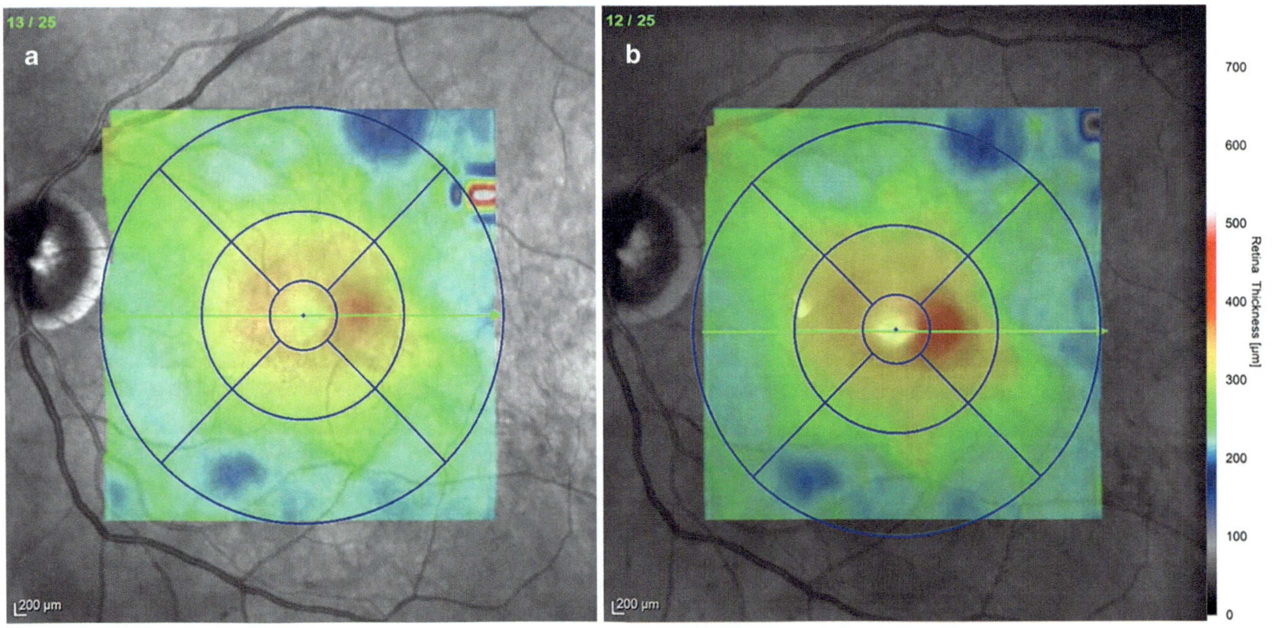

Fig. 14.27 Thickness map of the left eye after aflibercept (**a**) and 1 month prior (**b**) to injection showing improved intraretinal fluid temporal to the fovea

zumab monthly. Her presenting vision was 20/400 and 20/70 with correction in the setting of pseudophakic corneal edema of the right eye, cataract in the left eye, and DME in both eyes. She had incomplete treatment response and was then switched to aflibercept. She was slowly extended to 4–5-week intervals, then every 6 weeks, then every 8 weeks, and finally every 10 weeks. Upon re-evaluation, she was recently status post cataract surgery and posterior capsulotomy, and her vision was 20/20 in both eyes. She had parafoveal DME in both eyes (Fig. 14.29), and despite her excellent visual acuity, did not wish to stop injections. To decrease the burden of intravitreal injections, she was scheduled for focal/grid laser of both eyes (left eye first). Her focal laser treatment was performed with a power of 60 mW, duration of

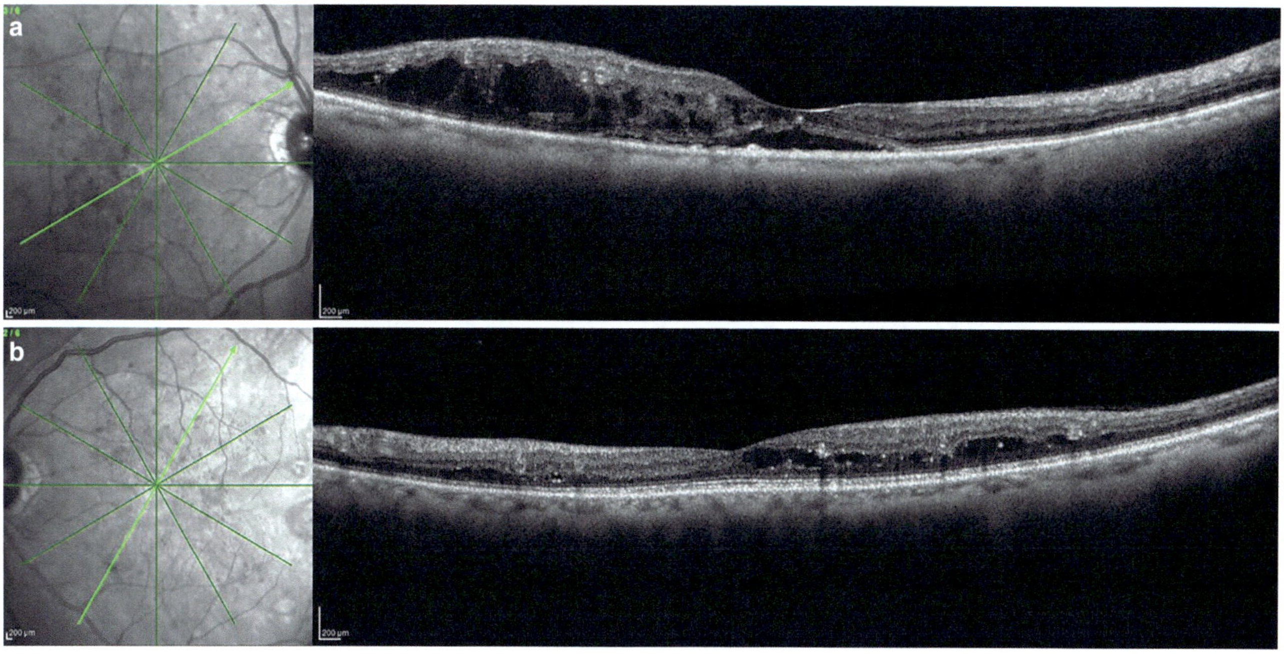

Fig. 14.28 Infrared (left image) and optical coherence tomography (right image) of the right (**a**) and left (**b**) eye showing intraretinal fluid and exudates in both eyes (right worse than left) with subretinal fluid in the right eye. This image was captured prior to treatment initiation with anti-VEGF

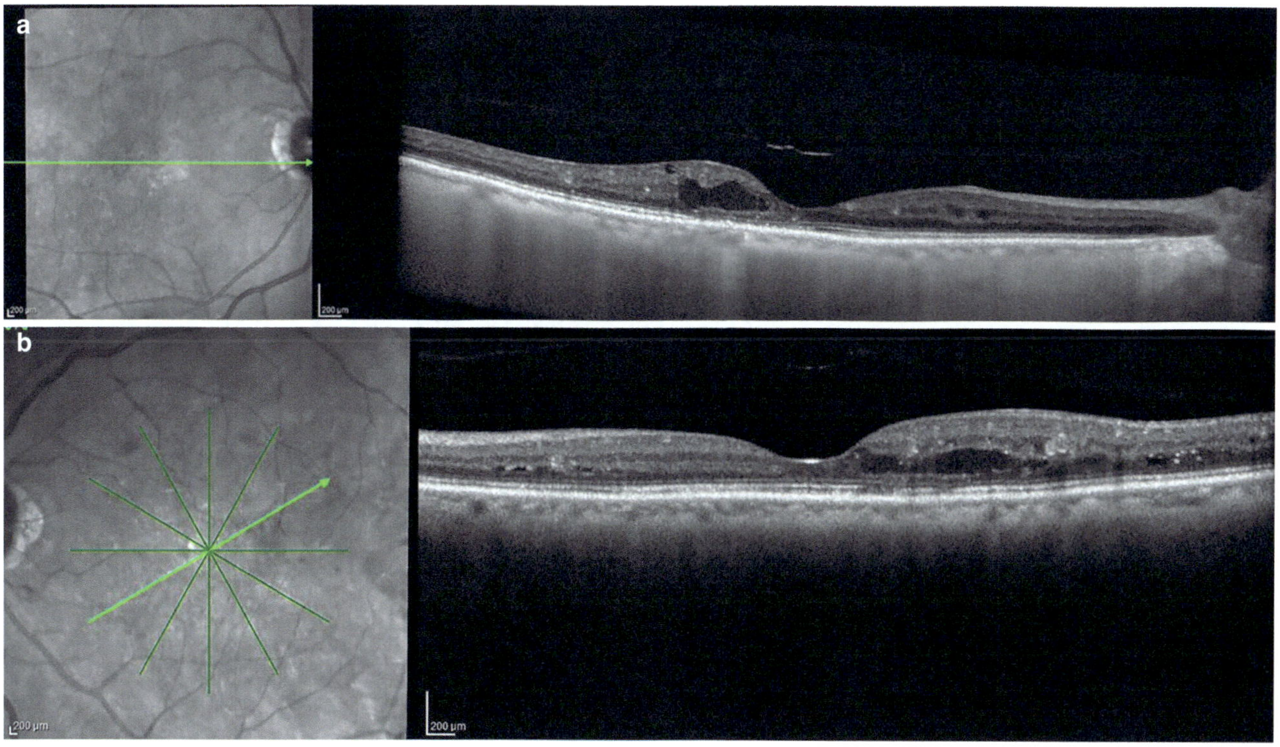

Fig. 14.29 Infrared (left image) and optical coherence tomography (right image) of the right (**a**) and left (**b**) eye showing non-foveal intraretinal fluid and exudates in both eyes

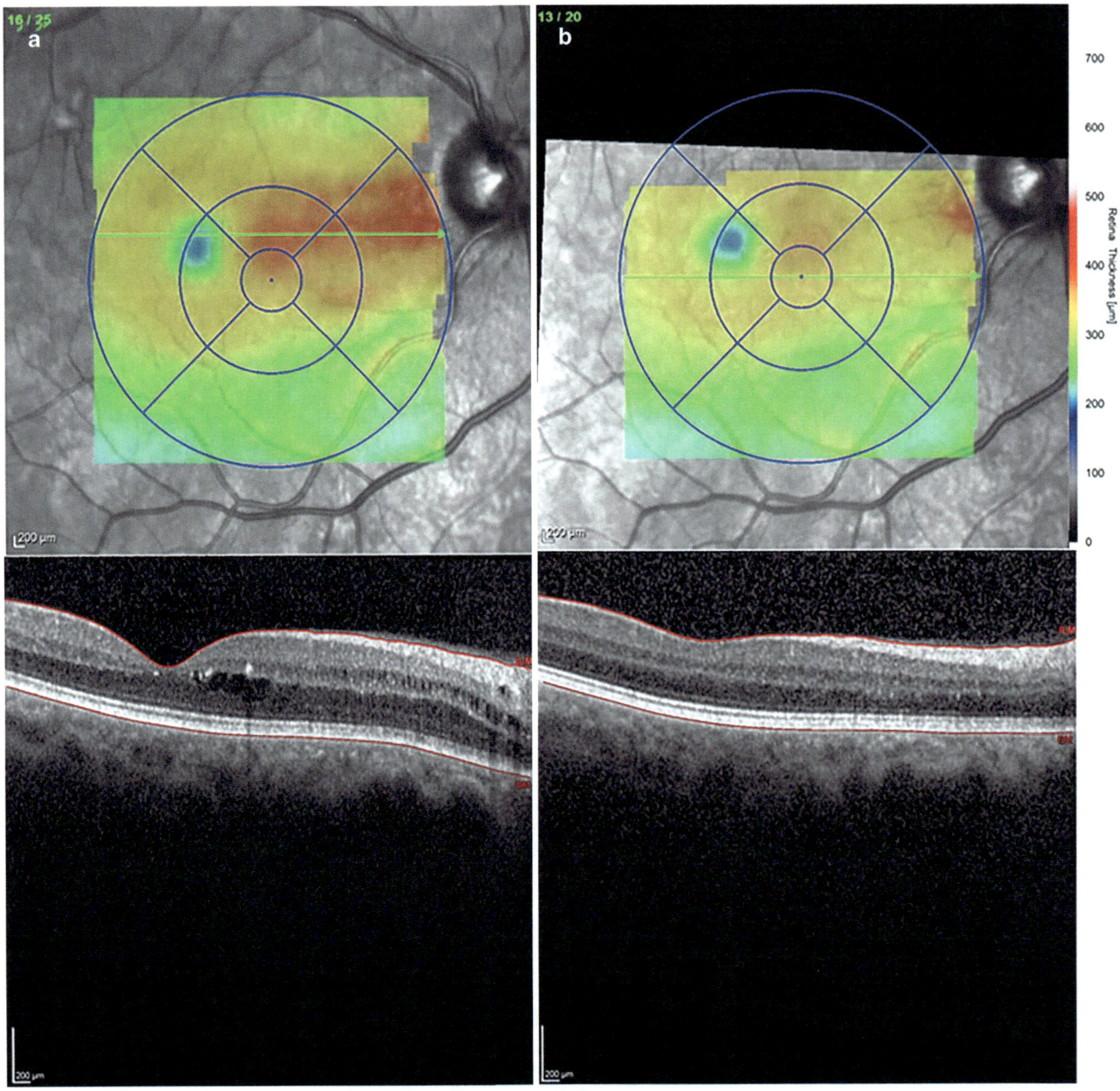

Fig. 14.30 Thickness map (top image) with optical coherence tomography (bottom image) of the right eye before (**a**) and after (**b**) topical prednisolone acetate 1% and ketorolac tromethamine with resolution of intraretinal fluid

0.1 s, and 24 spots in the left eye, and a power of 70 mW, duration of 0.1 s, and 22 spots in the right eye. She will continue aflibercept as a maintenance therapy in both eyes every 10 weeks for a total of three injections per eye, and then will return for re-evaluation 10 weeks after her last injection.

Case #7

A 65-year-old man with hypertension, hyperlipidemia, hypothyroidism, and secondary diabetes (last HbA1c of 6.7) in the setting of pancreatectomy was referred for cystic changes on OCT of the right eye. Vision upon presentation was 20/30 in both eyes uncorrected. Exam was notable for blunted foveal reflex with edema and thickening, and rare MAs of the right eye. OCT was notable for intraretinal fluid and hard exudates of the right eye. Given good vision, mild DME, and strong aversion to intravitreal injection, he was trialed conservatively on topical prednisolone acetate 1% and ketorolac tromethamine 4 times daily in the right eye. Four weeks later his vision uncorrected was 20/25 with pinhole to 20/20 in both eyes. His OCT showed improved intraretinal fluid in the right eye (Fig. 14.30). He will continue ketorolac four times daily and prednisolone four times daily for 1 month and then slowly taper the steroid to two times daily until follow-up in 6 weeks.

References

1. Flaxel CJ, Adelman RA, Bailey ST, et al. Diabetic retinopathy preferred practice pattern. Ophthalmology. 2020;127:66–145.
2. Browning DJ, Glassman AR, Aiello LP, et al. Relationship between optical coherence tomography measured central retinal thickness and visual acuity in diabetic macular edema. Ophthalmology. 2007;114(3):525–36.
3. Browning DJ, Apte RS, Bressler SB, et al. Association of the extent of diabetic macular edema as assessed by optical coherence tomography with visual acuity and retinal outcome variables. Retina. 2009;29(3):300–5.
4. Baker CW, Glassman AR, Beaulieu WT, et al. Effect of initial management with aflibercept vs laser photocoagulation vs observation on vision loss among patients with diabetic macular edema involving the center of the macula and good visual acuity: a randomized clinical trial. JAMA. 2019;321(19):1880–94.
5. Browning DJ, Stewart MW, Lee C. Diabetic macular edema: evidence-based management. Indian J Ophthalmol. 2018;66:1736–50.
6. Wells JA, Glassman AR, Ayala AR, et al. Aflibercept, bevacizumab, or ranibizumab for diabetic macular edema. N Engl J Med. 2015;372:1193–203.
7. Campochiaro PA, Haix G, Shah SM, et al. Sustained ocular delivery of fluocinolone acetonide by an intravitreal insert. Ophthalmology. 2010;117(7):1393–9.
8. Campochiaro PA, Brown DM, Pearson A, et al. Long-term benefit of sustained-delivery fluocinolone acetonide vitreous inserts for diabetic macular edema. Ophthalmology. 2011;118(4):626–35.
9. Campochiaro PA, Brown DM, Pearson A, et al. Sustained delivery fluocinolone acetonide vitreous inserts provide benefit for at least 3 years in patients with diabetic macular edema. Ophthalmology. 2012;119(10):2125–32.
10. Boyer DS, Yoon YH, Belfort R Jr, et al. Three-year, randomized, sham-controlled trial of dexamethasone intravitreal implant in patients with diabetic macular edema. Ophthalmology. 2014;121(10):1904–14.
11. Schmidt-Erfurth U, Garcia-Arumi J, Bandello F, et al. Guidelines for the management of diabetic macular edema by the European Society of Retina Specialists (EURETINA). Ophthalmologica. 2017;237:185–222.
12. Gale MJ, Scruggs BA, Flaxel CJ. Diabetic eye disease: a review of screening and management recommendations. Clin Experiment Ophthalmol. 2021;49:128–45.
13. Friberg TR. Subthreshold (invisible) modified grid diode laser photocoagulation and diffuse diabetic macular edema (DDME). Ophthalmic Surg Lasers. 1999;30:705.
14. Fong DS, Strauber SF, Aiello LP, et al. Comparison of the modified early treatment diabetic retinopathy study and mild macular grid laser photocoagulation strategies for diabetic macular edema. Arch Ophthalmol. 2007;125(4):469–80.
15. Kaur S, Yangzes S, Singh S, Sachdev N. Efficacy and safety of topical difluprednate in persistent diabetic macular edema. Int Ophthalmol. 2016;36(3):335–40.
16. Nakano S, Yamamoto T, Kirii E, Abe S, Yamashita H. Steroid eye drop treatment (difluprednate ophthalmic emulsion) is effective in reducing refractory diabetic macular edema. Graefes Arch Clin Exp Ophthalmol. 2010;248:805–10.
17. Goto SN, Yamamoto T, Kirii E, Abe S, Yamashita H. Treatment of diffuse diabetic macular oedema using steroid eye drops. Acta Ophthalmol. 2012;90:628–32.
18. Tanito M, Hara K, Takai Y, et al. Topical dexamethasone-cyclodextrin microparticle eye drops for diabetic macular edema. Invest Ophthalmol Vis Sci. 2011;52:7944–8.
19. Ohira A, Hara K, Jóhannesson G, et al. Topical dexamethasone γ-cyclodextrin nanoparticle eye drops increase visual acuity and decrease macular thickness in diabetic macular oedema. Acta Ophthalmol. 2015;93:610–5.
20. Pinna A, Blasetti F, Ricci GD, Boscia F. Bromfenac eyedrops in the treatment of diabetic macular edema: a pilot study. Eur J Ophthalmol. 2017;27(3):326–30.
21. Hariprasad SM, Callanan D, Gainey S, He YG, Warren K. Cystoid and diabetic macular edema treated with nepafenac 0.1%. J Ocul Pharmacol Ther. 2007;23(6):585–9.
22. Mohan S, Chawla G, Surya J, Raman R. Intravitreal anti-vascular endothelial growth factor with and without topical non-steroidal anti-inflammatory in centre-involving diabetic macular edema. Indian J Ophthalmol. 2021;69:3279–82.
23. Nikkhah H, Moez RN, Entezari M, et al. Topical ketorolac as an adjunctive treatment with intravitreal bevacizumab in the management of diabetic macular edema: a double-masked placebo-controlled randomized clinical trial. Graefes Arch Clin Exp Ophthalmol. 2021;259(10):2949–59.
24. Diabetic Retinopathy Clinical Research Network Writing Committee. Vitrectomy outcomes in eyes with diabetic macular edema and vitreomacular traction. Ophthalmology. 2010;117:1087–93.
25. Flaxel CJ, Edwards AR, Aiello LP, et al. Factors associated with visual acuity outcomes after vitrectomy for diabetic macular edema. Retina. 2010;30(9):1488–95.

Artificial Intelligence in the Management of Diabetic Macular Edema

15

Louis Cai, Andrew Jin, John W. Hinkle, David Xu, and Ajay E. Kuriyan

15.1 Introduction

Diabetic retinopathy (DR) is a leading cause of visual impairment, affecting nearly a third of all individuals with diabetes mellitus (DM) [1]. The worldwide prevalence of diabetes mellitus continues to increase rapidly and is expected to reach over 592 million by the year 2035 [2]. Screening for DR is necessary to prevent progression to vision threatening diabetic retinopathy (VTDR), which encompasses severe non-proliferative diabetic retinopathy (NPDR) and proliferative diabetic retinopathy (PDR) with or without the presence of diabetic macular edema (DME) [2].

Clinically significant macular edema (CSME) in DM or DME is present in approximately 7% of patients with DR, and is a treatable cause of VTDR [2]. It is characterized by retinal thickening and/or adjacent hard exudates that either involve the center of the macula (center involved) or threaten to involve it (non-center involved). Traditionally, clinical criteria were used to diagnose DME based on the presence of retinal thickening or hard exudates on fundoscopic exam [3]. More recently, the development of spectral domain optical coherence tomography (SD-OCT) has allowed clinicians to more accurately differentiate non-center involved DME (NCI-DME) and center involved DME (CI-DME), the latter of which represents a greater risk for vision loss [4].

L. Cai · J. W. Hinkle
Wills Eye Hospital, Philadelphia, PA, USA

Sidney Kimmel Medical College, Thomas Jefferson University, Philadelphia, PA, USA

A. Jin
Yale Eye Center, New Haven, CT, USA

D. Xu · A. E. Kuriyan (✉)
Wills Eye Hospital, Philadelphia, PA, USA

Sidney Kimmel Medical College, Thomas Jefferson University, Philadelphia, PA, USA

Mid Atlantic Retina, Philadelphia, PA, USA

As the burden of DR and its screening grows, it is increasingly important for clinicians to use technology to aid in decision making. Recent advances in artificial intelligence (AI), which encompass both traditional machine learning (ML) techniques and more recently deep learning (DL) techniques, have allowed computers to diagnose DR and identify DME without clinician supervision. One of the most promising developments in DL are convoluted neural networks (CNNs). Briefly, CNNs have network architectures that resemble layers of neurons to process information. Traditional CNNs output discrete labels (e.g., DME, no DME), while other neural network architectures can directly segment images—giving pixel level information in an image.

The terminology and statistical tests used in AI studies can seem inaccessible at first, but it is helpful to understand that the foundation for all AI algorithms is a classification question: "What are we asking the computer to identify?" In ophthalmology specifically, AI has been mostly utilized to process imaging (e.g., fundus photos, SD-OCT) and numerical/categorical variables (e.g., risk factors, best corrected visual acuity, mean central thickness) to make classifications. These classifications can be binary (e.g., the presence or absence of referrable DR), multi-categorical (e.g., AMD vs. DR vs. Normal), or numerical (e.g., risk of DR progression, visual acuity). Furthermore, classifications can be descriptive of a patient in the present (e.g., presence or absence of VTDR) or predictive of future changes (e.g., DME response to ranibizumab).

Finally, it is important to understand the sources of data for a study, which may come from datasets (e.g., Messidor), data pulled retrospectively from a population of patients, or data taken in a prospective fashion. Every AI algorithm will typically divide their data into training (to fit the model), validation (to provide unbiased assessment of model fit while tuning parameters), and testing (to assess performance of the model). Models are measured by their overall accuracy (total correct in classification), sensitivity (ability to correctly detect disease, i.e., true positives), specificity

S. Saxena et al. (eds.), *Diabetic Macular Edema*, https://doi.org/10.1007/978-981-19-7307-9_15

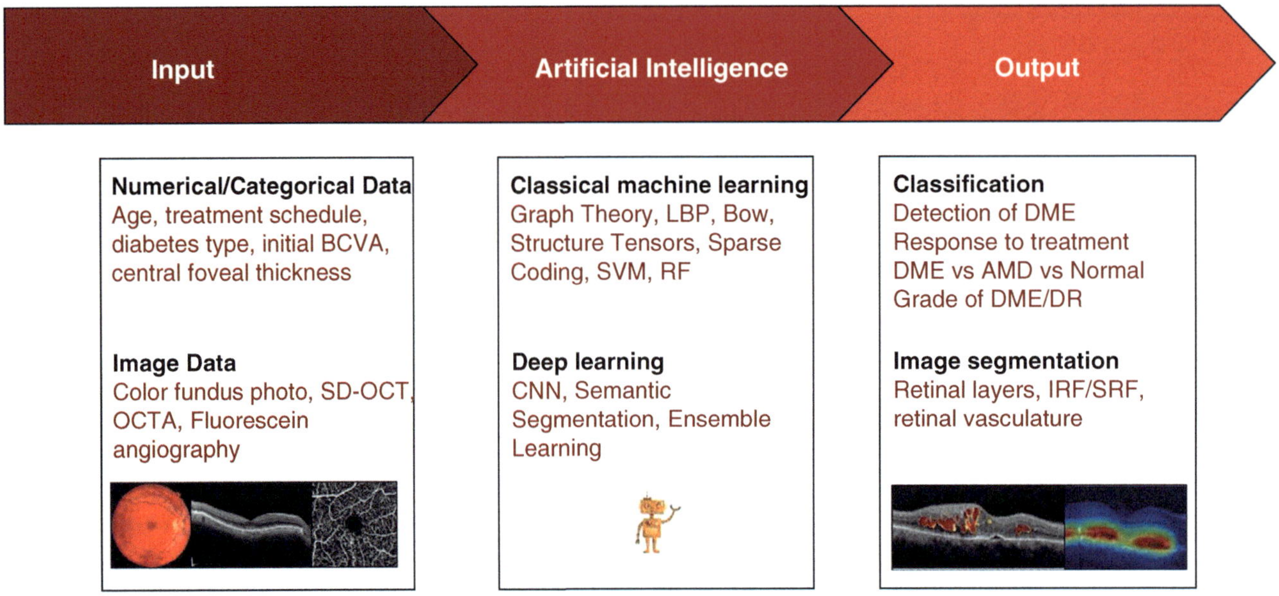

Fig. 15.1 A general framework for artificial intelligence algorithms for diabetic macular edema

(ability to detect the absence of disease, i.e., true negatives), and area under the receiver–operator curve (AUC), which is an aggregate metric of model performance. Figure 15.1 illustrates the general framework for artificial intelligence algorithms.

With this information in mind, it will be easier to begin assessing the value of the many AI studies in our field (See Table 15.1). In this chapter, we will give an overview of current applications of AI for the diagnosis and management of DME.

Table 15.1 Outcomes of studies utilizing artificial intelligence in the management of diabetic macular edema

Year	First author	Title	Classification problem	Data source (magnitude)	Algorithm type	Best performance
2011	Liu, Yu-Ying	Computerized macular pathology diagnosis in spectral domain optical coherence tomography scans based on multiscale texture and shape features [40]	Detecting macular hole, macular edema, and AMD	SD-OCT images (326 volumes)	Multiscale spatial pyramid, LBP histogram + PCA, non-linear SVM	AUC = 0.969 for ME
2014	Srinivasan, Pratul P	Fully automated detection of diabetic macular edema and dry age-related macular degeneration from optical coherence tomography images [41]	Detecting DME and AMD	SD-OCT images (45 volumes)	HOG, SVM	Acc = 100 for DME
2016	Hassan, Bilal	Structure tensor based automated detection of macular edema and central serous retinopathy using optical coherence tomography images [39]	Detecting DME and CSR	SD-OCT images (90 images)	Structure tensor, SVM	Acc = 97.8
2016	Abràmoff, Michael David	Improved automated detection of diabetic retinopathy on a publicly available dataset through integration of deep learning [7]	Detecting RDR (including DME)	Fundus photos. (1748 images, Messidor 2)	CNN	Se = 96.8, Sp = 87.0, AUC = 0.980
2016	Syed, Adeel M	Automated diagnosis of macular edema and central serous retinopathy through robust reconstruction of 3D retinal surfaces [42]	Detecting DME and CSR	SD-OCT images (90 volumes)	Structure tensor, 3D reconstruction, SVM	Acc = 98.9, Se = 100, Sp = 96.7%
2017	Sun, Yankui	Fully automated macular pathology detection in retina optical coherence tomography images using sparse coding and dictionary learning [72]	Detecting DME and AMD	SD-OCT images (45 volumes +678 images)	Sparse coding, dictionary learning, SVM	Acc = 100 for DME
2017	Alsaih, Khaled	Machine learning techniques for diabetic macular edema (DME) classification on SD-OCT images [38]	Detecting DME	SD-OCT images (32 volumes)	LBP, PCA, BoW, SVM	Se = 87.5, Sp = 87.5

(continued)

Table 15.1 (continued)

Year	First author	Title	Classification problem	Data source (magnitude)	Algorithm type	Best performance
2017	Lee, Cecilia S	Deep learning based, automated segmentation of macular edema in optical coherence tomography [53]	Segmentation of intraretinal fluid	SD-OCT (1289 images)	CNN	Dice coefficient = 0.911
2017	Gerendas, Bianca S	Computational image analysis for prognosis determination in DME [73]	Prediction of BCVA in DME (using segmentation of retinal layers and intraretinal cystoid fluid)	SD-OCT (629 volumes)	Graph theory, semantic segmentation (CNN based)	$R^2 = 0.23$ for BCVA at 1 year
2018	Schlegl, Thomas	Fully automated detection and quantification of macular fluid in OCT using deep learning [54]	Segmentation of intraretinal cystoid fluid (IRC) and subretinal fluid (SRF) in DME, AMD, and RVO	SD-OCT (1200 volumes)	Semantic segmentation (CNN based)	AUC = 0.94 for IRC. AUC = 0.92 for SRF
2018	Abràmoff, Michael D	Pivotal trial of an autonomous AI-based diagnostic system for detection of diabetic retinopathy in primary care offices [8]	Detecting RDR (including DME)	Fundus photos (900 prospective subjects)	CNN	Se = 87.2, Sp = 90.7
2018	Chen, shao-Chun	A novel machine learning algorithm to automatically predict visual outcomes in intravitreal ranibizumab-treated patients with diabetic macular edema [60]	Prediction of BCVA for DME treated with Ranibizumab	Baseline variables: sex, age, diabetes type, systemic conditions, treatment time tables (464 eyes)	ANN	$R = 0.81$ at 2 years
2018	Chan, Genevieve CY	Fusing results of several deep learning architectures for automatic classification of normal and diabetic macular edema in optical coherence tomography [48]	Detecting DME and AMD	SD-OCT (2 sets = 32 volumes & 83 volumes)	CNN, PCA, majority voting	Acc = 93.75
2019	Arcadu, Filippo	Deep learning predicts OCT measures of diabetic macular thickening from color fundus photographs [56]	Predicting OCT central subfield thickness (CST) and central foveal thickness (CFT)	Fundus photos (17,997)	CNN	$R^2 = 0.74$ CST and 0.54 for CFT
2019	Hassan, Bilal	Deep ensemble learning based objective grading of macular edema by extracting clinically significant findings from fused retinal imaging modalities [70]	Detecting ME. Segmenting retinal fluids, hard exudates, retinal blood vessels	SD-OCT (78,552 images). Fundus photos/FA (339 images)	CNN	Acc = 94.3% for detecting ME. Dice coefficient 0.91 for retinal fluids, 0.71 for hard exudates, 0.82 for blood vessels

2019	Sahlsten, Jaakko	Deep learning fundus image analysis for diabetic retinopathy and macular edema grading [21]	Detecting RDR, DME. Grading DR and DME	Fundus photos (41,122)	CNN	Acc = 0.94 for detecting and grading DR, Acc = 0.97 for detecting and grading DME
2020	Wang, Zhenhua	Detection of diabetic macular edema in optical coherence tomography image using an improved level set algorithm [45]	Detecting DME	SD-OCT (100 images)	Selective binary and Gaussian filtering regularized level set	Precision (positive predictive value) = 97.7. Se = 91.8, Sp = 99.2
2020	Varadarajan, Avinash V	Predicting optical coherence tomography-derived diabetic macular edema grades from fundus photographs using deep learning [23]	Detecting SD-OCT DME grades from fundus photographs	Fundus photos (8062)	CNN	Se = 85, Sp = 80 to detect ciDME. AUC = 0.81 to detecting IRF, AUC = 0.88 to detect SRF
2020	Rasti, Reza	Deep learning-based single-shot prediction of differential effects of anti-VEGF treatment in patients with diabetic macular edema [61]	Predicting DME response to anti-VEGF	SD-OCT (127 volumes)	CNN	AUC = 0.87, Se = 80.1, Sp = 85.5
2020	Jin, Kai	Automatic detection of non-perfusion areas in diabetic macular edema from fundus fluorescein angiography for decision making using deep learning [27]	Segmentation of non-perfusion areas	Fluorescein angiography (3013 images)	CNN	AUC = 0.89 for non-perfusion areas, 0.98 for microaneurysms, 0.98 for leakage classifier
2020	Zhang, Quan	Identifying diabetic macular edema and other retinal diseases by optical coherence tomography image and multiscale deep learning [67]	Detecting DME, Drusen, CNV	SD-OCT (38,057 images)	CNN	Acc = 94.5, Se = 97.7, Sp = 97
2020	Roberts, Philipp K	Quantification of fluid resolution and visual acuity gain in patients with diabetic macular edema using deep learning [62]	Examining intraretinal and subretinal fluid changes during DME treatment	SD-OCT (6945 volumes)	Semantic segmentation (CNN based)	Baseline SRF is associated with worse baseline VA ($P < 0.001$) and greater gain in VA at 4 weeks ($P = 0.02$). Both aflibercept and ranibizumab were associated with greater reduction of intraretinal fluid ($P < 0.001$)
2020	Guo, Yukun	Automated segmentation of retinal fluid volumes from structural and angiographic optical coherence tomography using deep learning [34]	Segmentation of retinal fluid	OCTA (51 volumes)	U-net CNN	F1 = 0.864 (OCTA alone). F1 = 0.892 (OCT = OCTA)

(continued)

Table 15.1 (continued)

Year	First author	Title	Classification problem	Data source (magnitude)	Algorithm type	Best performance
2020	Hwang, De-Kuang	Optical coherence tomography–based diabetic macula edema screening with artificial intelligence [51]	Detecting DME	SD-OCT (3495 images)	CNN	Acc = 93.1, Se = 96.5, Sp = 86.7)
2021	Tao, Zhifu	A joint model for macular edema analysis in optical coherence tomography images based on image enhancement and segmentation [46]	Segmentation of ME	SD-OCT (1000 images)	Selective binary and Gaussian filtering regularized level set	Acc = 99.7, Se = 96.0, Sp = 99.0, dice = 96.9
2021	Lin, Andrew C	Assessing the clinical utility of expanded macular OCTs using machine learning [69]	Determination of SD- OCT coverage area to detect DME, AMD, and POAG	SD-OCT (630,000 images)	CNN, random forest	Optimal macular OCT coverage was 4.25–4.50 mm for DME (21–28 B scans)
2021	Kang, Eugene Yu-Chuan	A multimodal imaging–based deep learning model for detecting treatment-requiring retinal vascular diseases: model development and validation study [71]	Detecting DME, nAMD, mCNV, BRVO, CRVO	SD-OCT (9316 images), Color fundus photos (5117 images), FA/ICG (20,922)	CNN	AUC for DME = 0.995
2021	Huang, Haifan	Algorithm for detection and quantification of hyperreflective dots on optical coherence tomography in diabetic macular edema [74]	Segmentation of hyperreflective dots (HRDs) in DME	SD-OCT (20 volumes). Original algorithm trained on 2560 images	CNN	Dice coefficient = 0.70 for total HRDs, 0.72 for hard exudates, 0.46 for small HRDs
2021	Liu, Baoyi	Automatic prediction of treatment outcomes in patients with diabetic macular edema using ensemble machine learning [63]	Prediction of central foveal thickness and BCVA in DME after anti-VEGF treatment	SD-OCT (304 volumes to train, 59 volumes to test)	Ensemble of four DL models and five classical ML models	R^2 = 0.74 for CFT, AUC = 0.94 to predict good anatomical response. R^2 = 0.68 for BCVA. With AUC = 0.81 to predict good functional response

Acc accuracy (in %), *AMD* age related macular degeneration, *ANN* artificial neural network, *AUC* area under the ROC curve, *BCVA* best corrected visual acuity, *BRVO* branch retinal vein occlusion, *CFT* central foveal thickness, *ciDME* center involving diabetic macular edema, *CNN* convolutional neural network, *CRVO* central retinal vein occlusion, Dice coefficient = Area of overlap * 2, *DL* deep learning, *DME* diabetic macular edema, F1 = 2*TP/[2*TP + FP + FN), *HOG* histogram oriented gradients, *HRD* hyperreflective dots, *LBP* local binary pattern, *ML* machine learning, *nAMD* neovascular AMD, OCT volume = approximately 128 B-scan slices, *PCA* principal component analysis, *R* = correlation coefficient, R^2 = coefficient of determination, *Se* sensitivity (in %), *Sp* specificity (in %), *SVM* support vector machine, *VA* visual acuity

15.2 Diabetic Retinopathy Screening

Telemedicine programs have improved access to DR screening, especially in the primary care setting [5]. In 2018, the FDA approved the IDx-DR software program for use in DR screening. This was the first software authorized for use in the USA that provides screening decisions based on a non-mydriatric fundus photograph without clinician interpretation [6]. These algorithms were based off initial studies by Abramoff et al. showing that DL (specifically CNNs) achieved sensitivities as high as 96.8% in identifying referrable DR (RDR, moderate NPDR or worse with/without DME) from image data sets [7]. This algorithm was later prospectively validated prospectively which led to FDA approval [8, 9]. Since then, similar algorithms around the world have been developed to identify referrable DR from fundus photos both retrospectively and prospectively with equally impressive accuracy, sensitivity, and specificity [10–20].

Researchers have also explored the performance of AI at other classification thresholds, including vision threatening diabetic retinopathy (VTDR), which includes severe non-proliferative DR (NPDR), proliferative DR (PDR), or the presence of DME. VTDR is less subtle than RDR, and Ting et al. used DL algorithm to screen 71,896 images with nearly 100% sensitivity and 91.1% specificity. Sahlsten et al. proposed an algorithm that used AI to grade fundus photos for both DR and DME severity on multi-level scales with an accuracy as high as 94.4% and 97.3%, respectively [21].

Sahlsten et al. also demonstrated that AI performance is dependent on the quality of images. Higher quality images, especially taken after pupil dilation, can train models more quickly and result in better performance. However, both imaging modality and mydriasis add another barrier to DR screening for patients and clinicians. Thankfully, DL algorithms have found reasonable success with non-mydriatic and even smartphone-based cameras [8, 22–24].

15.3 Assessing Impact of Diabetes on Retinal Vasculature

Fluorescein angiography can help identify areas of leakage corresponding to macular edema as well areas of non-perfusion. Recent work has shown CNNs can accurately segment vasculature, areas of nonperfusion, leakage, and microaneurysms on fluorescein angiograms [25–27]. One study using such machine learning approaches to identify retinal vessels found a correlation of visual acuity with macular vessel density. Of note, the macular non-perfusion was not associated with macular edema in this study, however, patients were required to have a minimal amount of macular edema to be enrolled in the study. These approaches will potentially allow for quantitative assessment of retinal vasculature on fluorescein angiography to better understand disease progression and the impact of treatments on the retinal vasculature.

Over the past decade, OCT angiography (OCT-A) has become increasingly used to image the retinal vasculature. Its chief advantages over traditional angiography with fluorescein or indocyanine green include less invasiveness and faster image acquisition. Researchers have shown that diabetes causes significant microangiopathic changes quantifiable by OCT-A including increased detection of microaneurysms and other vascular abnormalities [25], expansion of the foveal avascular zone [28], and increases in vascular tortuosity [29]. Diabetic macular edema also causes changes on OCT-A including lower vascular density, capillary nonperfusion in the superficial and deep capillary plexuses, and increased foveal avascular zone area [30, 31]. Deep learning algorithms with OCT-A are now being designed to aid in the diagnosis and management of diabetic retinopathy. Le et al. showed that a neural network trained on OCT-A diagnosed diabetic retinopathy with 87.27% accuracy, 83.76% sensitivity, and 90.82% specificity [32]. Similarly, Ryu et al. developed an AI classification algorithm using OCT-A that identified diabetic retinopathy with 91–98% accuracy, a sensitivity of 86–97% and a specificity of 94–99% [33]. Work is now being done in OCT-A and DME using machine learning methods. Guo et al. designed a deep learning model using OCT-A scans in conjunction with SD-OCT to automatically segment retinal fluid [34]. Future work is focused on guiding treatment based on deep learning algorithms.

15.4 Detecting Diabetic Macular Edema

Compared to stereoscopic examination, CI-DME is more easily diagnosed using SD-OCT imaging. Specifically, SD-OCT can quantify retinal thickness, cystoid macular edema, and subretinal fluid. Over the past two decades many groups have worked on automated methodologies to segment SD-OCT images, which were initially based on early machine learning techniques to both segment layers (e.g., graph theory, histogram of oriented gradients, bag of words, local binary pattern, structural tensors) and make classifications (support vector machine, random forest, Bayesian networks) [35–38].

One early example was the methodology proposed by Hasan et al. describing a method using two dimensional structure tensors to segment retinal layers/cyst fluid and subsequently passing the feature sets to support vector machine (SVM) classifiers [39]. Briefly, SVM algorithms consider the input of multiple variables to generate a hyperplane which divides a population of data points into two clusters. These and similar machine learning algorithms can classify normal, macular edema, and central serous retinopathy with performances as high as 98.88 accuracy, 100% sensitivity, and 96.66% specificity [38, 40–46].

Machine learning classification pipelines typically include four primary steps: (1) image pre-processing, (2) feature extraction, (3) feature representation, and (4) feature classification [38]. Image pre-processing includes identifying regions of interest, removing image noise, and standardizing image presentation. Aspects of image pre-processing often must be done manually and is more difficult with poor-quality images, making earlier machine learning algorithms less generalizable in real clinical practice.

On the other hand, deep learning, specifically fully convolutional neural networks, can bypass many manual pre-processing steps while still achieving equivalent, if not superior performance in detecting DME (accuracy 99.69%, sensitivity 99.53%, specificity 99.77%) [47–52]. One of the more promising features of DL is the ability to quantify intraretinal cystoid (IRC) fluid and subretinal fluid (SRF). Lee et al. demonstrated that a modified version of U-net autoencoder architecture can automatically segment intraretinal fluid [53]. This kind of architecture allows for classification of individual pixels in an image. Using this method, Schlegl et al. quantified the amount of IRC fluid (AUC = 0.94) and SRF (AUC = 0.92) on SD-OCT scans [54]. Both groups found that DL algorithms performed equivalently to clinician graders.

Not all clinics have access to SD-OCT imaging and there is interest in the ability of DL to diagnose DME from color fundus photos. This is inherently a more difficult problem, as fundus photos lack the ability to directly determine central thickness. Even among clinicians, there is a discordance in the prevalence of DME identified by fundus photographs or by SD-OCT imaging [55]. Despite this, CNNs can reach impressively high sensitivities (92.1%) and specificities (97.4%), especially with higher quality fundus photos (1092 × 1092) [21, 23, 56]. Being able to accurately identify DME from CFPs will potentially allow clinicians to identify more subtle causes of VTDR in lower resource settings.

15.5 Treatment of Diabetic Macular Edema

The treatment of diabetic macular edema has evolved greatly over the past few decades. The original ETDRS trial [3] established focal or macular grid laser for reducing the risk of vision loss. Since then, the rapid adoption of anti-VEGF agents for their superior efficacy and lower morbidity have revolutionized treatment paradigms for center involving macular edema. Other treatments include various steroid injectables. Currently, retina specialists base their practice pattern on a combination of established guidelines, clinical judgment, and patient preferences in the treatment of DME.

Recent advances in AI have attempted to characterize the natural history of DR and identify patients at higher risk of progression [57–59]. Similarly, researchers have investigated the possibility of DL to guide treatment in DME, with the ultimate goal of personalizing treatment based on baseline characteristics and imaging.

Extensive work has been done in examining the effect of anti-VEGF injections on macular edema, specifically its effect on central subfield thickness reduction and best corrected visual acuity (BCVA). The first paper published in this field examined approximately 500 eyes treated with ranibizumab for macular edema over 52, 78, and 104 weeks [60]. The study authors developed a neural network with baseline characteristics and found that baseline visual acuity, lens status, and the intravitreal injection time table to be most influential characteristics to impact visual acuity at 2 years for diabetic macular edema treated with ranibizumab [60]. Later work by Rasti et al. [61] examined 137 patients with diabetic macular edema on SD-OCT who received at least three sequential anti-VEGF injections. They designed a novel convolutional neural network that classified patients as responders versus non-responders to anti-VEGF injections (based on at least 10% reduction in retinal thickness) with 80.1% sensitivity, 85.0% specificity, and an AUC of 0.866. Identifying responders to anti-VEGF injections may aid in the choice of initial treatment modality or identifying patients that would benefit from switching to intravitreal corticosteroids. A study by Arcadu et al. showed their best model reached a sensitivity and specificity of 84% and 82% at 2 years in predicting treatment response to ranibizumab [57].

AI image segmentation has also been used to identify clinically meaningful features of an image, rather than whole-image classification. Oftentimes, the presence of macular edema among other OCT biomarkers is used as a proxy for overall macular health and visual function (i.e. BCVA) [62]. Macular thickness and visual acuity have a mild to moderate correlation in the absence of other pathology. Research in this area has used machine learning to segment intraretinal cystoid fluid volume and retinal thickness to predict BCVA [60]. DL segmentation of SD-OCT allows for quantification of response to treatment as well as correlation with visual acuity [63]. Work published by Roberts et al. found that SRF at baseline is associated with worse baseline BCVA but a greater gain in ETDRS score. Both aflibercept and ranibizumab were associated with greater reduction in IRF after first injection compared with bevacizumab. Overall, for the 570 study participants the mean IRF in the central 3 mm improved from 448.6 nL to 161.2 nL at 12 months, and the SRF improved from 36.9 nL to 4.4 nL [64]. Further study in this area may help guide treatment, such as forming a matrix of multiple factors including the type of retinal fluid that is responding to treatment and its impact on BCVA. While clinicians can use predictive models to get a general sense of disease prognosis, further work must be done to clarify how they should be used in treatment decisions.

15.6 Limitations of Artificial Intelligence for Diabetic Retinopathy

As research in this field continues to advance, artificial intelligence technology will likely change the way clinicians practice in the future. Deep learning has already been shown to be a cost-effective way to screen for diabetic retinopathy [65]. The FDA approval of IDx-Dr heralds a new era of using computers to assist clinical decision making and is the first step in changing treatment paradigms based on AI. However, real-world application of AI is currently limited by challenges not encountered in research settings.

A primary concern is capturing high-quality gradable imaging. Image quality, especially for color fundus photos, is dependent on pupil dilation, anterior/lenticular clarity, patient cooperation/understanding, and technician skill. In general, higher resolution images with less artifacts are better analyzed by AI. In the IDx-Dr study, 23.6% of patients needed to be dilated to obtain usable images and 8% of individuals were unable to be analyzed at all due to poor fundus photo quality [8]. This represents a significant portion of patients that are being excluded from ML algorithms independent of technical/software issues [66]. For AI-based DR screening programs, ungradable patients should all be referred for examination.

Furthermore, computer algorithms are limited to diagnosing pathology they have been trained on, and the robustness of their diagnosis depends on the accuracy of their training data. For common diseases such as diabetic retinopathy that have large, well-validated data sets, this is less of an issue. However, current image data sets do not encompass the breadth of pathology encountered in clinical settings, and rare diseases the algorithm has not previously encountered may be missed altogether. Work in this area is now expanding the output of CNNs to multi-categorical classifications (e.g: DME, choroidal neovascularization, drusen, normal) which have achieved accuracies as high as 99.6% for SD-OCTs [67–69]. Further work has been done to combine multimodal imaging to more accurately diagnose retinal diseases [70, 71]. Kang et al. combined SD-OCT, CFP, and FA imaging into montages to train CNNs to classify BRVO, CRVO, myopic CNV, neovascular AMD, and DME to relatively high accuracies (93%–98%) [71]. These strategies can improve the translatability of AI to the real-world setting.

15.7 Conclusion

Artificial intelligence algorithms can accurately identify diabetic macular edema using current imaging modalities. Furthermore, deep learning has provided more accurate segmentation which provides a better objective measurement of the anatomical changes seen in this disease. Algorithms can also predict response to treatments for diabetic macular edema. Further research needs to be done to translate these models into clinical tools that will help clinicians choose treatment modalities specific to each patient.

Financial Support None.

Conflict of Interest No conflicts of interest exist for any author.

References

1. Flaxel CJ, Adelman RA, Bailey ST, Fawzi A, Lim JI, Vemulakonda GA, et al. Diabetic retinopathy preferred practice pattern®. Ophthalmology. 2020;127(1):P66–145.
2. Yau JWY, Rogers SL, Kawasaki R, Lamoureux EL, Kowalski JW, Bek T, et al. Global prevalence and major risk factors of diabetic retinopathy. Diabetes Care. 2012;35(3):556–64.
3. Photocoagulation for diabetic macular edema. Early treatment diabetic retinopathy study report number 1. Early treatment diabetic retinopathy study research group. Arch Ophthalmol. 1985;103(12):1796–806.
4. Sikorski BL, Malukiewicz G, Stafiej J, Lesiewska-Junk H, Raczynska D. The diagnostic function of OCT in diabetic maculopathy. Mediators Inflamm. 2013;2013:434560.
5. Cuadros J, Bresnick G. EyePACS: an adaptable telemedicine system for diabetic retinopathy screening. J Diabetes Sci Technol. 2009;3(3):509–16.
6. Commissioner O of the FDA permits marketing of artificial intelligence-based device to detect certain diabetes-related eye problems [Internet]. FDA. 2020. https://www.fda.gov/news-events/press-announcementsfda-permits-marketing-artificial-intelligence-based-device-detect-certain-diabetes-related-eye. Accessed 1 Jan 2022.
7. Abràmoff MD, Lou Y, Erginay A, Clarida W, Amelon R, Folk JC, et al. Improved automated detection of diabetic retinopathy on a publicly available dataset through integration of deep learning. Invest Ophthalmol Vis Sci. 2016;57(13):5200–6.
8. Abràmoff MD, Lavin PT, Birch M, Shah N, Folk JC. Pivotal trial of an autonomous AI-based diagnostic system for detection of diabetic retinopathy in primary care offices. NPJ Digit Med. 2018;1:39.
9. Shah A, Clarida W, Amelon R, Hernaez-Ortega MC, Navea A, Morales-Olivas J, et al. Validation of automated screening for referable diabetic retinopathy with an autonomous diagnostic artificial intelligence system in a Spanish population. J Diabetes Sci Technol. 2020;15(3):655–63.
10. Gulshan V, Peng L, Coram M, Stumpe MC, Wu D, Narayanaswamy A, et al. Development and validation of a deep learning algorithm for detection of diabetic retinopathy in retinal fundus photographs. JAMA. 2016;316(22):2402–10.
11. Gargeya R, Leng T. Automated identification of diabetic retinopathy using deep learning. Ophthalmology. 2017;124(7):962–9.
12. Ting DSW, Cheung CY-L, Lim G, Tan GSW, Quang ND, Gan A, et al. Development and validation of a deep learning system for diabetic retinopathy and related eye diseases using retinal images from multiethnic populations with diabetes. JAMA. 2017;318(22):2211–23.
13. Xu K, Feng D, Mi H. Deep convolutional neural network-based early automated detection of diabetic retinopathy using fundus image. Molecules. 2017;22(12):2054.
14. Ramachandran N, Hong SC, Sime MJ, Wilson GA. Diabetic retinopathy screening using deep neural network. Clin Experiment Ophthalmol. 2018;46(4):412–6.
15. Bellemo V, Lim ZW, Lim G, Nguyen QD, Xie Y, Yip MYT, et al. Artificial intelligence using deep learning to screen for referable

and vision-threatening diabetic retinopathy in Africa: a clinical validation study. Lancet Digit Health. 2019;1(1):e35–44.
16. Bhaskaranand M, Ramachandra C, Bhat S, Cuadros J, Nittala MG, Sadda SR, et al. The value of automated diabetic retinopathy screening with the EyeArt system: a study of more than 100,000 consecutive encounters from people with diabetes. Diabetes Technol Ther. 2019;21(11):635–43.
17. Ruamviboonsuk P, Krause J, Chotcomwongse P, Sayres R, Raman R, Widner K, et al. Deep learning versus human graders for classifying diabetic retinopathy severity in a nationwide screening program. NPJ Digit Med. 2019;2:25.
18. He J, Cao T, Xu F, Wang S, Tao H, Wu T, et al. Artificial intelligence-based screening for diabetic retinopathy at community hospital. Eye. 2020;34(3):572–6.
19. Shah P, Mishra DK, Shanmugam MP, Doshi B, Jayaraj H, Ramanjulu R. Validation of deep convolutional neural network-based algorithm for detection of diabetic retinopathy—artificial intelligence versus clinician for screening. Indian J Ophthalmol. 2020;68(2):398–405.
20. Heydon P, Egan C, Bolter L, Chambers R, Anderson J, Aldington S, et al. Prospective evaluation of an artificial intelligence-enabled algorithm for automated diabetic retinopathy screening of 30 000 patients. Br J Ophthalmol. 2021;105(5):723–8.
21. Sahlsten J, Jaskari J, Kivinen J, Turunen L, Jaanio E, Hietala K, et al. Deep learning fundus image analysis for diabetic retinopathy and macular edema grading. Sci Rep. 2019;9(1):10750.
22. Natarajan S, Jain A, Krishnan R, Rogye A, Sivaprasad S. Diagnostic accuracy of community-based diabetic retinopathy screening with an offline artificial intelligence system on a smartphone. JAMA Ophthalmol. 2019;137(10):1182–8.
23. Varadarajan AV, Bavishi P, Ruamviboonsuk P, Chotcomwongse P, Venugopalan S, Narayanaswamy A, et al. Predicting optical coherence tomography-derived diabetic macular edema grades from fundus photographs using deep learning. Nat Commun. 2020;11:130.
24. Sosale B, Sosale AR, Murthy H, Sengupta S, Naveenam M. Medios—an offline, smartphone-based artificial intelligence algorithm for the diagnosis of diabetic retinopathy. Indian J Ophthalmol. 2020;68(2):391–5.
25. Ishibazawa A, Nagaoka T, Takahashi A, Omae T, Tani T, Sogawa K, et al. Optical coherence tomography angiography in diabetic retinopathy: a prospective pilot study. Am J Ophthalmol. 2015;160(1):35–44.e1.
26. Ding L, Bawany MH, Kuriyan AE, Ramchandran RS, Wykoff CC, Sharma G. A novel deep learning pipeline for retinal vessel detection in fluorescein angiography. IEEE Trans Image Process. 2020;29:6561. https://doi.org/10.1109/TIP.2020.2991530.
27. Jin K, Pan X, You K, Wu J, Liu Z, Cao J, et al. Automatic detection of non-perfusion areas in diabetic macular edema from fundus fluorescein angiography for decision making using deep learning. Sci Rep. 2020;10:15138.
28. Lu Y, Simonett JM, Wang J, Zhang M, Hwang T, Hagag AM, et al. Evaluation of automatically quantified foveal avascular zone metrics for diagnosis of diabetic retinopathy using optical coherence tomography angiography. Invest Ophthalmol Vis Sci. 2018;59(6):2212–21.
29. Zahid S, Dolz-Marco R, Freund KB, Balaratnasingam C, Dansingani K, Gilani F, et al. Fractal dimensional analysis of optical coherence tomography angiography in eyes with diabetic retinopathy. Invest Ophthalmol Vis Sci. 2016;57(11):4940–7.
30. Lee J, Moon BG, Cho AR, Yoon YH. Optical coherence tomography angiography of DME and its association with anti-VEGF treatment response. Ophthalmology. 2016;123(11):2368–75.
31. Mirshahi R, Riazi-Esfahani H, Khalili Pour E, Fadakar K, Yarmohamadi P, Alemzadeh SA, et al. Differentiating features of OCT angiography in diabetic macular edema. Sci Rep. 2021;11(1):23398.
32. Le D, Alam M, Yao CK, Lim JI, Hsieh Y-T, Chan RVP, et al. Transfer learning for automated OCTA detection of diabetic retinopathy. Transl Vis Sci Technol. 2020;9(2):35.
33. Ryu G, Lee K, Park D, Park SH, Sagong M. A deep learning model for identifying diabetic retinopathy using optical coherence tomography angiography. Sci Rep. 2021;11(1):23024.
34. Guo Y, Hormel TT, Xiong H, Wang J, Hwang TS, Jia Y. Automated segmentation of retinal fluid volumes from structural and angiographic optical coherence tomography using deep learning. Transl Vis Sci Technol. 2020;9(2):54.
35. Chiu SJ, Li XT, Nicholas P, Toth CA, Izatt JA, Farsiu S. Automatic segmentation of seven retinal layers in SDOCT images congruent with expert manual segmentation. Opt Express. 2010;18(18):19413–28.
36. Antony BJ, Abràmoff MD, Harper MM, Jeong W, Sohn EH, Kwon YH, et al. A combined machine-learning and graph-based framework for the segmentation of retinal surfaces in SD-OCT volumes. Biomed Opt Express. 2013;4(12):2712–28.
37. Carass A, Lang A, Hauser M, Calabresi PA, Ying HS, Prince JL. Multiple-object geometric deformable model for segmentation of macular OCT. Biomed Opt Express. 2014;5(4):1062–74.
38. Alsaih K, Lemaitre G, Rastgoo M, Massich J, Sidibé D, Meriaudeau F. Machine learning techniques for diabetic macular edema (DME) classification on SD-OCT images. Biomed Eng Online. 2017;16:68.
39. Hassan B, Raja G, Hassan T, Usman AM. Structure tensor based automated detection of macular edema and central serous retinopathy using optical coherence tomography images. J Opt Soc Am A Opt Image Sci Vis. 2016;33(4):455–63.
40. Liu Y-Y, Ishikawa H, Chen M, Wollstein G, Duker JS, Fujimoto JG, et al. Computerized macular pathology diagnosis in spectral domain optical coherence tomography scans based on multiscale texture and shape features. Invest Ophthalmol Vis Sci. 2011;52(11):8316–22.
41. Srinivasan PP, Kim LA, Mettu PS, Cousins SW, Comer GM, Izatt JA, et al. Fully automated detection of diabetic macular edema and dry age-related macular degeneration from optical coherence tomography images. Biomed Opt Express. 2014;5(10):3568–77.
42. Syed AM, Hassan T, Akram MU, Naz S, Khalid S. Automated diagnosis of macular edema and central serous retinopathy through robust reconstruction of 3D retinal surfaces. Comput Methods Programs Biomed. 2016;137:1–10.
43. Lemaître G, Rastgoo M, Massich J, Cheung CY, Wong TY, Lamoureux E, et al. Classification of SD-OCT volumes using local binary patterns: experimental validation for DME detection. J Ophthalmol. 2016;2016:e3298606.
44. Sidibé D, Sankar S, Lemaître G, Rastgoo M, Massich J, Cheung CY, et al. An anomaly detection approach for the identification of DME patients using spectral domain optical coherence tomography images. Comput Methods Programs Biomed. 2017;139:109–17.
45. Wang Z, Zhang W, Sun Y, Yao M, Yan B. Detection of diabetic macular edema in optical coherence tomography image using an improved level set algorithm. Biomed Res Int. 2020;2020:6974215.
46. Tao Z, Zhang W, Yao M, Zhong Y, Sun Y, Li X-M, et al. A joint model for macular edema analysis in optical coherence tomography images based on image enhancement and segmentation. Biomed Res Int. 2021;2021:6679556.
47. Sun Z, Sun Y. Automatic detection of retinal regions using fully convolutional networks for diagnosis of abnormal maculae in optical coherence tomography images. J Biomed Opt. 2019;24(5):1–9.
48. Chan GCY, Kamble R, Muller H, Shah SAA, Tang TB, Meriaudeau F. Fusing results of several deep learning architectures for automatic classification of normal and diabetic macular edema in optical coherence tomography. Annu Int Conf IEEE Eng Med Biol Soc. 2018;2018:670–3.
49. Perdomo O, Otalora S, Gonzalez FA, Meriaudeau F, Muller H. OCT-NET: 15th IEEE International Symposium on Biomedical

Imaging, ISBI 2018. In: 2018 IEEE 15th Int Symp Biomed Imaging ISBI 2018; 2018. p. 1423–6.
50. Kamble RM, Chan GCY, Perdomo O, Gonzralez FA, Kokare M, Muller H, et al. Automated diabetic macular edema (DME) analysis using fine tuning with inception-resnet-v2 on OCT images. Annu Int Conf IEEE Eng Med Biol Proc. 2018;2018:2715–8.
51. Hwang D-K, Chou Y-B, Lin T-C, Yang H-Y, Kao Z-K, Kao C-L, et al. Optical coherence tomography–based diabetic macula edema screening with artificial intelligence. J Chin Med Assoc. 2020;83(11):1034–8.
52. Wu Q, Zhang B, Hu Y, Liu B, Cao D, Yang D, et al. Detection of morphologic patterns of diabetic macular edema using a deep learning approach based on optical coherence tomography images. Retina. 2021;41(5):1110–7.
53. Lee CS, Tyring AJ, Deruyter NP, Wu Y, Rokem A, Lee AY. Deep-learning based, automated segmentation of macular edema in optical coherence tomography. Biomed Opt Express. 2017;8(7):3440–8.
54. Schlegl T, Waldstein SM, Bogunovic H, Endstraßer F, Sadeghipour A, Philip A-M, et al. Fully automated detection and quantification of macular fluid in OCT using deep learning. Ophthalmology. 2018;125(4):549–58.
55. Wang YT, Tadarati M, Wolfson Y, Bressler SB, Bressler NM. Comparison of prevalence of diabetic macular edema based on monocular fundus photography vs. optical coherence tomography. JAMA Ophthalmol. 2016;134(2):222–8.
56. Arcadu F, Benmansour F, Maunz A, Michon J, Haskova Z, McClintock D, et al. Deep learning predicts OCT measures of diabetic macular thickening from color fundus photographs. Invest Ophthalmol Vis Sci. 2019;60(4):852–7.
57. Arcadu F, Benmansour F, Maunz A, Willis J, Haskova Z, Prunotto M. Deep learning algorithm predicts diabetic retinopathy progression in individual patients. NPJ Digit Med. 2019;2:92.
58. Leontidis G, Al-Diri B, Hunter A. A new unified framework for the early detection of the progression to diabetic retinopathy from fundus images. Comput Biol Med. 2017;90:98–115.
59. Bora A, Balasubramanian S, Babenko B, Virmani S, Venugopalan S, Mitani A, et al. Predicting the risk of developing diabetic retinopathy using deep learning. Lancet Digit Health. 2021;3(1):e10–9.
60. Chen S-C, Chiu H-W, Chen C-C, Woung L-C, Lo C-M. A novel machine learning algorithm to automatically predict visual outcomes in intravitreal ranibizumab-treated patients with diabetic macular edema. J Clin Med. 2018;7(12):E475.
61. Rasti R, Allingham MJ, Mettu PS, Kavusi S, Govind K, Cousins SW, et al. Deep learning-based single-shot prediction of differential effects of anti-VEGF treatment in patients with diabetic macular edema. Biomed Opt Express. 2020;11(2):1139–52.
62. Li B, Zhang B, Chen Y, Li D. Optical coherence tomography parameters related to vision impairment in patients with diabetic macular edema: a quantitative correlation analysis. J Ophthalmol. 2020;2020:5639284.
63. Liu B, Zhang B, Hu Y, Cao D, Yang D, Wu Q, et al. Automatic prediction of treatment outcomes in patients with diabetic macular edema using ensemble machine learning. Ann Transl Med. 2021;9(1):43.
64. Roberts PK, Vogl W-D, Gerendas BS, Glassman AR, Bogunovic H, Jampol LM, et al. Quantification of fluid resolution and visual acuity gain in patients with diabetic macular edema using deep learning. JAMA Ophthalmol. 2020;138(9):945–53.
65. Tufail A, Rudisill C, Egan C, Kapetanakis VV, Salas-Vega S, Owen CG, et al. Automated diabetic retinopathy image assessment software: diagnostic accuracy and cost-effectiveness compared with human graders. Ophthalmology. 2017;124(3):343–51.
66. Scheetz J, Koca D, McGuinness M, Holloway E, Tan Z, Zhu Z, et al. Real-world artificial intelligence-based opportunistic screening for diabetic retinopathy in endocrinology and indigenous healthcare settings in Australia. Sci Rep. 2021;11:15808.
67. Zhang Q, Liu Z, Li J, Liu G. Identifying diabetic macular edema and other retinal diseases by optical coherence tomography image and multiscale deep learning. Diabetes Metab Syndr Obes. 2020;13:4787–800.
68. Tsuji T, Hirose Y, Fujimori K, Hirose T, Oyama A, Saikawa Y, et al. Classification of optical coherence tomography images using a capsule network. BMC Ophthalmol. 2020;20(1):114.
69. Lin AC, Lee CS, Blazes M, Lee AY, Gorin MB. Assessing the clinical utility of expanded macular OCTs using machine learning. Transl Vis Sci Technol. 2021;10(6):32.
70. Hassan B, Hassan T, Li B, Ahmed R, Hassan O. Deep ensemble learning based objective grading of macular edema by extracting clinically significant findings from fused retinal imaging modalities. Sensors. 2019;19(13):2970.
71. Kang EY-C, Yeung L, Lee Y-L, Wu C-H, Peng S-Y, Chen Y-P, et al. A multimodal imaging–based deep learning model for detecting treatment-requiring retinal vascular diseases: model development and validation study. JMIR Med Inform. 2021;9(5):e28868.
72. Sun Y, Li S, Sun Z. Fully automated macular pathology detection in retina optical coherence tomography images using sparse coding and dictionary learning. J Biomed Opt. 2017;22(1):16012.
73. Gerendas BS, Bogunovic H, Sadeghipour A, Schlegl T, Langs G, Waldstein SM, et al. Computational image analysis for prognosis determination in DME. Vision Res. 2017;139:204–10.
74. Huang H, Zhu L, Zhu W, Lin T, Los LI, Yao C, et al. Algorithm for detection and quantification of hyperreflective dots on optical coherence tomography in diabetic macular edema. Front Med. 2021;8:688986.

16 Endpoints of Anti-Vascular Endothelial Growth Factor Clinical Trials for Diabetic Macular Edema

Aditya Verma, Yamini Attiku, and Srinivas R. Sadda

16.1 Overview of Diabetic Macular Edema

Diabetic macular edema (DME) is a vision-threatening microvascular complication arising in patients suffering from long standing diabetes mellitus (DM) [1, 2]. It manifests as retinal thickening within the macular region, due to accumulation of fluid in intraretinal and sometimes subretinal locations [3]. As the understanding regarding the pathophysiology of diabetic retinopathy (DR) has evolved over the years, it is now apparent that neuronal loss secondary to apoptosis may occur independently of the visible vascular manifestations [4]. The complex interplay of microvascular damage, neuronal injury (leading to early photoreceptor loss), oxidative stress, and inflammation has now been established to play a key role in the development of changes associated with DME [4].

Over the years, various definitions have been suggested describing several patho-anatomical aspects of DME. Clinically significant macular edema (CSME) was one the earliest phenotypes, defined in the landmark trial Early Treatment of Diabetic Retinopathy Study (ETDRS), demonstrating the efficacy of focal laser to treat DME [5]. CSME, evaluated using slit-lamp bio-microscopy, was defined based on the presence of retinal thickening and/or associated hard exudates either involving or threatening the foveal center. At that time, color fundus photos and fundus fluorescein angiography (FFA) were the primary diagnostic technologies utilized for assessing severity of retinopathy and planning management (Fig. 16.1). Although it was understood that the treatment options and visual outcomes may differ in eyes with DME involving the foveal center, laser still stood the test of time as the gold standard in management of DME until about a decade ago [5–7]. The wide availability of optical coherence tomography (OCT) changed the outlook of how the clinicians would perceive DME, and the management strategies changed significantly. The term center-involved DME (CI-DME) came into vogue to describe edema when the thickening involved the foveal center (Fig. 16.2) [8]. The terms focal and diffuse DME were coined to differentiate the leakage of the fluorescein dye as seen on FFA arising from microaneurysms (focal) or hyperpermeable capillaries (diffuse) [9, 10]. These terms have been used ambiguously in the literature owing to the presence of both components in different proportions in most cases of DME. Subclinical DME has been used to bridge the gap between clinically visible DME and the thickening which is noted on OCT with no clinically recognizable edema on biomicroscopy [11]. Persistent (DME that persists despite adequate treatment); recurrent (DME that resolves with treatment but recurs later); and recalcitrant (persistent DME despite multiple treatment sessions) have been used to describe the treatment outcome related forms of DME [9].

The majority of patients with DME maintain good visual acuity, at least early in the course of the disease [12]. This was also evident in the ETDRS trial with approximately 40% of eyes with a visual acuity of 20/20 [5, 13]. These eyes were not offered any treatment as the optimal therapeutic strategy for these eyes was not known to the clinicians at that time. This trend, however, has changed over the years based on the results of large clinical trials, and clinicians now prefer to initiate the treatment of DME with anti-vascular endothelial growth factor (VEGF) agents even when the visual acuity is good [7, 14, 15]. The treatment armamentarium underwent a paradigm shift beginning in 2010, when anti-VEGF agents were introduced, and they have largely replaced laser photocoagulation as the mainstay of therapy for DME [6, 7, 16–19].

A. Verma · Y. Attiku
Doheny Eye Institute, Pasadena, CA, USA

S. R. Sadda (✉)
Department of Ophthalmology, David Geffen School of Medicine at UCLA, University of California, Los Angeles, CA, USA
e-mail: SSadda@doheny.org

S. Saxena et al. (eds.), *Diabetic Macular Edema*, https://doi.org/10.1007/978-981-19-7307-9_16

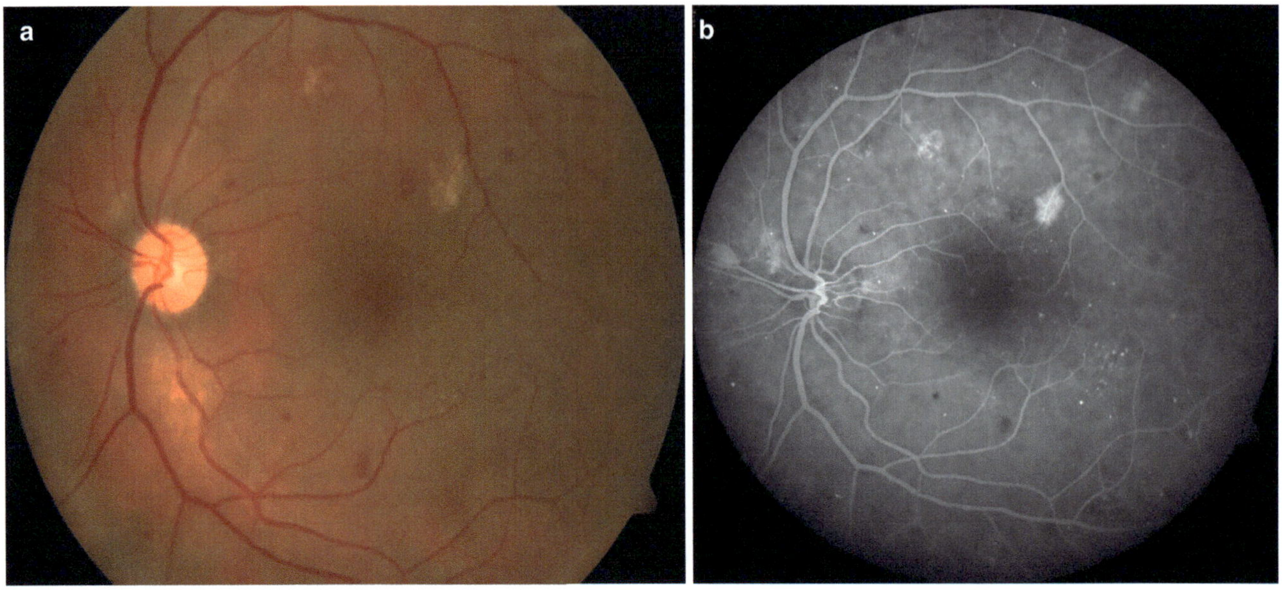

Fig. 16.1 Color fundus photo (**a**) and the corresponding fundus fluorescein angiogram (FFA, **b**) of the left eye showing scattered intraretinal hemorrhages over the posterior pole, with a few microaneurysms and hard exudate infero-temporal to the macula. FFA demonstrates blocked fluorescence due to hemorrhages and punctate hyperfluorescence related to microaneurysms

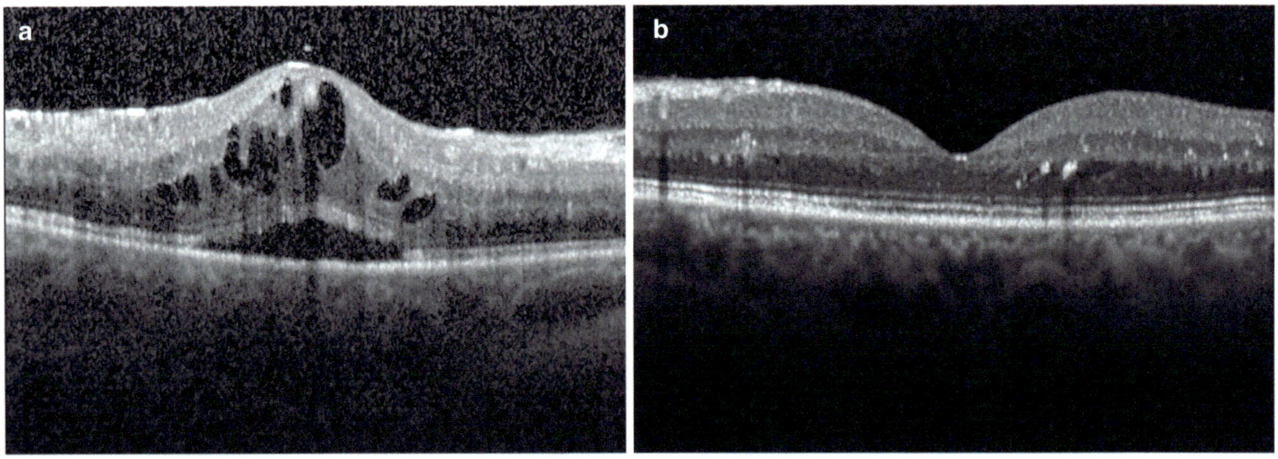

Fig. 16.2 Optical coherence tomography B scans of two eyes with different severities and distributions of diabetic macular edema (DME). (**a**) Center-involved (CI) DME with both intraretinal cystoid spaces and subretinal fluid. (**b**) Subtle cystoid spaces with a few cystoid spaces and intraretinal hyper-reflective foci (hard exudates) temporal to the fovea

16.2 Outcomes of a Clinical Trial

Endpoints of a clinical trial are defined as the quantifiable measures or variables used to assess the objectives of the study [20]. The primary endpoint for which the study is powered is used to assess the key objective of the study. The fundamental principle of a study design is to pre-define the primary and secondary endpoints, failure of which can introduce bias and opportunities for misinterpretation. In those trials where the primary endpoint is undesirable (death/loss of tissue), or when the number of events being studies is very small, a surrogate endpoint (surrogate biomarker) is used which is a measure of effect of an intervention, that may correlate with the "true" primary endpoint [21]. Regardless, it is obvious that the endpoints of a study should directly highlight the outcome, should be measurable as well as reproducible, and should be translatable into clinical practice. Understandably, the clinically relevant outcomes of a study should encompass both the structural and functional aspects of the effect of intervention being studied on the disease. However, there may be fallacies and practical challenges which may challenge these end points. We shall discuss these relevant issues in the context of anti-VEGF trials for DME in this chapter.

16.3 Endpoints of Anti-VEGF Trial for DME

Anti-VEGF agents are among the most highly researched drugs in ophthalmic practice, especially in the context of exudative diseases such as DME and neovascular AMD. Visual acuity and central macular thickness measurements have remained as standardized definitions to measure outcomes of most of these trials (Table 16.1) [7, 16, 17, 22–37]. Best corrected visual acuity (BCVA) as assessed by ETDRS letter score (developed by Baily and Lovie) is used extensively in clinical research over the standard Snellen's visual acuity assessment [38, 39]. Analysis of EDTRS letter score can be converted into a logarithmic minimal angle of resolution score (logMAR) suitable for quantitative statistical analysis [40, 41]. Various trials have applied visual acuity measurements in terms of the mean change in BCVA, the mean change in the ETDRS letter score, proportion of eyes gaining a standard unit of vision (for example, 10-letter or 2-lines) from the baseline over a prescribed course of treatment, and a decrease of a standard letter score from baseline as a result of a particular treatment.

A number of OCT biomarkers have been found to be associated with visual acuity in DME, apart from clinical features such as duration of edema, retinal perfusion, vitreomacular surface abnormalities, and morphology of edema [42]. These include the integrity of the ellipsoid zone, disorganization of retinal inner layers (DRIL, defined as involvement of ≥50% of the 1 mm region centered at the fovea), and the choroidal thickness [43–46]. However, it is the central macular thickness that has stood the test of time to assess the severity and efficacy of treatment strategies for DME.

Over the years, there has been a debate about thickening in the macular region that best correlates with visual acuity. The macular thickening described by the term CSME has now been largely replaced by thickening specific to the foveal region (central 1000 μ diameter, the central subfield [CSF] thickness), sometimes simply referred to as the foveal thickness. In contrast, the central point thickness, which is determined only by six data points, has a higher chance of being affected by minor eye movements, and is therefore, not considered as a reliable indicator of the foveal thickness [47]. OCT instrument software can provide automated CSF

Table 16.1 A summary of major clinical trials in diabetic macular edema with pre-defined primary and secondary end-points for each study

Intervention	Duration	Primary end point	Secondary end point
Macugen Diabetic Retinopathy Study Group: A phase II randomized double-masked trial of Pegaptanib for diabetic macular edema [22]	36 weeks	Change in BCVA (number of letters and lines gained or lost and proportions of subjects maintaining baseline VA or gaining 5 letters, 10 letters, or 15 letters) Change in CRT Proportion of subjects with the need for additional therapy with photocoagulation between weeks 12 and 36	Safety outcomes
DRCR-Protocol H: A phase II randomized clinical trial of intravitreal bevacizumab for diabetic macular edema [23]	24 weeks	Change in central subfield thickness Change in BCVA	Adverse effects
READ-2 study: Primary end point (6 months) results of the ranibizumab for edema of the mAcula in diabetes [24]	6 months	Mean change in BCVA	Mean change in central subfield thickness Adverse events
DRCR Protocol I: Randomized trial evaluating ranibizumab plus prompt or deferred laser or triamcinolone plus prompt laser for DME [7]	1 year	Mean change in BCVA Safety outcomes	Change in central subfield thickness Effect of treatment on level of retinopathy
READ-2 study: Two-year outcomes of the ranibizumab for edema of the mAcula in diabetes [25]	2 years	Mean change in BCVA	Mean change in central subfield thickness Mean number of RBZ injections
RESOLVE study: Safety and efficacy of ranibizumab in diabetic macular edema—A 12-month, randomized, controlled, double-masked, multicenter phase II study [26]	12 months	Mean change in BCVA Mean change in CRT Safety outcomes	

(continued)

Table 16.1 (continued)

Intervention	Duration	Primary end point	Secondary end point
RESTORE study: Ranibizumab monotherapy or combined with Laser versus laser monotherapy for diabetic macular edema [16]	12 months	Mean change in BCVA from baseline to month 1–12 Safety outcomes	Mean BCVA letter score change from baseline to month 12 Proportion of patients who gained ≥10 and ≥15 letters in BCVA Patients with BCVA letter score ≥73 at month 1 Mean change in CRT over time Proportion of patients with CRT <275 μ
A phase 2/3, multicenter, randomized, double-masked, 2-year trial of pegaptanib sodium for the treatment of diabetic macular edema [27]	2 years	Proportion of subjects with a 10-letter (2-line) improvement from baseline in VA at week 54	Proportion of subjects with a 10-letter improvement from baseline in VA at week 102 Changes from baseline in mean VA over time; and, at weeks 54 and 102 Proportion of subjects with a 15-letter (3-line) improvement in VA Proportion of subjects with a change in degree of retinopathy of two steps based on the retinopathy scale Proportion of subjects with a decrease in retinal thickness at the center point by 25% and 50% Proportion of subjects requiring focal or grid laser Change in NEI-VFQ-25 and EQ-5D from baseline Safety endpoints
DRCR Protocol J: Randomized trial evaluating short-term effects of intravitreal ranibizumab or triamcinolone acetonide on macular edema following focal/grid laser for diabetic macular edema in eyes also receiving PRP [28]	14 weeks	Mean change in BCVA from baseline	Mean change in central subfield thickness Ocular adverse effects
DA VINCI: Phase 2 primary results of VEGF Trap-Eye in patients with DME [29]	24 weeks	Mean change in BCVA	Proportion of patients who gained at least 15 ETDRS letters in BCVA compared with baseline Change from baseline in CRT Number of focal laser treatments received
RISE and RIDE: Ranibizumab for diabetic macular edema—results from 2 Phase III randomized trials [17]	24 months	Proportion of patients gaining 15 letters in BCVA from baseline	Mean change from baseline BCVA score over time Proportion of patients with BCVA Snellen equivalent of ≥20/40 Mean change from baseline BCVA score over time in patients with focal edema as assessed on FA Proportion of patients losing 15 letters in BCVA score from baseline Mean change from baseline in central subfield thickness over time Proportion of patients with a three-step progression from baseline in ETDRS retinopathy severity on FP Proportion of patients with resolution of leakage on FA Mean number of macular laser treatments over time
DRCR Protocol I: Intravitreal ranibizumab for diabetic macular edema with prompt vs. deferred laser treatment: 3-year randomized trial results [30]	3 years	Mean change in BCVA Safety outcomes	Percentage of eyes with a ≥10 letter gain Percentage of eyes with a ≥10 letter loss Median numbers of injections Percentage of eyes with central subfield thickness ≥250 μ

Table 16.1 (continued)

Intervention	Duration	Primary end point	Secondary end point
BOLT study: A 2-year prospective randomized controlled trial of intravitreal bevacizumab or laser therapy in the management of diabetic macular edema [31]	2 years	Difference in ETDRS BCVA between arms	Mean change in BCVA Proportion gaining at least 15 and at least 10 ETDRS letters Losing fewer than 15 and at least 30 letters Change in CMT ETDRS retinopathy severity Safety outcomes
DRCR protocol T: Aflibercept, bevacizumab, or ranibizumab for diabetic macular edema [32]	1 year	Mean improvement in the visual-acuity letter score	Change in central subfield thickness Safety outcomes
DRCR Protocol I: Repeated intravitreous Ranibizumab injections for diabetic macular edema and the risk of sustained elevation of intraocular pressure or the need for ocular hypotensive treatment [33]	3 years	Cumulative probability of sustained IOP elevation through 3 years of follow-up	
DRCR Protocol I: Persistent macular thickening after ranibizumab treatment for diabetic macular edema with vision impairment [34]	3 years	Cumulative 3-year probabilities of chronic persistent DME (failure to achieve a central subfield thickness <250 μ and at least a 10% reduction from the 24-week visit on at least two consecutive study visits) Cumulative 3-year probabilities of at least 10 letters (2 lines) gain or loss of visual acuity among those eyes	
Protocol T: Persistent macular thickening following intravitreous aflibercept, bevacizumab, or ranibizumab for central-involved diabetic macular edema with vision impairment—A secondary analysis of a randomized clinical trial [35]	2 years	age of eyes with persistent DME at each visit through 24 weeks Probability of chronic persistent DME through 2 years At least 10 letters (2 lines) gain or loss of visual acuity among eyes with persistent DME	
DRCR Protocol V: To compare vision loss at 2 years among eyes initially managed with aflibercept, laser photocoagulation, or observation [36]	2 years	At least a 5-letter visual acuity decrease from baseline at 2 years	Mean change in VA from baseline VA of at least 84 letters (Snellen equivalent of 20/20) Loss of at least 10 and at least 15 letters of VA Gain of at least 5 letters of VA Mean change in CST from baseline Proportion of eyes with at least 10% CST change from baseline Proportion of eyes with at least a 10% decrease in CST from baseline 1 and 2 log-step worsening and improvement in CST Mean change in OCT retinal volume from baseline
DRCR Protocol T Extension Study: Participants were assigned randomly to aflibercept, bevacizumab, or ranibizumab with protocol-defined follow-up and retreatment for 2 years. Thereafter, participants were managed at clinician discretion and recalled for a 5-year visit [37]	5 years	Mean number of anti-VEGF injections from year 2 to 5 Mean change in VA letter score Change in central subfield thickness	Change in diabetic retinopathy severity level Adverse events

thickness values, and while these may be susceptible to segmentation error, their performance has improved over time, and has reduced the previous subjectivity over assessing for the presence of macular edema. Not surprisingly, CSF thickness is utilized as the primary eligibility criterion, defining recurrent/persistent/recalcitrant DME, and retreatment criterion in trials studying the effects of anti-VEGF agents in DME.

16.4 Limitations of Endpoints in the Pre-(High-Definition) OCT Era

Anti-VEGF agents for DME are indicated in the setting of edema (thickening due to fluid accumulation), and therefore, a precise endpoint to estimate their efficacy would be to analyze the retinal volume rather than central macular thickness [48]. However, studies have proven otherwise. CSF thickness has not been found to correlate with retinal volume (Fig. 16.3). With advantages like easy computation, good reproducibility, and being a better analytical tool, CSF has been identified as a useful endpoint to define anatomical thickness outcomes [47, 49–51]. Furthermore, it is the macular thickness, rather than the presence of macular edema, which correlates well with visual acuity [52, 53]. Researchers have identified the minimum scan density required to generate a reliable macular thickness map using OCT [54]. Having to only correct segmentation errors on a limited number of scans, may make manual segmentation a practical solution for managing segmentation errors in the context of clinical trials. Another relevant method for assessing the efficacy of anti-VEGF therapy is to compare all B scans in the macular region in terms of reduction of cystic spaces (hypo-reflective areas), which would essentially measure the dry retinal volume, indicating the drying capacity of the intravitreal drugs [55]. However, it is a reasonable assumption that these methods are useful research tools but may lose their practical efficacy in the clinical settings.

Studies have also shown a rather modest correlation between the visual acuity and CSF thickness [56, 57]. OCT biomarkers showing a good correlation with visual acuity are the photoreceptor outer segment length and DRIL (Figs. 16.3 and 16.4) [41, 58–62]. Although these approaches appear to be scientifically relevant, they may not be practical in a clinical setting, unless automated instrument software is introduced.

Similarly, BCVA assessment, due to its subjectivity, may not be an accurate assessment of the functional outcomes of anti-VEGF agents in DME. As neurodegeneration appears to set in early in the course of disease, researchers have adopted

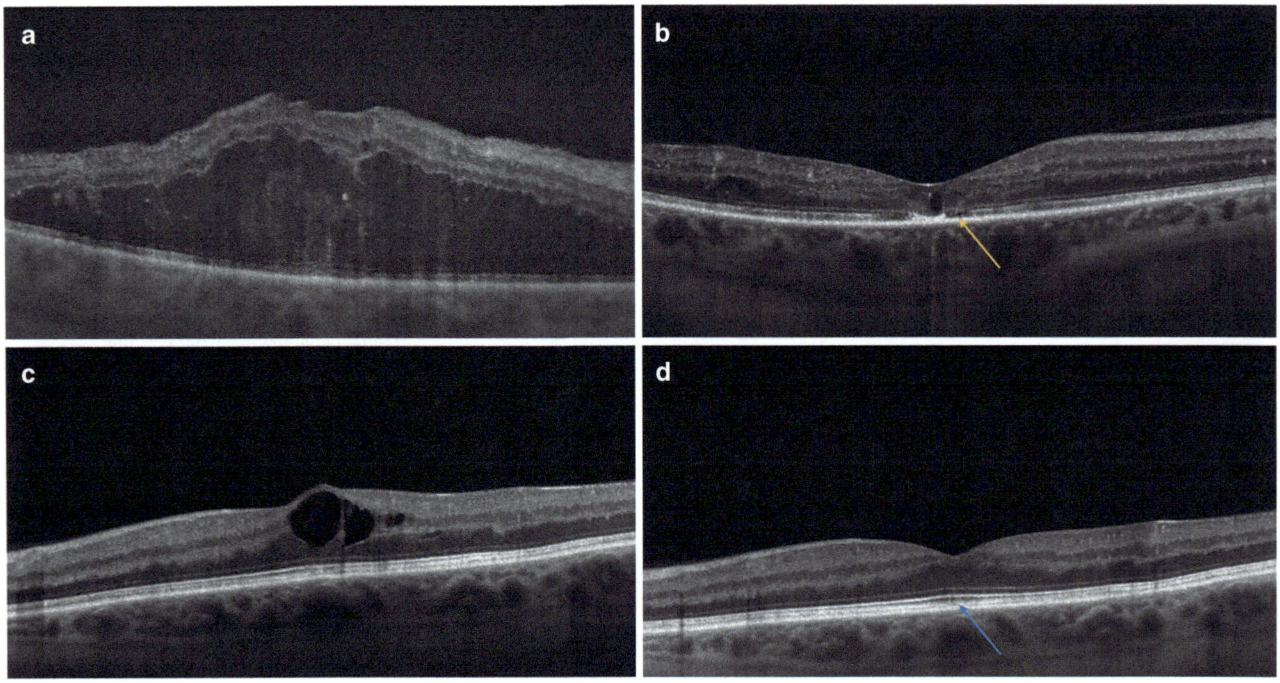

Fig. 16.3 Differential response of anti-vascular endothelial growth factor (VEGF) therapy for diabetic macular edema (DME). Although the marked center-involved diabetic macular edema in (**a**) was dramatically reduced by anti-VEGF therapy (**b**), the final visual outcome was poor due to some disruption of the ellipsoid zone (yellow arrow). In contrast, in the eye with DME shown in (**c**), anti-VEGF therapy was associated with a good visual outcome (**d**) and the outer retinal bands were noted to be intact (blue arrow)

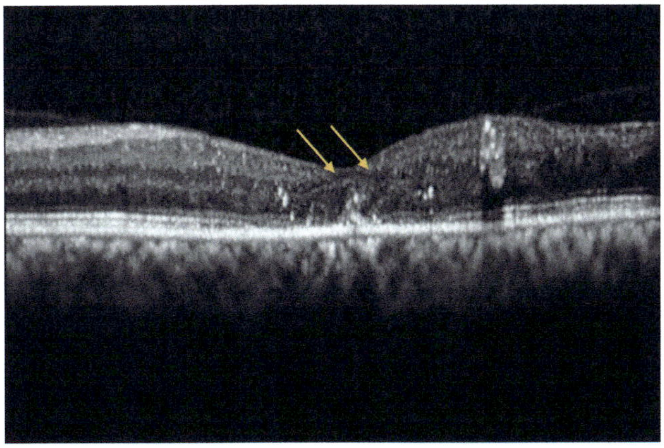

Fig. 16.4 Optical coherence tomography B scan of an eye with DME after anti-VEGF therapy, demonstrating the disruption of retinal inner layers (DRIL). Note that the boundaries between ganglion cell layer and the outer plexiform layer cannot be identified in at least 50% of 1 mm region centered at the fovea

various techniques to assess the functional correlates in these eyes. Apart from the extensive SD-OCT based observations, scanning laser polarimetry to assess the retinal nerve fiber layer thickness, microperimetry and electrophysiological and clinical studies have also been employed for this purpose [63–70]. Furthermore, the outer retinal disorganization characterized by loss of outer segment reflectivity using SD-OCT has been shown to correlate well with visual acuity and thus overall photoreceptor integrity in these eyes [71].

16.5 Newer Biomarkers for DME

Over the last decade, investigators have identified novel structural and functional biomarkers to assess the efficacy of treatment of eyes with DME using anti-VEGF agents. This became relevant owing to the development of novel therapeutic strategies compelling the researchers to foster precise patho-anatomic features of DME. This has been feasible with the exceptional improvements in OCT mechanics and reading software (structural), as well as advancements in the psychophysical and electrophysical testing (functional) [72, 73]. Furthermore, as OCT has been found to have a reliable correlation with FFA findings of cystic spaces in eyes with DME, researchers have essentially targeted the structural features in such eyes as seen by OCT to assess the response to therapy [46, 74]. Being novel, these correlates have so far been used in isolated clinical studies and case series rather than larger prospective trials. Can they qualify as standard primary endpoints of a trial using anti-VEGF agents? What is their efficacy over a research platform versus a clinic? Do they fare better when compared with the time-tested conventional visual acuity and retinal thickness?

16.5.1 Structural Biomarkers

As discussed earlier, various structural alterations in retina layers have been investigated in terms of treatment outcomes in eyes with DME [42–46]. Earlier investigators attempted to described sequential development of clinical stages of DME and subsequent SRF formation with specific pathological alterations in various layers [75]. Thereafter, it is only since the last decade that various additional features have been reported using advanced OCT imaging. These include hyper-reflective foci, photoreceptor outer segment length, external limiting membrane integrity, DRIL, and quantification of retinal cystic spaces and subretinal fluid (SRF) [43–46, 76, 77]. Sun et al. reported a good correlation of DRIL extent (and to a lesser extent, reduced cone outer segment tip (COST) visibility) with visual acuity at baseline in eyes with DME (Fig. 16.4), and that the changes in DRIL could predict future changes in visual acuity in these eyes [60]. They also reported an independent association of DRIL, CSF thickness, presence of SRF and COST visibility with visual acuity when these patients were followed over time. An increase in DRIL, CSF thickness, and reduced COST visibility were found to be good predictors of future visual acuity in the same study. Das et al. further evaluated the association of DRIL with other OCT biomarkers and reported that the outer retinal layer disruption, i.e., disrupted external limiting membrane (ELM) and ellipsoid zone (EZ), as well as the presence of epiretinal membrane and increased thickness at the fovea were found to have higher odds of having DRIL [62]. They also reported poor visual acuity in eyes with outer retinal alterations. This finding may suggest that the retinal alterations can occur in varied proportions in these eyes and may have varied effects of visual acuity. However, DRIL has been reported in association with macular ischemia, even in eyes without DME, and therefore, cannot be taken as a standalone biomarker when assessing the effects of anti-VEGF in these eyes [78].

Another interesting feature that has been described in association with DME is the presence of hyper-reflective foci (HRF) in different retinal layers. First described by Bolz et al. in 2009, they have been reported throughout the retinal layers (Fig. 16.5), reminiscent of small intraretinal protein, and/or lipid deposits secondary to vascular hyperpermeability [75]. Other investigators have suggested that these foci may indicate RPE migration or photoreceptor debris and are associated with disrupted ELM and/or EZ and decreased visual acuity [79]. Not surprisingly, although these HRF show a dynamic rearrangement after the treatment with anti-VEGF agents, the HRF distributed in the outer retinal layers are significantly associated with the final visual acuity, and disruption of the ELM and EZ [80–82]. The presence of SRF, as well as the presence of HRF within the SRF have

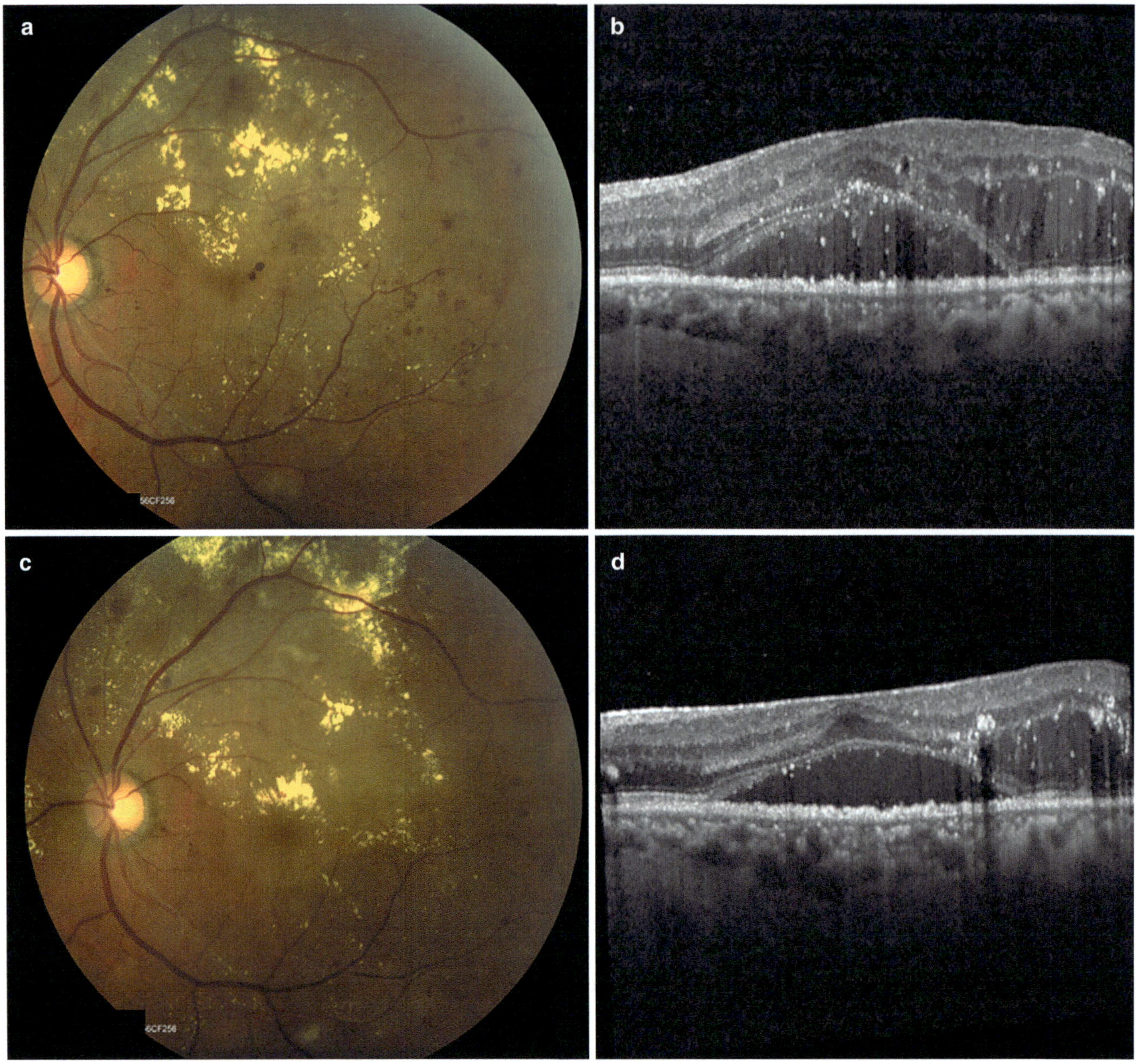

Fig. 16.5 Color fundus photos showing extensive hard exudates (**a**), and corresponding macular OCT B scan (**b**) showing intraretinal and subretinal fluid with extensive hyper-reflective foci (HRF) distributed in the retinal layers and the subretinal space. Following anti-VEGF treatment, accumulation of hard exudates in the fovea is observed (**c**), with partial resolution of the intraretinal and subretinal fluid (**d**) and larger aggregates of HRF closer to the foveal center

been found to be poor prognostic factors after treatment with anti-VEGF agents in such eyes with subsequent subfoveal hard exudate accumulation [83–85].

On the contrary, some investigators have reported an association of HRF at baseline with favorable visual outcomes and a greater decrease in the CSF thickness after treatment with anti-VEGF agents [86]. Since the eyes with HRF in outer retinal layers had a greater disruption of the EZ and these eyes showed a greater improvement with treatment, they hypothesized that foveal photoreceptor restoration in such cases may partly explain the greater extent of visual improvement when compared with eyes without the evidence of baseline HRF. Such foveal restoration, associated with decreased EZ and ELM line disruption, was reported in a study by Mori et al. [87]. Interestingly, the shortening of disrupted ELM was also associated with baseline visual acuity and CSF thickness in their study. Although the resolution of HRF and reduction of the EZ and ELM disruption have been linked to favorable visual acuity in these reports, interplay of other structural correlates, especially at the level of photoreceptors and RPE cannot be disregarded as additional events which may influence these results.

Presence of SRF in eyes with DME has been associated with greater inflammatory load (Fig. 16.5) [87, 88]. Various sub-analysis reports from large trials indicated that the baseline SRF correlated with good visual acuity and resolution of macular edema when treated with ranibizumab (RISE and RIDE, READ-3) [83, 89]. Furthermore, post-hoc analysis in VIVID and VISTA-DME trials suggested that baseline SRF had no role in determining the visual outcomes when treated with aflibercept [90]. Deák et al. reported that the majority of the structural alterations seen in eyes with DME showed a significant negative correlation with the retinal function as assessed using microperimetry, with the serous detachment (SRF) and large outer nuclear layer cysts having the greatest impact [77]. Yet, there are reports which suggest a negative impact of SRF on the visual acuity gains in these eyes [91, 92]. As discussed previously, the presence of HRF in the SRF significantly alters the visual outcomes in these eyes [84]. Yoshitake et al. in their study reported better visual gains in eyes with SRF which had additional HRF on univariate analysis [86]. It can be stated with confidence that resolution of SRF correlates with the greater quantum of VEGF load and therefore, better visual acuity outcomes when treated with anti-VEGF agents. However, the presence of HRF may tilt the balance to either side depending upon the origin of these foci, with those secondary to vessel hyperpermeability appearing to have better visual acuity gains as compared to those which are originate from photoreceptors/RPE migration. With evidence of microglial origin, these HRF have been reported to represent inflammatory load in eyes with DME [93, 94]. This was also suggested in a study by Rübsam et al. in which smaller HRF responded to steroid treatment better as compared with the larger ones, suggesting that smaller foci may have an inflammatory onset as compared with the larger ones which may signify organized exudates [95]. As the authors suggested, we also believe that HRF may represent a dynamic phenomenon, with a migration towards the outer retina based on the disease severity as well as systemic profile of the patient. When associated with SRF, it may be the initial effect of SRF resolution which may equate with good visual acuity gains. With migration towards the subretinal space, the beneficial effects of treatment may transfigure towards more guarded outcomes, with proportionally larger expanse of outer retinal defects [79–82, 96]. These reports suggest that HRF may have diverse pathophysiological origins (based on morphological characteristics and location, as reported by Vujosevic et al.), and their relevance needs to be investigated as a biomarker for retinal structural integrity [97]. Nonetheless, there is recent evidence indicating that eyes with HRF may have earlier recurrence of macular edema when treated with steroid implants, suggesting frequent follow ups in such eyes [98].

Intraretinal cystoid spaces (RCS) are the hallmark structural alterations in DME, resulting from increased vascular permeability secondary to inner blood–retinal barrier breakdown [99]. Majority of trials have designated resolution of these RCS and decreasing CSF thickness as the primary end points when assessing the efficacy of anti-VEGF agents in eyes with DME, as they are directly associated with photoreceptor damage [100]. Larger cysts in the outer retinal layers have been shown to have negative impact macular microperimetry as they are responsible for EZ and photoreceptor loss [101, 102]. Resolution of these RCS in the outer retinal layers has been shown to occur with anti-VEGF agents with resultant improvement in visual acuity and retinal sensitivity in macular region [101]. In contrast, those RCS with increased reflectivity signals have been shown to respond poorly to the anti-VEGF agents, as these have been associated with severe inner blood-retinal barrier loss [103]. Investigators have hypothesized these hyper-reflective signals as suspended scattering particles in motion using OCT angiography (OCTA) as a result of Brownian motion of particles within these fluid pockets, which can result in the formation of hard exudates at a later date [104]. With the limited evidence available in literature, it is certain that these RCS with hyper-reflective signals may be associated with poorer visual outcomes in such eyes treated with anti-VEGF agents.

There are less well investigated structural features that have been reported to have a bearing on the visual acuity in eyes with DME. Bridging retinal processes between the cystic cavities is one such feature [105]. Authors hypothesized that eyes without the evidence of such processes may develop thinning and atrophy after treatment with anti-VEGF agents [106]. Studies have also shown that the photoreceptor outer segment length (measured between the IS/OS junction and the RPE) correlates better with the visual acuity as compared with the macular thickness in eyes with DME [43].

OCTA is a novel imaging technique used to analyze the retinal and choroidal microvasculature in a depth resolved fashion (Fig. 16.6). Since visual acuity may not show expected improvement in some eyes treated adequately with anti-VEGF agents with satisfactory resolution of edema, investigators have tried to identify independent OCTA-based prognostic indicators in such eyes [107]. Baseline parafoveal vessel density (VD) in the superficial capillary plexus (SCP) was shown as an independent predictor for visual improvement in these eyes [108]. Others have suggested the VD at the deep capillary plexus (DCP) and FAZ at the SCP as adequate predictors of visual function and monitor response to treatment [109]. Tang et al. reported a worse visual acuity with lower VD at the level of DCP. This becomes relevant as DCP contributes about 10–15% of the oxygen supply to photoreceptors and is the first layer to be affected in DME, OCTA evaluation could predict visual acuity changes at an early stage facilitating aggressive treatment strategies and monitoring response to treatment [110]. Although there is insufficient data regarding the OCTA-based endpoints in

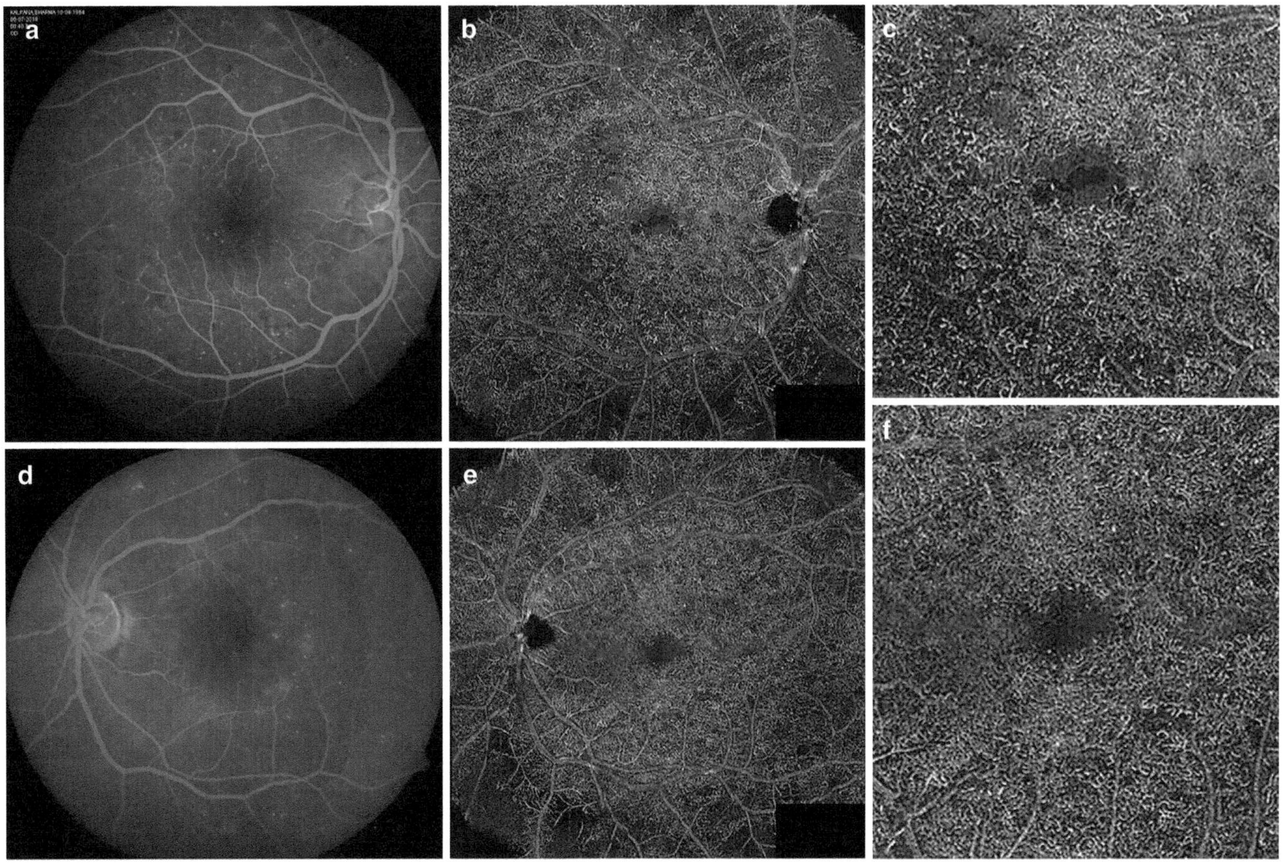

Fig. 16.6 Fundus fluorescein angiogram (FFA) and the corresponding optical coherence tomography montaged images (OCTA) of the right eye (**a**, **b**, and **c**) and left eye (**d**, **e**, and **f**) of a patient with diabetic retinopathy showing extensive microvascular alterations in the superficial capillary plexus across the posterior pole, with disrupted foveal avascular zone and scattered microaneurysms (**c**, **f**). In contrast to the FFA images, OCTA only demonstrates a subset of microaneurysms and does not demonstrate leakage

eyes with DME treated with anti-VEGF agents, it can be stated with a high level of confidence that the changes noted on the parafoveal angioarchitecture may correlate with the functional outcomes better that the structural biomarkers as seen on OCT, as described previously.

Nonetheless, it is clear at present that no single structural corelate can be a surrogate in isolation to predict the retinal integrity and the ultimate outcomes of anti-VEGF therapy in eyes with DME.

16.5.2 Functional Biomarkers

The outcomes as reported by clinical trials for DME may not correlate well with the actual functional outcomes as perceived by the patients. Assessment of visual gains by visual letter score on ETDRS scale may not be sufficient to quantify the functional success of anti-VEGF therapy. With the concept of neuronal degeneration early in the course of disease, there is mounting evidence that functional deterioration takes place much earlier than actually perceived by the clinicians [63–70, 111, 112]. Furthermore, hypoxic insult in early stages of DR has been associated with delayed dark adaptation, diminished color discrimination sensitivity, and a decline in achromatic contrast sensitivity [113].

Electroretinogram (ERG) has been a prime focus of interest by many investigators in the treatment outcomes of DME. It measures the electrical currents generated by retinal neurons and glial cells thereby assessing the functional status of retinal neural tissues. Treatment with anti-VEGF agents has been shown to increase the implicit times in eyes with DME, the changes occurring as early as 2 h following the injection [114]. This increase in the implicit times has been hypothesized as a stress response of the retinal neurons with initiation of the treatment, which gets stabilized with time [115]. Multifocal ERG (mf-ERG) measures local cone-driven responses from the macular region utilizing contrast-reversing stimulus. Baget-Bernaldiz et al. reported a good correlation of the mf-ERG responses with the morphological types of DME, at baseline and after treatment with ranibizumab over a period of 1 year [116]. The response density was increased in all eyes after the injection, with best responses seen in eyes with spongiform edema, well-preserved EZ and ELM at baseline, and absence of hard exudates. The improvements in the response density of P1 wave was significantly correlated with the baseline preserved EZ and ELM in R1 and R2 rings, corresponding to the foveal region (up to 5°). The resolution of macular thickness correlated significantly with the improvements in response density in R1.

The Lucentis in Diabetic Macular Edema: A Treatment Evaluation (LUCIDATE) study was designed as a randomized trial to assess the structural and functional outcomes of ranibizumab versus laser treatment in eyes with DME [117]. The retinal sensitivity on microperimetry showed a good improvement in the central 4° (the region mainly affected by macular edema), and smaller improvements in the central 12° of macula. Ranibizumab-treated eyes also showed an improvement in both protan and tritan axis of color contrast over 48 weeks. The pattern ERG data showed a mild decline in the P50 component (amplitudes and implicit times) at 12 and 24 weeks, but stabilization by 48 weeks in ranibizumab-treated group as compared to a consistent decline in the laser group. 34% of eyes in the ranibizumab-treated group and 18% of the laser group showed mild to moderate improvements in mf-ERG amplitudes. These results suggested that the functional improvements tend to stabilize over time when treated with long-term anti-VEGF therapy.

These studies suggest that the functional improvement in eyes with DME treated with anti-VEGF therapy are dependent upon the structural alterations and are seen mainly in the central foveal region. Of note, the decrease in retinal sensitivity patterns in eyes with DME have been known to corelate with the disruption of EZ in the same way as visual acuity does [45, 118].

In summary, advances in diagnostic technologies, in particular OCT and OCTA, have facilitated the development of an extensive portfolio of biomarkers to better characterize and monitor patients in clinical trials of DME. These novel biomarkers and endpoints are of particular importance in this era of pharmacotherapeutics and personalized medicine.

Acknowledgement We would like to acknowledge the contributions made by Dr. Giulia Corradetti, a research fellow affiliated with the Doheny Eye Institute and the Department of Ophthalmology, David Geffen School of Medicine at UCLA, who provided invaluable insights for some important aspects of this chapter.

Financial Disclosures AV: None;

YA: None;

SRS: Consultant: Amgen, Allergan, Genentech/Roche, Iveric, Oxurion, Novartis, Regeneron, Bayer, 4DMT, Centervue, Heidelberg, Optos, Merck, Apellis, Pfizer, Biogen, Boerhinger Ingelheim.

Speaker Fees: Nidek, Novartis; Research support: Carl Zeiss Meditec.

Research Instruments: Nidek, Topcon, Heidelberg, Carl Zeiss Meditec, Optos, Centervue.

References

1. Johnson MW. Etiology and treatment of macular edema. Am J Ophthalmol. 2009;147(1):11–21.e1.
2. Ciulla TA, Amador AG, Zinman B. Diabetic retinopathy and diabetic macular edema: pathophysiology, screening, and novel therapies. Diabetes Care. 2003;26(9):2653–64.
3. Albert D, Miller J, Azar D, Young LH. Albert and Jakobiec's principles and practice of ophthalmology, vol. 2. 3rd ed. North York, ON: Saunders Elsevier; 2008. p. 1793–996.
4. Das A, McGuire PG, Rangasamy S. Diabetic macular edema: pathophysiology and novel therapeutic targets. Ophthalmology. 2015;122(7):1375–94.
5. Early Treatment Diabetic Retinopathy Study research group. Photocoagulation for diabetic macular edema. Early treatment diabetic retinopathy study report number 1. Arch Ophthalmol. 1985;103(12):1796–806.
6. Michaelides M, Kaines A, Hamilton RD, et al. A prospective randomized trial of intravitreal bevacizumab or laser therapy in the management of diabetic macular edema (BOLT study) 12-month data: report 2. Ophthalmology. 2010;117(6):1078–1086.e2.
7. Elman MJ, Aiello LP, Beck RW, et al. Randomized trial evaluating ranibizumab plus prompt or deferred laser or triamcinolone plus prompt laser for diabetic macular edema. Ophthalmology. 2010;117(6):1064–1077.e35.
8. Diabetic Retinopathy Clinical Research Network. Relationship between optical coherence tomography-measured central retinal thickness and visual acuity in diabetic macular edema. Ophthalmology. 2007;114(3):525–36.
9. Browning DJ, Stewart MW, Lee C. Diabetic macular edema: evidence-based management. Indian J Ophthalmol. 2018;66(12):1736–50.
10. Verma LK, Vivek MB, Kumar A, et al. A prospective controlled trial to evaluate the adjunctive role of posterior subtenon triamcinolone in the treatment of diffuse diabetic macular edema. J Ocul Pharmacol Ther. 2004;20(4):277–84.
11. Brown JC, Solomon SD, Bressler SB, et al. Detection of diabetic foveal edema: contact lens biomicroscopy compared with optical coherence tomography. Arch Ophthalmol. 2004;122(3):330–5.
12. Bressler NM, Varma R, Doan QV, et al. Underuse of the health care system by persons with diabetes mellitus and diabetic macular edema in the United States. JAMA Ophthalmol. 2014;132(2):168–73.
13. Early Treatment Diabetic Retinopathy Study Research Group. Early treatment diabetic retinopathy study design and baseline patient characteristics: ETDRS report number 7. Ophthalmology. 1991;98(5 suppl):741–56.
14. American Society of Retina Specialists. Preferences and trends survey 2014. Chicago, IL: American Society of Retina Specialists; 2014.
15. Brown DM, Nguyen QD, Marcus DM, RIDE and RISE Research Group, et al. Long-term outcomes of ranibizumab therapy for diabetic macular edema: the 36-month results from two phase III trials: RISE and RIDE. Ophthalmology. 2013;120(10):2013–22.
16. Mitchell P, Bandello F, Schmidt-Erfurth U, et al. The RESTORE study: ranibizumab monotherapy or combined with laser versus laser monotherapy for diabetic macular edema. Ophthalmology. 2011;118(4):615–25.
17. Nguyen QD, Brown DM, Marcus DM, et al. Ranibizumab for diabetic macular edema: results from 2 phase III randomized trials: RISE and RIDE. Ophthalmology. 2012;119(4):789–801.
18. Brown DM, Schmidt-Erfurth U, Do DV, et al. Intravitreal aflibercept for diabetic macular edema: 100-week results from the VISTA and VIVID studies. Ophthalmology. 2015;122(10):2044–52.

19. American Society of Retina Specialists. Preferences and trends survey 2018. Chicago, IL: American Society of Retina Specialists; 2018.
20. Evans S. When and how can endpoints be changed after initiation of a randomized clinical trial? PLoS Clin Trials. 2007;2(4):e18.
21. De Gruttola VG, Clax P, DeMets DL, et al. Considerations in the evaluation of surrogate endpoints in clinical trials: summary of a National Institutes of Health workshop. Control Clin Trials. 2001;22(5):485–502.
22. Macugen Diabetic Retinopathy Study Group. A phase II randomized double-masked trial of pegaptanib, an anti-vascular endothelial growth factor aptamer, for diabetic macular edema. Ophthalmology. 2005;112(10):1747–57.
23. Diabetic Retinopathy Clinical Research Network. A phase II randomized clinical trial of intravitreal bevacizumab for diabetic macular edema. Ophthalmology. 2007;114(10):1860–7.
24. Nguyen QD, Shah SM, Heier JS, et al. Primary end point (six months) results of the ranibizumab for edema of the macula in diabetes (READ-2) study. Ophthalmology. 2009;116(11):2175–81.
25. Nguyen QD, Shah SM, Khwaja AA, et al. Two-year outcomes of the ranibizumab for edema of the mAcula in diabetes (READ-2) study. Ophthalmology. 2010;117(11):2146–51.
26. Massin P, Bandello F, Garweg JG, et al. Safety and efficacy of ranibizumab in diabetic macular edema (RESOLVE study): a 12-month, randomized, controlled, double-masked, multicenter phase II study. Diabetes Care. 2010;33(11):2399–405.
27. Sultan MB, Zhou D, Loftus J, et al. A phase 2/3, multicenter, randomized, double-masked, 2-year trial of pegaptanib sodium for the treatment of diabetic macular edema. Ophthalmology. 2011;118(6):1107–18.
28. Diabetic Retinopathy Clinical Research Network. Randomized trial evaluating short-term effects of intravitreal ranibizumab or triamcinolone acetonide on macular edema after focal/grid laser for diabetic macular edema in eyes also receiving panretinal photocoagulation. Retina. 2011;31(6):1009–27.
29. Do DV, Schmidt-Erfurth U, Gonzalez VH, et al. The DA VINCI study: phase 2 primary results of VEGF trap-eye in patients with diabetic macular edema. Ophthalmology. 2011;118(9):1819–26.
30. Elman MJ, Qin H, Aiello LP, et al. Intravitreal ranibizumab for diabetic macular edema with prompt versus deferred laser treatment: three-year randomized trial results. Ophthalmology. 2012;119(11):2312–8.
31. Rajendram R, Fraser-Bell S, Kaines A, et al. A 2-year prospective randomized controlled trial of intravitreal bevacizumab or laser therapy (BOLT) in the management of diabetic macular edema: 24-month data: report 3. Arch Ophthalmol. 2012;130(8):972–9.
32. Wells JA, Glassman AR, Ayala AR, et al. Aflibercept, bevacizumab, or ranibizumab for diabetic macular edema. N Engl J Med. 2015;372(13):1193–203.
33. Bressler SB, Almukhtar T, Bhorade A, et al. Repeated intravitreous ranibizumab injections for diabetic macular edema and the risk of sustained elevation of intraocular pressure or the need for ocular hypotensive treatment. JAMA Ophthalmol. 2015;133(5):589–97.
34. Bressler SB, Ayala AR, Bressler NM, et al. Diabetic retinopathy clinical research network. Persistent macular thickening after ranibizumab treatment for diabetic macular edema with vision impairment. JAMA Ophthalmol. 2016;134(3):278–85.
35. Bressler NM, Beaulieu WT, Glassman AR, et al. Persistent macular thickening following intravitreous aflibercept, bevacizumab, or ranibizumab for central-involved diabetic macular edema with vision impairment: a secondary analysis of a randomized clinical trial. JAMA Ophthalmol. 2018;136(3):257–69.
36. Baker CW, Glassman AR, Beaulieu WT, et al. Effect of initial management with aflibercept vs laser photocoagulation vs observation on vision loss among patients with diabetic macular edema involving the center of the macula and good visual acuity: a randomized clinical trial. JAMA Ophthalmol. 2019;329(19):1880–94.
37. Glassman AR, Wells JA III, Josic K, et al. Five-year outcomes after initial aflibercept, bevacizumab, or ranibizumab treatment for diabetic macular edema (protocol T extension study). Ophthalmology. 2020;127(9):1201–10.
38. Kniestedt C, Stamper RL. Visual acuity and its measurement. Ophthalmol Clin North Am. 2003;16(2):155–70.
39. Ranibizumab (Lucentis): visual impairment due to choroidal neovascularization secondary to pathologic myopia [Internet]. Ottawa (ON): Canadian Agency for Drugs and Technologies in Health; 2015. Appendix 4, validity of outcome measures. https://www.ncbi.nlm.nih.gov/books/NBK349531.
40. Holladay JT, Prager TC. Snellen equivalent for the bailey-lovie acuity chart. Arch Ophthalmol. 1989;107(7):955.
41. Gangnon RE, Davis MD, Hubbard LD, et al. A severity scale for diabetic macular edema developed from ETDRS data. Invest Ophthalmol Vis Sci. 2008;49(11):5041–7.
42. Blumenkranz MS, Haller JA, Kuppermann BD, et al. Correlation of visual acuity and macular thickness measured by optical coherence tomography in patients with persistent macular edema. Retina. 2010;30(7):1090–4.
43. Forooghian F, Stetson PF, Meyer SA, et al. Relationship between photoreceptor outer segment length and visual acuity in diabetic macular edema. Retina. 2010;30(1):63–70.
44. Otani T, Yamaguchi Y, Kishi S. Correlation between visual acuity and foveal microstructural changes in diabetic macular edema. Retina. 2010;30(5):774–80.
45. Maheshwary AS, Oster SF, Yuson RM, et al. The association between disruption of the photoreceptor inner segment-outer segment junction and visual acuity in diabetic macular edema. Am J Ophthalmol. 2010;150(1):63–7.e1.
46. Alasil T, Keane PA, Updike JF, et al. Relationship between optical coherence tomography retinal parameters and visual acuity in diabetic macular edema. Ophthalmology. 2010;117(12):2379–86.
47. Chan A, Duker JS. A standardized method for reporting changes in macular thickening using optical coherence tomography. Arch Ophthalmol. 2005;123(7):939–43.
48. You QS, Tsuboi K, Guo Y, et al. Comparison of central macular fluid volume with central subfield thickness in patients with diabetic macular edema using optical coherence tomography angiography. JAMA Ophthalmol. 2021;139(7):734–41.
49. Patel JI, Hykin PG, Schadt M, et al. Pars plana vitrectomy for diabetic macular oedema: OCT and functional correlations. Eye (Lond). 2006;20(6):674–80.
50. Browning DJ, Glassman AR, Aiello LP, et al. Diabetic retinopathy clinical research network. Optical coherence tomography measurements and analysis methods in optical coherence tomography studies of diabetic macular edema. Ophthalmology. 2008;115(8):1366–71, 1371.e1.
51. Davis MD, Bressler SB, Aiello LP, et al. Diabetic Retinopathy Clinical Research Network Study Group. Comparison of time-domain OCT and fundus photographic assessments of retinal thickening in eyes with diabetic macular edema. Invest Ophthalmol Vis Sci. 2008;49(5):1745–52.
52. Nussenblatt RB, Kaufman SC, Palestine AG, Davis MD, Ferris FL III. Macular thickening and visual acuity: measurement in patients with cystoid macular edema. Ophthalmology. 1987;94(9):1134–9.
53. Stark WJ Jr, Maumenee AE, Fagadau W, et al. Cystoid macular edema in pseudophakia. Surv Ophthalmol. 1984;28:442–51.
54. Nittala MG, Konduru R, Ruiz-Garcia H, Sadda SR. Effect of OCT volume scan density on thickness measurements in diabetic macular edema. Eye. 2011;25(10):1347–55.
55. Nittala MG, Velaga SB, Hu Z, Sadda SR. Relationship between dry retinal volume and visual acuity in diabetic macular edema. Ophthalmic Surg Lasers Imaging Retina. 2018;49(7):510–5.

56. Bressler SB, Odia I, Maguire MG, et al. Factors associated with visual acuity and central subfield thickness changes when treating diabetic macular edema with anti-vascular endothelial growth factor therapy: an exploratory analysis of the protocol T randomized clinical trial. JAMA Ophthalmol. 2019;137(4):382–9.
57. Ou WC, Brown DM, Payne JF, Wykoff CC. Relationship between visual acuity and retinal thickness during anti-vascular endothelial growth factor therapy for retinal diseases. Am J Ophthalmol. 2017;180:8–17.
58. Eliwa TF, Hussein MA, Zaki MA, Raslan OA. Outer retinal layer thickness as good visual predictor in patients with diabetic macular edema. Retina. 2018;38(4):805–11.
59. Wong RL, Lee JW, Yau GS, Wong IY. Relationship between outer retinal layers thickness and visual acuity in diabetic macular edema. Biomed Res Int. 2015;2015:981471.
60. Sun JK, Lin MM, Lammer J, et al. Disorganization of the retinal inner layers as a predictor of visual acuity in eyes with center-involved diabetic macular edema. JAMA Ophthalmol. 2014;132(11):1309–16.
61. Fickweiler W, Schauwvlieghe AM, Schlingemann RO, et al. Predictive value of optical coherence tomographic features in the bevacizumab and ranibizumab in patients with diabetic macular edema (BRDME) study. Retina. 2018;38(4):812–9.
62. Das R, Spence G, Hogg RE, Stevenson M, Chakravarthy U. Disorganization of inner retina and outer retinal morphology in diabetic macular edema. JAMA Ophthalmol. 2018;136(2):202–8.
63. Tang Z, Chan MY, Leung WY, et al. Assessment of retinal neurodegeneration with spectral-domain optical coherence tomography: a systematic review and meta-analysis. Eye. 2021;35(5):1317–25.
64. De Faria JL, Russ H, Costa VP. Retinal nerve fibre layer loss in patients with type 1 diabetes mellitus without retinopathy. Br J Ophthalmol. 2002;86(7):725–8.
65. Ozdek S, Lonneville YH, Onol M, Yetkin I, Hasanreisoğlu BB. Assessment of nerve fiber layer in diabetic patients with scanning laser polarimetry. Eye. 2002;16(6):761–5.
66. Verma A, Rani PK, Raman R, et al. Is neuronal dysfunction an early sign of diabetic retinopathy? Microperimetry and spectral domain optical coherence tomography (SD-OCT) study in individuals with diabetes, but no diabetic retinopathy. Eye. 2009;23(9):1824–30.
67. Verma A, Raman R, Vaitheeswaran K, et al. Does neuronal damage precede vascular damage in subjects with type 2 diabetes mellitus and having no clinical diabetic retinopathy? Ophthalmic Res. 2012;47(4):202–7.
68. Huang J, Li Y, Chen Y, et al. Multifocal electroretinogram can detect the abnormal retinal change in early stage of type2 DM patients without apparent diabetic retinopathy. J Diabetes Res. 2021;2021:1.
69. Kim YH, Yun C, Kim JT, et al. The correlation between retinal sensitivity assessed by microperimetry and contrast sensitivity in diabetic macular oedema. Br J Ophthalmol. 2014;98(12):1618–24.
70. Sokol S, Moskowitz A, Skarf B, et al. Contrast sensitivity in diabetics with and without background retinopathy. Arch Ophthalmol. 1985;103(1):51–4.
71. Guyon B, Elphege E, Flores M, et al. Retinal reflectivity measurement for cone impairment estimation and visual assessment after diabetic macular edema resolution (RECOVER-DME). Invest Ophthalmol Vis Sci. 2017;58(14):6241–7.
72. Kostanyan T, Wollstein G, Schuman JS. New developments in optical coherence tomography. Curr Opin Ophthalmol. 2015;26(2):110–5.
73. Laishram M, Srikanth K, Rajalakshmi AR, Nagarajan S, Ezhumalai G. Microperimetry—a new tool for assessing retinal sensitivity in macular diseases. J Clin Diagn Res. 2017;11(7):NC08–11.
74. Bolz M, Ritter M, Schneider M, et al. A systematic correlation of angiography and high-resolution optical coherence tomography in diabetic macular edema. Ophthalmology. 2009;116(1):66–72.
75. Soliman W, Sander B, Jorgensen TM. Enhanced optical coherence patterns of diabetic macular oedema and their correlation with the pathophysiology. Acta Ophthalmol Scand. 2007;85(6):613–7.
76. Bolz M, Schmidt-Erfurth U, Deák G, et al. Optical coherence tomographic hyperreflective foci: a morphologic sign of lipid extravasation in diabetic macular edema. Ophthalmology. 2009;116(5):914–20.
77. Deák GG, Bolz M, Ritter M, et al. A systematic correlation between morphology and functional alterations in diabetic macular edema. Invest Ophthalmol Vis Sci. 2010;51(12):6710–4.
78. Radwan SH, Soliman AZ, Tokarev J, et al. Association of disorganization of retinal inner layers with vision after resolution of center-involved diabetic macular edema. JAMA Ophthalmol. 2015;133(7):820–5.
79. Uji A, Murakami T, Nishijima K, et al. Association between hyperreflective foci in the outer retina, status of photoreceptor layer, and visual acuity in diabetic macular edema. Am J Ophthalmol. 2012;153(4):710–7.
80. Framme C, Schweizer P, Imesch M, Wolf S, Wolf-Schnurrbusch U. Behavior of SD-OCT-detected hyperreflective foci in the retina of anti-VEGF-treated patients with diabetic macular edema. Invest Ophthalmol Vis Sci. 2012;53(9):5814–8.
81. Pemp B, Deák G, Prager S, et al. Distribution of intraretinal exudates in diabetic macular edema during anti-vascular endothelial growth factor therapy observed by spectral domain optical coherence tomography and fundus photography. Retina. 2014;34(12):2407–15.
82. Kang JW, Chung H, Chan KH. Correlation of optical coherence tomographic hyperreflective foci with visual outcomes in different patterns of diabetic macular edema. Retina. 2016;36(9):1630–9.
83. Sophie R, Lu N, Campochiaro PA. Predictors of functional and anatomic outcomes in patients with diabetic macular edema treated with ranibizumab. Ophthalmology. 2015;122(7):1395–401.
84. Ota M, Nishijima K, Sakamoto A, et al. Optical coherence tomographic evaluation of foveal hard exudates in patients with diabetic maculopathy accompanying macular detachment. Ophthalmology. 2010;117(10):1996–2002.
85. Otani T, Kishi S. Tomographic findings of foveal hard exudates in diabetic macular edema. Am J Ophthalmol. 2001;131(1):50–4.
86. Yoshitake T, Murakami T, Suzuma K, e al. Hyperreflective foci in the outer retinal layers as a predictor of the functional efficacy of ranibizumab for diabetic macular edema. Sci Rep. 2020;10(1):1–8.
87. Mori Y, Suzuma K, Uji A, et al. Restoration of foveal photoreceptors after intravitreal ranibizumab injections for diabetic macular edema. Sci Rep. 2016;6(1):1–1.
88. Chung YR, Kim YH, Ha SJ, et al. Role of inflammation in classification of diabetic macular edema by optical coherence tomography. J Diabetes Res. 2019;2019:8164250.
89. Aggarwal K, Agarwal A, Afridi R, et al. Visual outcome of patients in Ranibizumab for edema of the mAcula in diabetes (READ-3) study based on the characteristics of edema on optical coherence tomography. Invest Ophthalmol Vis Sci. 2016;57(12):2089.
90. Korobelnik JF, Lu C, Katz TA, et al. Effect of baseline subretinal fluid on treatment outcomes in VIVID-DME and VISTA-DME studies. Ophthalmol Retina. 2019;3(8):663–9.
91. Seo KH, Yu SY, Kim M, Kwak HW. Visual and morphologic outcomes of intravitreal ranibizumab for diabetic macular edema based on optical coherence tomography patterns. Retina. 2016;36(3):588–95.
92. Giocanti-Aurégan A, Hrarat L, Qu LM, et al. Functional and anatomical outcomes in patients with serous retinal detachment in dia-

betic macular edema treated with ranibizumab. Invest Ophthalmol Vis Sci. 2017;58(2):797–800.
93. Lee H, Jang H, Choi YA, Kim HC, Chung H. Association between soluble CD14 in the aqueous humor and hyperreflective foci on optical coherence tomography in patients with diabetic macular edema. Invest Ophthalmol Vis Sci. 2018;59(2):715–21.
94. Midena E, Pilotto E, Bini S. Hyperreflective intraretinal foci as an OCT biomarker of retinal inflammation in diabetic macular edema. Invest Ophthalmol Vis Sci. 2018;59(13):5366.
95. Rübsam A, Wernecke L, Rau S, et al. Behavior of SD-OCT detectable hyperreflective foci in diabetic macular edema patients after therapy with anti-VEGF agents and dexamethasone implants. J Diabetes Res. 2021;2021:8820216.
96. Chatziralli IP, Sergentanis TN, Sivaprasad S. Hyperreflective foci as an independent visual outcome predictor in macular edema due to retinal vascular diseases treated with intravitreal dexamethasone or ranibizumab. Retina. 2016;36(12):2319–28.
97. Vujosevic S, Bini S, Torresin T, et al. Hyperreflective retinal spots in normal and diabetic eyes: B-scan and en face spectral domain optical coherence tomography evaluation. Retina. 2017;37(6):1092–103.
98. Kim KT, Kim DY, Chae JB. Association between hyperreflective foci on spectral-domain optical coherence tomography and early recurrence of diabetic macular edema after intravitreal dexamethasone implantation. J Ophthalmol. 2019;2019:3459164.
99. Fine BS, Brucker AJ. Macular edema and cystoid macular edema. Am J Ophthalmol. 1981;92(4):466–81.
100. Yanoff M, Fine BS, Brucker AJ, Eagle RC Jr. Pathology of human cystoid macular edema. Surv Ophthalmol. 1984;28:505–11.
101. Reznicek L, Cserhati S, Seidensticker F, et al. Functional and morphological changes in diabetic macular edema over the course of anti-vascular endothelial growth factor treatment. Acta Ophthalmol. 2013;91(7):e529–36.
102. Murakami T, Nishijima K, Akagi T, et al. Optical coherence tomographic reflectivity of photoreceptors beneath cystoid spaces in diabetic macular edema. Invest Ophthalmol Vis Sci. 2012;53(3):1506–11.
103. Liang MC, Vora RA, Duker JS, Reichel E. Solid-appearing retinal cysts in diabetic macular edema: a novel optical coherence tomography finding. Retin Cases Brief Rep. 2013;7(3):255–8.
104. Kashani AH, Green KM, Kwon J, et al. Suspended scattering particles in motion: a novel feature of OCT angiography in exudative maculopathies. Ophthalmol Retina. 2018;2(7):694–702.
105. Al Faran A, Mousa A, Al Shamsi H, Al Gaeed A, Ghazi NG. Spectral domain optical coherence tomography predictors of visual outcome in diabetic cystoid macular edema after bevacizumab injection. Retina. 2014;34(6):1208–15.
106. Pelosini L, Hull CC, Boyce JF, et al. Optical coherence tomography may be used to predict visual acuity in patients with macular edema. Invest Ophthalmol Vis Sci. 2011;52(5):2741–8.
107. Moein HR, Novais EA, Rebhun CB, et al. Optical coherence tomography angiography to detect macular capillary ischemia in patients with inner retinal changes after resolved diabetic macular edema. Retina. 2018;38(12):2277–84.
108. Hsieh YT, Alam MN, Le D, et al. OCT angiography biomarkers for predicting visual outcomes after ranibizumab treatment for diabetic macular edema. Ophthalmol Retina. 2019;3(10):826–34.
109. AttaAllah HR, Mohamed AAM, Ali MA. Macular vessels density in diabetic retinopathy: quantitative assessment using optical coherence tomography angiography. Int Ophthalmol. 2019;39(8):1845–59.
110. Tang FY, Chan EO, Sun Z, et al. Clinically relevant factors associated with quantitative optical coherence tomography angiography metrics in deep capillary plexus in patients with diabetes. Eye Vis (Lond). 2020;7(1):1–11.
111. Ghirlanda G, Di Leo MA, Caputo S, Cercone S, Greco AV. From functional to microvascular abnormalities in early diabetic retinopathy. Diabetes Metab Rev. 1997;13(1):15–35.
112. Barber AJ. A new view of diabetic retinopathy: a neurodegenerative disease of the eye. Prog Neuropsychopharmacol Biol Psychiatry. 2003;27(2):283–90.
113. Arden GB, Jyothi S, Hogg CH, Lee YF, Sivaprasad S. Regression of early diabetic macular oedema is associated with prevention of dark adaptation. Eye. 2011;25(12):1546–54.
114. Terauchi G, Shinoda K, Sakai H, et al. Retinal function determined by flicker ERGs before and soon after intravitreal injection of anti-VEGF agents. BMC Ophthalmol. 2019;19(1):1–9.
115. Kozak I, Centeno J. The effect of anti-VEGF injection loading dose in diabetic macular edema as measured by hand-held ERG system. Invest Ophthalmol Vis Sci. 2021;62(8):603.
116. Baget-Bernaldiz M, Romero-Aroca P, Bautista-Perez A, Mercado J. Multifocal electroretinography changes at the 1-year follow-up in a cohort of diabetic macular edema patients treated with ranibizumab. Doc Ophthalmol. 2017;135(2):85–96.
117. Comyn O, Sivaprasad S, Peto T, et al. A randomized trial to assess functional and structural effects of ranibizumab versus laser in diabetic macular edema (the LUCIDATE study). Am J Ophthalmol. 2014;157(5):960–70.
118. Yohannan J, Bittencourt M, Sepah YJ, et al. Association of retinal sensitivity to integrity of photoreceptor inner/outer segment junction in patients with diabetic macular edema. Ophthalmology. 2013;120(6):1254–61.

Nutrient Supplementation in Diabetic Macular Edema

17

Malvika Singh, Akshay Mohan, Anupriya Chaubey, and Sandeep Saxena

17.1 Introduction

A report by International Diabetes Federation Atlas stated that in 2019 that diabetes mellitus (DM) affects 463 million people around the globe. It is estimated that this global burden will reach 578 million by 2030 and about 700 million by 2045. Majority of DM cases, estimated at 80–95% of the total diabetic population, are contributed by type-2 diabetes.

The prevalence rate of diabetic retinopathy (DR) in patients with type 2 DM in India is reported to increase from 12% to 37%. In 2019, In India, it is estimated that nearly 77 million people are affected by DM ranking India as second in the world among the number of people with diabetes [1]. As the life expectancy of people is increasing, along with the growing population, the burden of disease in India is presently facing an uncertain future.

The pathophysiology of vision loss in DR is an intricate process. A decrease in visual acuity (VA) in the spectrum of DR can be due to severe NPDR (NPDR), diabetic macular edema (DME), and retinal neovascularization. Several studies have been conducted to investigate the risk factors associated with DR and to recognize both modifiable and non-modifiable risk factors for the presence and severity of DR [2, 3].

The basis for prevention of onset of DR and its progression to advanced stages can be done by identification of modifiable risk factors and their control.

Modifiable risk factors include the blood glucose level, blood pressure, serum lipids, obesity, alcohol, and smoking. The early recognition and treatment of these modifiable risk factors such as hyperglycemia and hypertension have played a major role in halting or decelerating the prevention and progression of DR spectrum of diseases. It has paved way for preventive approach in the treatment of disease in patients who are at high risk of developing and progression of DR. Understanding the role of nutrition is key for modifying and augmenting treatment, which is related to both supplementation as well as counseling, for those suffering from DME.

M. Singh (✉) · A. Mohan · A. Chaubey · S. Saxena
Department of Ophthalmology, King George's Medical University, Lucknow, India

17.2 Macronutrients

17.2.1 Carbohydrates

Pathogenesis of DME and DR are centered around the process of hyperglycemia. Hyperglycemia, at a point in time, is quantified by increased blood or serum levels of glucose. Long-term glycemic control is indicated by blood levels of glycosylated hemoglobin (HbA1c). A diet with foods containing high glycemic indices are associated with impaired blood glucose control and leads to an increase in predisposition towards DR and DME. Risk of DR incidence and progression may be increased by a high total caloric intake [4]. This agrees with clinical and experimental evidence which suggests that a higher caloric intake will increase the metabolic burden and oxidative stress in diabetic persons, which may cause the oxidative stress-susceptible retina to develop DR [5, 6].

17.2.2 Fats

Carnitine is vital for the transport of long chain fatty acids into mitochondria for β-oxidation. Studies have shown that there is an increased levels of an acylcarnitine and dehydroxycarnitine, in patients with DR compared with patients with DM who do not have DR. However, studies are conflicting with respect to plasma carnitine in patients of type 2 DM. Conclusive evidence is lacking whether carnitine levels are associated with complications of diabetes or not. One study has demonstrated that carnitine metabolites are elevated in both PDR and age-related macular degeneration, which suggests that changes in fatty acid metabolism are related to neovascularization or ischemia [7]. Experimental

S. Saxena et al. (eds.), *Diabetic Macular Edema*, https://doi.org/10.1007/978-981-19-7307-9_17

studies have suggested polyunsaturated fatty acids (PUFA) intake to be protective against DR [8, 9] through anti-inflammatory and antiangiogenic properties [10], however, current evidence remains inconclusive on this subject [4, 11].

17.2.3 Proteins and Co-Factors

17.2.3.1 Amino-Levulinic Acid

5-aminolevulinic acid (ALA) is an endogenous non-proteinogenic amino acid. It is the first compound in the porphyrin synthesis pathway. Administration of ALA in diabetic rats has been shown to ameliorate nuclear translocation factor κB (NF-κB) activation, scavenging of reactive oxygen species (ROS), decreasing level of vascular endothelial growth factor (VEGF) in the retina, and protection of the retina against ischemic injury. In an experimental study done on rats, ALA has been shown to protect the mitochondria against oxidative damage by preventing dysfunction of the mitochondria, preventing apoptosis of capillary cells present in the retina, and development of DR [12]. In addition, it has been seen that ALA has beneficial effects on contrast sensitivity in patients with DM [13].

17.2.3.2 Coenzyme Q10

Coenzyme Q10 is a fat soluble antioxidant also known as ubiquinone. By virtue of its electron carrying property, it has a key role in oxidative phosphorylation of mitochondria [14]. Several studies have demonstrated its beneficial effects on the endothelial function in patients with type 2 DM, patients with cardiovascular diseases and in animal models of diabetic nephropathy [15]. Coenzyme Q10 can reduce oxidative stress due to its influence on the mitochondrial respiratory chain or by recoupling endothelial nitric oxide synthase. Coenzyme Q10 supplementation with or without vitamin E supplementation may be associated with an improvement in visual acuity and central macular thickness in patients with NPDR [16].

17.2.3.3 Lipoic Acid (LA, Alpha Lipoic Acid, Thioctic Acid)

Lipoic acid is another important cofactor for mitochondrial metabolism. LA is required to generate acetyl Co-A, the key compound of Krebs cycle, the core of the energy-generating aerobic metabolism of cells [17]. LA has several other roles in the cell, namely, scavenging of ROS, enhancing the effects of endogenous antioxidant compounds such as vitamin C, E, and glutathione, by recycling. LA supplementation has been shown to increase available glutathione [18]. LA administration has been shown to have protect the retinal cells, particularly the ganglion cells and pigment epithelial cells from ischemia and apoptosis [19]. LA has also been shown to decrease hyperglycemia and hyperglycemic vascular endothelial dysfunction in patients with type 2 DM [20]. In animal models of DR, it has been shown to reduce VEGF expression and protect the retinal ganglion cells and capillaries VEGF induced damage [12]. It has also been shown that supplementation of LA was associated with increased contrast sensitivity in patients with DM [13]. LA appears to be safe and well-tolerated at 600 mg/day as a dietary supplement.

17.2.3.4 *N*-Acetyl Cysteine

N-Acetyl Cysteine (NAC) is a thiol antioxidant and a precursor to glutathione [21]. Glutathione is neuroprotective and retina protective [22]. The availability of cysteine is often the rate limiter for glutathione synthesis, and thus supplementation of NAC increases the net levels of glutathione, which is useful in various disease states which are characterized by increased oxidative stress and ischemia [23]. In animal models of DR, it has been shown that long-term administration of NAC reduces the levels of ROS in the retinal mitochondria, and decreases the expression of VEGF and PDR [24]. NAC restores the tight junctions and thus reduces vascular leakage [25]. Ischemia induced apoptosis of ganglion cells, photoreceptor cells and retinal pigment epithelial (RPE) cell, are reduced when NAC is present [26]. It has also been shown to reduce the expression of VEGF, icariin-1, free radical species, ischemia, and thus improve the structural changes of DR [22]. Animal models also suggest that it may have a role in decreasing retinal detachment in PDR [27]. Therefore, NAC is beneficial at the cellular level to prevent the apoptosis of retinal neuron and photoreceptor cells.

17.2.3.5 Trimethylglycine

Trimethylglycine (TMG, Betaine) is a trimethylated dietary amino acid derivative which is primarily found in sugar beets. Betaine is not included as a vitamin as it can be synthesized in the mitochondria in small amounts by methylating choline. Therefore, betaine has no established RDA, but choline has an RDA. Diets across the world are frequently low in both [28, 29]. Betaine works with methylfolate to keep serum homocysteine low and methionine optimal levels [30]. Betaine is used as a secondary treatment for elevated homocysteine levels in patients who do not respond adequately to B6, B9, and B12 supplementation [31]. The human average dietary intake of betaine is 500–2000 mg/day.

17.2.3.6 Arginine

The association between arginine metabolism and DR is complex. Arginine is a key molecule in several overlapping pathways with several metabolic end products. In the urea cycle, arginine is cleaved by arginase to form ornithine and urea. Ornithine is then converted back to arginine through the intermediate citrulline, completing the cycle.

Alternatively, ornithine may also be metabolized to proline through the intermediate glutamic γ-semialdehyde [32]. In patients with PDR, increased levels of ornithine, citrulline, proline, and arginine have been found in the vitreous, [33]. In several animal models of DR, retinal endothelial cells cultured in high glucose found elevated arginase activity, which also implicates that derangement in the arginine metabolism may be a mediator of DR [34].

Arginine also has a role as a substrate for NO synthase enzyme, which catalyzes a reaction that produces NO and citrulline. NO is a vasodilator that plays a critical role in maintenance of a healthy vascular endothelium. This NO synthase enzyme is inhibited by asymmetric dimethylarginine (ADMA), which has been reported to be elevated in the plasma, serum, and aqueous humor [35, 36] of DR patients. This suggests that dysregulations in the arginine metabolism may be linked through urea cycle metabolites, as well as through ADMA and NO.

17.2.3.7 Homocysteine

Homocysteine has been discussed further in the chapter along with folate and cobalamine.

17.3 Micronutrients

17.3.1 Vitamins

17.3.1.1 Vitamin A

Carotenoids are biosynthesized by linkage of two C20 geranylgeranyl diphosphate molecules to make C40-based isoprenoids of the tetraterpene family [36]. Stahl and Sies have divided carotenoids into two groups: pro-vitamin A (e.g., α-carotene, β-carotene, and β-cryptoxanthin) and the non-pro-vitamin A compounds [37]. Jomova and Valko have divided carotenoids into three groups: carotenes, xanthophylls, and lycopenes [38].

β-carotene, α-carotene, lycopene, lutein, and cryptoxanthin are dietary carotenoids which have been found in human blood [39]. β-carotenes have greater pro-vitamin A potential as compared to α-carotene or β-cryptoxanthin because of the presence of a β-ionone ring linked to a chain of 11 carbons [40].

Lutein and zeaxanthin are the major macular xanthophylls present in the macula lutea which are derived from dietary sources, and mesozeaxanthin, another macular xanthophyll is synthesized from lutein in the retina [41]. These carotenoids are dipolar, terminally dihydroxylated carotenoids. The peak concentrations of these xanthophylls appear at the center of the fovea [42].

Carotenoids are able to accept electrons from ROS due to the presence of conjugated double bonds, they hence are able to neutralize these free radicals, isomerize and help in oxidation [43]. Light absorbing properties and chemical reactivity properties of carotenoids are attributed to the single bonds and alternating double bonds present in the nucleus of polyene chain that make a conjugated system which contains delocalized π-electrons. Different structural configurations and shapes are possible because of the various isomerism possible around the carbon double bonds and the possible rotations around the carbon single bonds in the polyene chain. Due to the steric hindrance between methyl groups, *cis* isomers are structurally more unstable as compared to the *trans* isomers. Carotenoids absorb light in the wavelength range of 400–500 nm of the spectrum, which promotes one of the conjugated double bond π-electrons to occupy the previously unoccupied π^* antibonding orbital [44].

Carotenoids have various therapeutic benefits in DR through multiple cellular and molecular pathways. Antioxidants such as ascorbate, tocopherol, and carotenoids are known to protect from oxidative damage [45]. Carotenoids have a role in the neutralization of free radicals, scavenging of ROS, modulation of gene expression, reduction of inflammation, and prevention of diabetes-related microvascular complications, which includes not only DR but also diabetic nephropathy, and neuropathy [46].

Macular pigments such as lutein, zeaxanthin and mesozeaxanthin also contribute to the protection of retinal tissues in DM due to their potent antioxidant and anti-inflammatory effects. It has been demonstrated that type 2 DM patients have lower levels of macular xanthophylls as compared to healthy controls [47]. Lutein supplementation has been known to prevent oxidative damage to the retina [48]. In an animal model of DR, long-term administration of lutein reduced inflammation, and retinal vascular damage [49]. Short-term lutein administration has also been shown to downregulate the production of ROS and upregulate the effect of superoxide dismutase enzyme, reducing the inflammation and protecting the retina from oxidative damage [50]. Several signaling pathways have been implicated in the carotenoid-mediated protection of the retina in DR, including VEGF, PKC, nuclear factor erythroid 2-related factor 2, and Rho/Rho-associated coiled-coil containing protein kinase. An in vitro study has shown that co-administration of lutein and zeaxanthin decreased VEGF-induced oxidative stress in the retinal endothelium [51]. Lutein has also been found to modulate the sirtuin-1 signaling pathway thus inhibiting premature senescence in RPE cells [52].

The recommended dietary intake level of carotenoids is 6–14 mg/day to reduce the risk of macular degeneration and cataract [53].

17.3.1.2 Vitamin B

B vitamins are a class of essential water-soluble cofactors that regulate key cellular metabolic processes in a number of pathways critical to all cells of the body. They have various homeostatic roles for intermediate metabolism, particularly the one carbon cycle, which is important for the maintenance of the healthy vascular endothelium, as well as for mitochondrial quenching of free radicals, conduction of white matter tract signaling, regulation of blood pressure, attention, memory, sleep, and mood. These are functions are critical functions for normal neural, vascular, and visual function [54].

In the human body, the retina has the highest metabolic activity and metabolic stress. The inner retina is highly vulnerable to damage cause by ischemia [55, 56].

Vitamin B1 (Thiamin) is a potent scavenger of free radicals that is involved in the regulation of intracellular glucose and prevention of the activation of the polyol pathway which is thought to induce DR in rats and humans [57, 58]. High levels of thiamin can protect the vascular endothelium from injury caused by advanced glycation end products [59, 60]. Supplementation of thiamin at high doses of 50–100 mg/day is safe and useful for vascular damage in DM and neuroprotection. Toxicity of thiamin is so low that no upper limit has been established. Thiamin supplementation is thus a useful low-risk low-cost supplementation in the treatment of DR [61].

Vitamin B2 (Riboflavin) is a flavin adenine dinucleotide which is essential for intermediate metabolic reactions, energy production, and normal mitochondrial function [62]. Riboflavin is an essential cofactor for the synthesis of L-methylfolate, which lowers homocysteine levels. Dietary supplementation with riboflavin increases L-methylfolate synthesis, lowering homocysteine levels and blood pressure [63]. In a murine model, it was found that riboflavin supplementation was associated with an increase in glucose uptake and amelioration of oxidative stress [64]. Riboflavin supplementation has also been shown to increase brain derived neurotrophic factor (BDNF) expression in a murine model [65]. BDNF is higher in prediabetics than diabetics, which suggests neuroprotective benefits of BDNF [66]. Optimal riboflavin dosages are not established for DR and toxicity is minimal as no upper limit is established that long-term treatment with 400 mg/day is safe and may be beneficial [67].

Vitamin B3 is also known as niacin. High dose supplementation of niacin may be involved in the causation or aggravation of DM. Dose of niacin that is used for lipid control is 1000–3000 mg/day, with uncertain benefit and an increased risk of insulin resistance and impairment of glucose tolerance, hepatic toxicity, and possible all-cause mortality [68]. There is an additional increased risk of cystoid macular edema with high dose niacin supplementation [69]. However, in an animal model of DM, niacin supplementation was associated with an increase in endothelial growth factors, promotion of sprouting, migration, and survival of endothelial cells and mediated vascular remodeling following occlusion of the middle cerebral artery [70]. Therefore, the recommended dietary allowances (RDA) for niacin should be strictly followed (14–30 mg/day) [71].

Vitamin B5 (Pantothenic Acid) is involved in fatty acid metabolism, particularly in the Kreb's cycle. It is abundant naturally in foods and does not usually require additional supplementation [72].

Vitamin B6 (Pyridoxal 5′ Phosphate, PLP, P5P) is a cofactor required for key metabolic processes, including one carbon cycle [73]. The National Health and Nutrition Examination Survey based on the US population suggested that inadequate serum B6 levels were present in 10–40% of subjects despite widespread use of vitamins [74]. When methyltetrahydrofolate receptor (MTHFR) polymorphisms are present, deficiencies in B6 increases serum homocysteine levels which is a risk factor for DR [75, 76]. Vitamin B6 deficiency contributes to the autoimmunity of pancreatic islet cells resulting in type I DM [77]. In a large cohort study of type 2 DM which monitored vitamin B6 intake and the development of DR found that lower intake of B6 was associated with an increased incidence of DR [78]. There are several forms of B6 of which the nature derived active form is P5P which is safe in recommended doses. Other forms such as pyridoxine, even in pharmacological doses, may induce peripheral neuropathy similar to B6 deficiency. Supplementation with B6 in P5P is safest and may reduce the risk of developing DM and DR [79].

Vitamin B7 (Biotin) Glucose kinase (GCK) activity is particularly reduced in type 2 DM, which correlates negatively with HbA1c levels [80]. Animal models show that biotin regulates GCK and that biotin supplementation improves postprandial glucose response by affecting GCK and PCK1 [81]. Biotin is safe and inexpensive, without an assigned upper limit and can be used in DM [82].

17.3.1.3 Vitamin B9, B12 and Homocysteine

Homocysteine is a biomarker for increased risk of complications of DM, since retinopathy, nephropathy, and cardiovascular disease have all been linked to high homocysteine levels. It has been suggested that a relatively small increase in the plasma homocysteine concentration, in the order of 1 μmol/L, may be a useful trigger for intensification of treatment of the major risk factors for diabetes complications (blood pressure, blood glucose, and blood lipids) to prevent a patient without DR, developing retinopathy. Timely identification of individuals at greater risk of the vascular complications of diabetes is crucial and it is preferable to have a high degree of caution and in the treatment of patients who have homocysteine levels in the upper limit of the normal range [83].

A study has demonstrated a correlation between increased serum levels of homocysteine and retinal nerve fiber layer thinning in the patients with DM. This study also found that increased serum levels of homocysteine correlated with an increased severity of retinopathy [84].

L-methylfolate is known to improve the ischemic consequences caused due to the reduced function polymorphisms of the MTHFR gene in patients with DM. MTHFR polymorphisms cause a decrease in tetrahydrofolate methylation, which results in decreased availability of L-methylfolate, methylcobalamin, and the elevation in the levels of homocysteine. This further causes elevation of blood pressure which damages small vessels [85]. MTHFR polymorphisms are risk factors for the progression of various retinal vascular diseases, including DR [86].

A decrease in the levels of homocysteine results in an improve in the retinal blood flow due to an improvement in homocysteine-induced narrowing of retinal artery [87]. Since folic acid as well as L-methylfolate lower homocysteine levels, their use seems to improve retinal blood flow, resulting in the improvement of DR [88]. Studies have shown that L-methylfolate is a better choice as compared to folic acid with reduced toxicity and better penetration of the retina and central nervous system [89].

17.3.1.4 Vitamin C and E

Vitamin C and E like Vitamin A have antioxidant properties. Some evidences have showed that Vitamin C and E protects retina against DR through free radical scavenging, reducing ROS production, suppressing lipid peroxidation, and reducing leukocyte adhesion in retinal vessels [90–92].

In an animal model of DR, the mixture of Vitamin C and E in diet showed a reduction in retinal neovascularization by improving antioxidant defense system and decreasing ROS levels. However, administration of Vitamin C and E with other antioxidants may lead to a better response than sole intake of Vitamin C or E due to decreased activation of protein kinase C, and decreased production of nitric oxide (NO) and subsequent reduction in formation of microvascular lesions in the retina [93].

A high level of vitamin C is present in the vitreous humor is maintained by a sodium-dependent ascorbate transporter (SLC23A2) located in the pigmented layer of the ciliary epithelium [94]. This indicates that under high oxidative stress, vitamin C acts as an antioxidant and has a protective effect on the retina, even in physiologically normal conditions [95].

Studies have shown that serum vitamin C levels are low in patients with DM in persons without diabetes [96]. Vitreous vitamin C is physiologically higher in eyes without DM than in eyes with DM. It has been shown that retinal ischemia might be related to depleted vitreous vitamin C levels in patients having PDR. In this condition, due to increased oxidative stress, vitreous vitamin C gets consumed faster. The vitreous humor regulates intraocular oxygen tension by metabolizing molecular oxygen in an ascorbate-dependent manner [97]. The vitreous humor may also be involved in the development of cataract and primary open angle glaucoma in patients with DM, and vitamin C may be related in the pathogenesis of the above [98]. It has been seen that serum level of vitamin C are lower in patients with T2DM and DR than healthy individuals [99].

Since, reported beneficial effects may be related to intake of fruits and vegetables as a main source of mixture of micronutrients and possibility of a synergistic interaction between different antioxidative supplements, it is reasonable that patients may respond better to a mixture mode of dietary antioxidants than sole intake [100]. Therefore, that along with selecting a suitable type and appropriate dosage of supplements as well as selecting antioxidants in combination with each other can be helpful. The beneficial effects of combination of Vitamin C with E have been seen in several complications of diabetes [91, 93]. However, evidence is lacking in terms of establishing role of dietary supplementation of vitamin C and E in patients of DME or its severity with DR and DME [101].

17.3.1.5 Vitamin D

In animal models of DM, Vitamin D deficiency has been shown to impair insulin synthesis and secretion [102, 103]. Vitamin D3 has been shown to decrease diabetes induced ROS production and exert a protective effect against cell apoptosis and retinal vascular damage in association with the inhibition of the ROS/TXNIP/NLRP3 inflammasome pathway [104, 105]. Vitamin D has antiangiogenic and anti-inflammatory effects and a subsequent suppressive role in the pathogenesis of DR. In an animal model of DR, it has been demonstrated that the active metabolite of vitamin D, calcitriol is a potent inhibitor of retinal neovascularization [106]. Vitamin D inhibits VEGF induced endothelial cell sprouting, elongation and proliferation [107]. In human cancer cells, it has been shown that vitamin D exerts its antiangiogenic activity by inhibiting the transcription of hypoxia-inducible factor (HIF-1) [108]. Vitamin D exerts an anti-inflammatory effect by inhibiting the proliferation of pro-inflammatory cytokines, natural killer cells and lymphocytes. Vitamin D also inhibits the production of the metalloproteinase, MMP-9, which are released by inflammatory cells [109]. Vitamin D inhibition increases the risk of DM. Among patients of DM, vitamin D deficiency is found to be associated with a higher risk of DR [104].

It has been shown that serum levels of vitamin D is associated with RPE alterations, disorganization of retinal inner layers and ellipsoid zone (EZ) disruption on spectral-domain optical coherence tomography in patients with DME [110, 111].

17.3.2 Minerals

17.3.2.1 Zinc

Zinc is important for DNA synthesis, cell division, as well as for the metabolism of proteins and carbohydrates. Moderate deficiency of zinc is common in normal population [112, 113]. Zinc deficiency is known to be associated with progression of chronic diseases such as DM, metabolic syndrome, and associated diabetic microvascular complications including DR [114, 115]. Low serum zinc levels have been shown to be correlated with the duration of DM, increased HbA1c levels, hypertension, and microvascular complications of DM. With increased duration of DM and severity of DR, serum zinc levels have been seen to fall progressively [115]. A trial of zinc supplementation in a murine model of type 2 DM has shown to improved insulin resistance, glucose intolerance, hypertension, and obesity [116]. A possible mechanism for this may be protection against lipid peroxidation and pericyte protection by zinc. Increasing zinc can also decreased VEGF levels and reduced ischemic inflammation [114]. Further studies are needed to establish optimum zinc levels for the treatment of DR.

17.3.2.2 Calcium

Retinal photoreceptor apoptosis has been seen to be associated with impaired serum ionized calcium homeostasis in diabetic retinopathy. It has been seen that EZ disruption is positively associated with serum total calcium and ionized calcium [117]. EZ disruption is associated with decreased VA in patients with DME [118].

17.3.2.3 Magnesium

Current evidence is inconclusive on establishing a role of dietary supplementation of magnesium in patients of DME or its severity with DR [101].

17.4 Naturaceuticals

A search for alternative treatments for DM and DR has been ongoing. A promising option for early-stage NPDR comes from nutraceuticals. In vitro and in vivo studies have revealed that a variety of nutraceuticals may offer anti-inflammatory and antioxidant effects that can improve the diabetes-driven molecular processes that cause vitreoretinopathy, acting as upstream regulators [119]. Based on several studies done in the area, it is rational to assert that a single compound that affects a single target will have limited effect in the prevention of progression of multifactorial diseases. Several studies have shown that the use of a combination of constituents with synergistic multitarget effects may offer a more powerful approach for the prevention of diseases, including retinal neurodegeneration [120, 121].

Curcumin, a non-flavonoid polyphenol that is the main active compound of *Curcuma longa*, is widely known for its anti-inflammatory and antioxidant properties. Many studies have shown its marked protective effect on retinal cells against oxidative stress and inflammation [122, 123].

Curcumin has been known to decrease the levels of cytokines in the vitreous of patients with DM. The synergism of curcumin with other bioactive molecules like those present in turmeric are well known. Together, they generate high concentrations of free curcuminoids in the plasma. The combination of curcumin, homotaurine, and vitamin D3 downregulate pro-inflammatory cytokine genes TNFα and IL6 and cyclinD1 gene expression [124].

17.5 Diet

Several studies have suggested that adherence to a diet high in fruit, vegetable, and fish intake, Mediterranean diet may protect against the development of DR, although evidence is limited [48, 125]. The role of diet in the development of DR needs more attention [126]. Greater focus on reducing total caloric intake as well as the *quality* of carbohydrates, may be more beneficial in the prevention of development and progression of DM [127].

The ingestion of dietary fibers tends to modulate the postprandial glucose response [128], and is thus proposed to reduce glucose-induced damage to the retina [129]. Oily-fish is a rich source of Vitamin D and LCω3-PUFAs [130, 131].

Moderate consumption of alcohol has been suggested to be protective against DR by increasing insulin sensitivity [132] and decreasing platelet aggregation [133]. These associations have been reported by cross-sectional studies only, with no longitudinal studies reporting clear conclusions. Research on the effect of beverages such as tea, coffee, milk [125, 133, 134] on DR remains limited.

Diet intake for DR can be suggested by the existing American Diabetic Association (ADA) guidelines for DM management. ADA recognizes the beneficial effects of the Mediterranean diet, diets rich in fruits and vegetables, and lower caloric intakes for people with DM. The ADA states insufficient evidence for the benefits of antioxidant supplementation [135] or an ideal amount of protein intake for diabetic individuals. It recommends DM patients to monitor their sodium and carbohydrate intake [136]. It also recommends PUFAs and monounsaturated fatty acids over trans fats and saturated fats [135], and also recommends moderate alcohol consumption, should a person wish to drink [137] for diabetic patients.

17.6 Conclusion

Our knowledge of nutrition in DME is only partial and ever growing. More studies are required to explore individual compounds and understand the underlying pathophysiology. As most of the available literature is in view of DM and diabetic retinopathy as a whole, DME becomes an area of possible research. A high degree of suspicion and a holistic view on the treatment of patients in necessary for the best possible care that can be provided to those suffering from DME.

References

1. Diabetes Federation International. IDF Diabetes Atlas Ninth edition 2019 [Internet]. Brussels: International Diabetes Federation; 2019. p. 1. http://www.idf.org/about-diabetes/facts-figures.
2. Zhang X, Saaddine JB, Chou CF, Cotch MF, Cheng YJ, Geiss LS, et al. Prevalence of diabetic retinopathy in the United States, 2005-2008. JAMA. 2010;304:649–56.
3. Hammes HP, Welp R, Kempe HP, Wagner C, Siegel E, Holl RW, et al. Risk factors for retinopathy and DME in type 2 diabetes-results from the German/Austrian DPV database. PLoS One. 2015;10:e0132492.
4. Roy MS, Janal MN. High caloric and sodium intakes as risk factors for progression of retinopathy in type 1 diabetes mellitus. Arch Ophthalmol. 2010;128(1):33–9.
5. Archer DB. Bowman lecture 1998. Diabetic retinopathy: some cellular, molecular and therapeutic considerations. Eye (Lond). 1999;13(4):497–523.
6. Skrha J, Kunesova M, Hilgertova J, Weiserova H, Krizova J, Kotrlikova E. Short-term very low calorie diet reduces oxidative stress in obese type 2 diabetic patients. Physiol Res. 2005;54(1):33–9.
7. Sumarriva K, Uppal K, Ma C, Herren DJ, Wang Y, Chocron IM, et al. Arginine and carnitine metabolites are altered in diabetic retinopathy. Invest Ophthalmol Vis Sci. 2019;60(8):3119–26.
8. Connor KM, SanGiovanni JP, Lofqvist C, Aderman CM, Chen J, Higuchi A, et al. Increased dietary intake of omega-3-polyunsaturated fatty acids reduces pathological retinal angiogenesis. Nat Med. 2007;13(7):868–73.
9. Sapieha P, Chen J, Stahl A, Seaward MR, Favazza TL, Juan AM, et al. Omega-3 polyunsaturated fatty acids preserve retinal function in type 2 diabetic mice. Nutr Diabetes. 2012;2:e36.
10. Lottenberg AM, Afonso Mda S, Lavrador MS, Machado RM, Nakandakare ER. The role of dietary fatty acids in the pathology of metabolic syndrome. J Nutr Biochem. 2012;23(9):1027–40.
11. Sala-Vila A, Díaz-López A, Valls-Pedret C, Cofán M, García-Layana A, Lamuela-Raventós RM, et al. Dietary marine ω-3 fatty acids and incident sight-threatening retinopathy in middle-aged and older individuals with type 2 diabetes: prospective investigation from the PREDIMED trial. JAMA Ophthalmol. 2016;134(10):1142–9.
12. Kowluru RA, Odenbach S. Effect of long-term administration of alpha-lipoic acid on retinal capillary cell death and the development of retinopathy in diabetic rats. Diabetes. 2004;53(12):3233–8.
13. Gebka A, Serkies-Minuth E, Raczynska D. Effect of the administration of alpha-lipoic acid on contrast sensitivity in patients with type 1 and type 2 diabetes. Mediators Inflamm. 2014;2014:131538.
14. Littarru GP, Langsjoen P. Coenzyme Q10 and statins: biochemical and clinical implications. Mitochondrion. 2007;7:S168–74.
15. Hamilton SJ, Chew GT, Watts GF. Coenzyme Q10 improves endothelial dysfunction in statin-treated type 2 diabetic patients. Diabetes Care. 2009;32:810–2.
16. Roig-Revert MJ, Lleó-Pérez A, Zanón-Moreno V, Vivar-Llopis B, Marín-Montiel J, Dolz-Marco R, et al. Valencia study on diabetic retinopathy (VSDR). Enhanced oxidative stress and other potential biomarkers for retinopathy in type 2 diabetics: beneficial effects of the nutraceutic supplements. Biomed Res Int. 2015;2015:408180.
17. Solmonson A, DeBerardinis RJ. Lipoic acid metabolism and mitochondrial redox regulation. J Biol Chem. 2018;293(20):7522–30.
18. Park S, Karunakaran U, Jeoung NH, Jeon JH, Lee IK. Physiological effect and therapeutic application of alpha lipoic acid. Curr Med Chem. 2014;21(32):3636–45.
19. Voloboueva LA, Liu J, Suh JH, Ames BN, Miller SS. (R)-alpha-lipoic acid protects retinal pigment epithelial cells from oxidative damage. Invest Ophthalmol Vis Sci. 2005;46(11):4302–10.
20. Ansar H, Mazloom Z, Kazemi F, Hejazi N. Effect of alpha-lipoic acid on blood glucose, insulin resistance and glutathione peroxidase of type 2 diabetic patients. Saudi Med J. 2011;32(6):584–8.
21. Pei Y, Liu H, Yang Y, Yang Y, Jiao Y, Tay FR, et al. Biological activities and potential oral applications of N-acetylcysteine: progress and prospects. Oxid Med Cell Longev. 2018;2018:2835787.
22. Aoyama K, Wang F, Matsumura N, Kiyonari H, Shioi G, Tanaka K, et al. Increased neuronal glutathione and neuroprotection in GTRAP3-18-deficient mice. Neurobiol Dis. 2012;45(3):973–82.
23. Atkuri KR, Mantovani JJ, Herzenberg LA, Herzenberg LA. N-Acetylcysteine—a safe antidote for cysteine/glutathione deficiency. Curr Opin Pharmacol. 2007;7(4):355–9.
24. Zhu Y, Zhang XL, Zhu BF, Ding YN. Effect of antioxidant N-acetylcysteine on diabetic retinopathy and expression of VEGF and ICAM-1 from retinal blood vessels of diabetic rats. Mol Biol Rep. 2012;39(4):3727–35.
25. Mohamed R, Sharma I, Ibrahim AS, Saleh H, Elsherbiny NM, Fulzele S, et al. Hyperhomocysteinemia alters retinal endothelial cells barrier function and angiogenic potential via activation of oxidative stress. Sci Rep. 2017;7(1):11952.
26. Gerona G, Lopez D, Palmero M, Maneu V. Antioxidant N-acetylcysteine protects retinal pigmented epithelial cells from long-term hypoxia changes in gene expression. J Ocul Pharmacol Ther. 2010;26(4):309–14.
27. Lei H, Velez G, Cui J, Samad A, Maberley D, Matsubara J, et al. Nacetylcysteine suppresses retinal detachment in an experimental model of proliferative vitreoretinopathy. Am J Pathol. 2010;177(1):132–40.
28. Choline-Health Professional Fact Sheet. National Institutes of Health. 2020. https://ods.od.nih.gov/factsheets/Choline-HealthProfessional/. Accessed 24 Feb 2020.
29. Drews K, Rozycka A, Barlik M, Klejewski A, Kurzawinska G, Wolski H, et al. Polymorphic variants of genes involved in choline pathway and the risk of intrauterine fetal death. Ginekol Pol. 2017;88(4):205–11.
30. Obeid R. The metabolic burden of methyl donor deficiency with focus on the betaine homocysteine methyltransferase pathway. Nutrients. 2013;5(9):3481–95.
31. Wilcken DE, Wilcken B, Dudman NP, Tyrrell PA. Homocystinuria—the effects of betaine in the treatment of patients not responsive to pyridoxine. N Engl J Med. 1983;309(8):448–53.
32. Morris SM. Arginine metabolism: boundaries of our knowledge. J Nutr. 2007;137:1602S–9S.
33. Paris LP, Johnson CH, Aguilar E, Usui Y, Cho K, Hoang LT, et al. Global metabolomics reveals metabolic dysregulation in ischemic retinopathy. Metabolomics. 2016;12:15.
34. Narayanan SP, Rojas M, Suwanpradid J, Toque HA, Caldwell RW, Caldwell RB. Arginase in retinopathy. Prog Retin Eye Res. 2013;36:260–80.

35. Malecki MT, Undas A, Cyganek K, Mirkiewicz-Sieradzka B, Wolkow P, Osmenda G, et al. Plasma asymmetric dimethylarginine (ADMA) is associated with retinopathy in type 2 diabetes. Diabetes Care. 2007;30:2899–901.
36. Namitha KK, Negi PS. Chemistry and biotechnology of carotenoids. Crit Rev Food Sci Nutr. 2010;50:728–60.
37. Sugai M, Ohta A, Ogata Y, Nakanishi M, Ueno S, Kawata T, et al. Asymmetric dimethylarginine (ADMA) in the aqueous humor of diabetic patients. Endocr J. 2007;54:303–9.
38. Jomova K, Valko M. Health protective effects of carotenoids and their interactions with other biological antioxidants. Eur J Med Chem. 2013;70:102–10.
39. Nakagawa K, Kiko T, Hatade K, Asai A, Kimura F, Sookwong P, et al. Development of a high-performance liquid chromatography-based assay for carotenoids in human red blood cells: application to clinical studies. Anal Biochem. 2008;381:129–34.
40. Saini RK, Nile SH, Park SW. Carotenoids from fruits and vegetables: chemistry, analysis, occurrence, bioavailability and biological activities. Food Res Int. 2015;76:735–50.
41. Subczynski W, Wisniewska A, Widomska J. Location of macular xanthophylls in the most vulnerable regions of photoreceptor outer-segment membranes. Arch Biochem Biophys. 2010;504:61–6.
42. Hammond BR Jr, Wooten BR, Snodderly DM. Individual variations in the spatial profile of human macular pigment. J Opt Soc Am A Opt Image Sci Vis. 1997;14:1187–96.
43. Rutz JK, Borges CD, Zambiazi RC, da Rosa CG, da Silva MM. Elaboration of microparticles of carotenoids from natural and synthetic sources for applications in food. Food Chem. 2016;202:324–33.
44. Britton G. Structure and properties of carotenoids in relation to function. FASEB J. 1995;9:1551–8.
45. Ames B, Shigenaga M, Hagen T. Oxidants, antioxidants, and the degenerative diseases of aging. Proc Natl Acad Sci U S A. 1993;90:7915–22.
46. Murillo A, Fernandez M. Potential of dietary non-provitamin a carotenoids in the prevention and treatment of diabetic microvascular complications. Adv Nutr. 2016;7:14–24.
47. Scanlon G, Loughman J, Farrell D, McCartney D. A review of the putative causal mechanisms associated with lower macular pigment in diabetes mellitus. Nutr Res Rev. 2019;32:247–64.
48. Sasaki M, Ozawa Y, Kurihara T, Kubota S, Yuki K, Noda K, et al. Neurodegenerative influence of oxidative stress in the retina of a murine model of diabetes. Diabetologia. 2010;53:971–9.
49. Wang W, Tam KC, Ng TC, Goit RK, Chan KLS, Lo ACY. Long-term lutein administration attenuates retinal inflammation and functional deficits in early diabetic retinopathy using the Ins2Akita/+ mice. BMJ Open Diabetes Res Care. 2020;8:e001519.
50. Kamoshita M, Toda E, Osada H, Narimatsu T, Kobayashi S, Tsubota K, et al. Lutein acts via multiple antioxidant pathways in the photo-stressed retina. Sci Rep. 2016;6:1–10.
51. Keegan G, Pardhan S, Chichger H. Lutein and zeaxanthin attenuates VEGF-induced neovascularisation in human retinal microvascular endothelial cells through a Nox4-dependent pathway. Exp Eye Res. 2020;197:108104.
52. Hwang JS, Han SG, Lee CH, Seo HG. Lutein suppresses hyperglycemia-induced premature senescence of retinal pigment epithelial cells by up-regulating SIRT1. J Food Biochem. 2018;42:e12495.
53. Harikumar K, Nimita C, Preethi K, Kuttan R, Shankaranarayana M, Deshpande J. Toxicity profile of lutein and lutein Ester isolated from Marigold flowers (Tagetes erecta). Int J Toxicol. 2008;27:1–9.
54. Shi C, Wang P, Airen S, Brown C, Liu Z, Townsend JH, Wang J, Jiang H. Nutritional and medical food therapies for diabetic retinopathy. Eye Vis (Lond). 2020;7:33.
55. Raichle ME, Gusnard DA. Appraising the brain's energy budget. Proc Natl Acad Sci U S A. 2002;99(16):10237–9.
56. Kurihara T, Westenskow PD, Gantner ML, Usui Y, Schultz A, Bravo S, et al. Hypoxia-induced metabolic stress in retinal pigment epithelial cells is sufficient to induce photoreceptor degeneration. Elife. 2016;5:e14319.
57. Okai Y, Higashi-Okai K, Sato EF, Konaka R, Inoue M. Potent radical scavenging activities of thiamin and thiamin diphosphate. J Clin Biochem Nutr. 2007;40(1):42–8.
58. Luong KV, Nguyen LT. The impact of thiamine treatment in the diabetes mellitus. J Clin Med Res. 2012;4(3):153–60.
59. Beltramo E, Berrone E, Buttiglieri S, Porta M. Thiamine and benfotiamine prevent increased apoptosis in endothelial cells and pericytes cultured in high glucose. Diabetes Metab Res Rev. 2004;20(4):330–6.
60. Booth AA, Khalifah RG, Hudson BG. Thiamine pyrophosphate and pyridoxamine inhibit the formation of antigenic advanced glycation end products: comparison with aminoguanidine. Biochem Biophys Res Commun. 1996;220(1):113–9.
61. Thiamin-Health Professional Fact Sheet. National Institutes of Health. 2020. https://ods.od.nih.gov/factsheets/Thiamin-HealthProfessional/. Accessed 19 Feb 2020.
62. Riboflavin-Health Professional Fact Sheet. National Institutes of Health. 2020. https://ods.od.nih.gov/factsheets/Riboflavin-HealthProfessional/. Accessed 6 Mar 2020. Shi et al. Eye and Vision 2020;7:33.
63. McNulty H, Strain JJ, Hughes CF, Ward M. Riboflavin, MTHFR genotype and blood pressure: a personalized approach to prevention and treatment of hypertension. Mol Aspects Med. 2017;53:2–9.
64. Moat SJ, Ashfield-Watt PA, Powers HJ, Newcombe RG, McDowell IF. Effect of riboflavin status on the homocysteine-lowering effect of folate in relation to the MTHFR (C677T) genotype. Clin Chem. 2003;49(2):295–302.
65. Naghashpour M, Amani R, Sarkaki A, Ghadiri A, Samarbafzadeh A, Jafarirad S, et al. Brain-derived neurotrophic and immunologic factors: beneficial effects of riboflavin on motor disability in murine model of multiple sclerosis. Iran J Basic Med Sci. 2016;19(4):439–48.
66. Liu W, Han X, Zhou X, Zhang S, Cai X, Zhang L, et al. Brain derived neurotrophic factor in newly diagnosed diabetes and prediabetes. Mol Cell Endocrinol. 2016;429:106–13.
67. Mohn ES, Erdman JW Jr, Kuchan MJ, Neuringer M, Johnson EJ. Lutein accumulates in subcellular membranes of brain regions in adult rhesus macaques: relationship to DHA oxidation products. PLoS One. 2017;12(10):e0186767.
68. Kuvin JT, Ramet ME, Patel AR, Pandian NG, Mendelsohn ME, Karas RH. A novel mechanism for the beneficial vascular effects of high-density lipoprotein cholesterol: enhanced vasorelaxation and increased endothelial nitric oxide synthase expression. Am Heart J. 2002;144(1):165–72.
69. Domanico D, Verboschi F, Altimari S, Zompatori L, Vingolo EM. Ocular effects of niacin: a review of the literature. Med Hypothesis Discov Innov Ophthalmol. 2015;4(2):64–71.
70. Yan T, Chopp M, Ye X, Liu Z, Zacharek A, Cui Y, et al. Niaspan increases axonal remodeling after stroke in type 1 diabetes rats. Neurobiol Dis. 2012;46(1):157–64.
71. Niacin-Health Professional Fact Sheet. National Institutes of Health. 2020. https://ods.od.nih.gov/factsheets/Niacin-HealthProfessional/. Accessed 6 Mar 2020.
72. Pantothenic Acid-Health Professional Fact Sheet. 2020. https://ods.od.nih.gov/factsheets/PantothenicAcid-HealthProfessional/. Accessed 2 Mar 2020.
73. Vitamin B6-Health Professional Fact Sheet. 2020. https://ods.od.nih.gov/factsheets/VitaminB6-HealthProfessional/. Accessed 24 Feb 2020.

74. Morris MS, Picciano MF, Jacques PF, Selhub J. Plasma pyridoxal 5′-phosphate in the US population: the National Health and nutrition examination survey, 2003-2004. Am J Clin Nutr. 2008;87(5):1446–54.
75. Lei X, Zeng G, Zhang Y, Li Q, Zhang J, Bai Z, et al. Association between homocysteine level and the risk of diabetic retinopathy: a systematic review and meta-analysis. Diabetol Metab Syndr. 2018;10:61.
76. Kowluru RA, Mohammad G, Sahajpal N. Faulty homocysteine recycling in diabetic retinopathy. Eye Vis (Lond). 2020;7:4.
77. Rubi B. Pyridoxal 5′-phosphate (PLP) deficiency might contribute to the onset of type I diabetes. Med Hypotheses. 2012;78(1):179–82.
78. Horikawa C, Aida R, Kamada C, Fujihara K, Tanaka S, Tanaka S, et al. Vitamin B6 intake and incidence of diabetic retinopathy in Japanese patients with type 2 diabetes: analysis of data from the Japan diabetes complications study (JDCS). Eur J Nutr. 2019;58:281.
79. Vrolijk MF, Opperhuizen A, Jansen EHJM, Hageman GJ, Bast A, Haenen GRMM. The vitamin B6 paradox: supplementation with high concentrations of pyridoxine leads to decreased vitamin B6 function. Toxicol In Vitro. 2017;44:206–12.
80. Haeusler RA, Camastra S, Astiarraga B, Nannipieri M, Anselmino M, Ferrannini E. Decreased expression of hepatic glucokinase in type 2 diabetes. Mol Metab. 2015;4(3):222–6.
81. Xiang X, Liu Y, Zhang X, Zhang W, Wang Z. Effects of biotin on blood glucose regulation in type 2 diabetes rat model. Wei Sheng Yan Jiu. 2015;44(2):185–9, 195.
82. Biotin-Health Professional Fact Sheet. National Institutes of Health. 2020. https://ods.od.nih.gov/factsheets/Biotin-HealthProfessional/. Accessed 19 Feb 2020.
83. Brazionis L, Rowley K, Itsiopoulos C, Harper CA, O'Dea K. Homocysteine and diabetic retinopathy. Diabetes Care. 2008;31(1):50–6.
84. Srivastav K, Saxena S, Mahdi AA, Shukla RK, Meyer CH, Akduman L, et al. Increased serum level of homocysteine correlates with retinal nerve fiber layer thinning in diabetic retinopathy. Mol Vis. 2016;22:1352–60.
85. Heifetz EM, Birk RZ. MTHFR C677T polymorphism affects normotensive diastolic blood pressure independently of blood lipids. Am J Hypertens. 2015;8(3):387–92.
86. Chen D, Wang J, Dan Z, Shen X, Ci D. The relationship between methylenetetrahydrofolate reductase C677T polymorphism and diabetic retinopathy: a meta-analysis in multiethnic groups. Ophthalmic Genet. 2018;39(2):200–7.
87. Gopinath B, Wang JJ, Flood VM, Burlutsky G, Wong TY, Mitchell P. The associations between blood levels of homocysteine, folate, vitamin B12, and retinal vascular caliber. Am J Ophthalmol. 2009;148(6):902–9.
88. Wang J, Brown C, Shi C, Townsend J, Gameiro GR, Wang P, et al. Improving diabetic and hypertensive retinopathy with a medical food containing L-methylfolate: a preliminary report. Eye Vis (Lond). 2019;6:21.
89. Huang W, Prasad PD, Kekuda R, Leibach FH, Ganapathy V. Characterization of N5-methyltetrahydrofolate uptake in cultured human retinal pigment epithelial cells. Invest Ophthalmol Vis Sci. 1997;38(8):1578–87.
90. Rahimi R, Nikfar S, Larijani B, Abdollahi M. A review on the role of antioxidants in the management of diabetes and its complications. Biomed Pharmacother. 2005;59:365–73.
91. Khodaeian M, Tabatabaei-Malazy O, Qorbani M, Farzadfar F, Amini P, Larijani B. Effect of vitamins C and E on insulin resistance in diabetes: a meta-analysis study. Eur J Clin Invest. 2015;45(11):1161–74.
92. Tabatabaei-Malazy O, Nikfar S, Larijani B, Abdollahi M. Influence of ascorbic acid supplementation on type 2 diabetes mellitus in observational and randomized controlled trials; a systematic review with meta-analysis. J Pharm Pharm Sci. 2014;17(4):554–82.
93. Kowluru RA, Tang J, Kern TS. Abnormalities of retinal metabolism in diabetes and experimental galactosemia, VII, effect of long-term administration of antioxidants on the development of retinopathy. Diabetes. 2001;50:1938–42.
94. Tsukaguchi H, Tokui T, Mackenzie B, Berger UV, Chen XZ, Wang Y, et al. A family of mammalian Na+−dependent L-ascorbic acid transporters. Nature. 1999;399(6731):70–5.
95. Traber MG, Stevens JF. Vitamins C and E: beneficial effects from a mechanistic perspective. Free Radic Biol Med. 2011;51(5):1000–13.
96. Will JC, Byers T. Does diabetes mellitus increase the requirement for vitamin C? Nutr Rev. 1996;54(7):193–202.
97. Shui YB, Holekamp NM, Kramer BC, Crowley JR, Wilkins MA, Chu F, et al. The gel state of the vitreous and ascorbate-dependent oxygen consumption: relationship to the etiology of nuclear cataracts. Arch Ophthalmol. 2009;127(4):475–82.
98. Holekamp NM. The vitreous gel: more than meets the eye. Am J Ophthalmol. 2010;149(1):32–6.
99. Park SW, Ghim W, Oh S, Kim Y, Park UC, Kang J, et al. Association of vitreous vitamin C depletion with diabetic macular ischemia in proliferative diabetic retinopathy. PLoS One. 2019;14(6):e0218433.
100. Tabatabaei-Malazy O, Larijani B, Abdollahi M. A novel management of diabetes by means of strong antioxidants' combination. J Med Hypotheses Ideas. 2013;7:25–30.
101. Tabatabaei-Malazy O, Ardeshirlarijani E, Namazi N, Nikfar S, Jalili RB, Larijani B. Dietary antioxidative supplements and diabetic retinopathy; a systematic review. J Diabetes Metab Disord. 2019;18(2):705–16.
102. Jude S, Amalraj A, Kunnumakkara AB, Divya C, Löffler BM, Gopi S. Development of validated methods and quantification of curcuminoids and curcumin metabolites and their pharmacokinetic study of oral administration of complete natural turmeric formulation (Cureit™) in human plasma via UPLC/ESI-Q-TOF-MS spectrometry. Molecules. 2018;23:2415.
103. Snijder M, van Dam R, Visser M, Deeg D, Seidell J, Lips P, et al. Vitamin D and diabetes. Diabetologia. 2005;48:1247–57.
104. Luo BA, Gao F, Qin LL. The association between vitamin D deficiency and diabetic retinopathy in type 2 diabetes: a meta-analysis of observational studies. Nutrients. 2017;9:307.
105. Lu L, Lu Q, Chen W, Li J, Li C, Zheng Z. Vitamin D3 protects against diabetic retinopathy by inhibiting high-glucose-induced activation of the ROS/TXNIP/NLRP3 inflammasome pathway. J Diabetes Res. 2018;2018:8193523.
106. Albert DM, Scheef EA, Wang S, Mehraein F, Darjatmoko SR, Sorenson CM, et al. Calcitriol is a potent inhibitor of retinal neovascularization. Invest Ophthalmol Vis Sci. 2007;48:2327–34.
107. Mantell DJ, Owens PE, Bundred NJ, Mawer EB, Canfeld AE. 1alpha,25- dihydroxyvitamin D(3) inhibits angiogenesis in vitro and in vivo. Circ Res. 2000;87:214–20.
108. Ben-Shoshan M, Amir S, Dang DT, Dang LH, Weisman Y, Mabjeesh NJ. 1alpha,25-dihydroxyvitamin D3 (calcitriol) inhibits hypoxia-inducible factor-1/vascular endothelial growth factor pathway in human cancer cells. Mol Cancer Ther. 2007;6:1433–9.
109. Bahar-Shany K, Ravid A, Koren R. Upregulation of MMP-9 production by TNF alpha in keratinocytes and its attenuation by vitamin D. J Cell Physiol. 2010;22:729–37.
110. Nadri G, Saxena S, Stefanickova J, Ziak P, Benacka J, Gilhotra JS, Kruzliak P. Disorganization of retinal inner layers correlates with ellipsoid zone disruption and retinal nerve fiber layer thinning in diabetic retinopathy. J Diabetes Complications. 2019;33(8):550–3.
111. Saxena S, Nadri G, Kaur A, Mahdi A, Ahmad K, Garg P. Low serum vitamin D levels correlate with disorganization of retinal

inner layers, ellipsoid zone disruption and retinal pigment epithelium alterations in diabetic retinopathy. Invest Ophthalmol Vis Sci. 2019;60(9):5321.
112. Derouiche S, Kechrid Z. Zinc supplementation overcomes effects of copper on zinc status, carbohydrate metabolism and some enzyme activities in diabetic and nondiabetic rats. Can J Diabetes. 2016;40(4):342–7.
113. Zinc-Health Professional Fact Sheet. National Institutes of Health. 2020. https://ods.od.nih.gov/factsheets/Zinc-HealthProfessional/. Accessed 6 Mar 2020.
114. Miao X, Sun W, Miao L, Fu Y, Wang Y, Su G, et al. Zinc and diabetic retinopathy. J Diabetes Res. 2013;2013:425854.
115. Luo YY, Zhao J, Han XY, Zhou XH, Wu J, Ji LN. Relationship between serum zinc level and microvascular complications in patients with type 2 diabetes. Chin Med J (Engl). 2015;128(24):3276–82.
116. Adachi Y, Yoshida J, Kodera Y, Kiss T, Jakusch T, Enyedy EA, et al. Oral administration of a zinc complex improves type 2 diabetes and metabolic syndromes. Biochem Biophys Res Commun. 2006;351(1):165–70.
117. Ankita SS, Nim DK, Stefanickova J, Ziak P, Stefanicka P, et al. Retinal photoreceptor apoptosis is associated with impaired serum ionized calcium homeostasis in diabetic retinopathy: an in-vivo analysis. J Diabetes Complications. 2019;33(3):208–11.
118. De S, Saxena S, Kaur A, Mahdi AA, Misra A, Singh M, Meyer CH, Akduman L. Sequential restoration of external limiting membrane and ellipsoid zone after intravitreal anti-VEGF therapy in diabetic macular oedema. Eye (Lond). 2021;35(5):1490–5.
119. Duh EJ, Sun JK, Stitt AW. Diabetic retinopathy: current understanding, mechanisms, and treatment strategies. JCI Insight. 2017;2:e93751.
120. Rossino MG, Casini G. Nutraceuticals for the treatment of diabetic retinopathy. Nutrients. 2019;11:771.
121. Davinelli S, Maes M, Corbi G, Zarrelli A, Willcox DC, Scapagnini G. Dietary phytochemicals and neuro-inflammaging: from mechanistic insights to translational challenges. Immun Ageing. 2016;13:16.
122. Barber AJ. A new view of diabetic retinopathy: a neurodegenerative disease of the eye. Prog Neuro-Psychoph. 2003;27:283–90.
123. Nucci C, Russo R, Martucci A, Giannini C, Garaci F, Floris R, et al. New strategies for neuroprotection in glaucoma, a disease that affects the central nervous system. Eur J Pharmacol. 2016;787:119–26.
124. Filippelli M, Campagna G, Vito P, Zotti T, Ventre L, Rinaldi M, et al. Anti-inflammatory effect of curcumin, Homotaurine, and vitamin D3 on human vitreous in patients with diabetic retinopathy. Front Neurol. 2021;11:592274.
125. Millen AE, Sahli MW, Nie J, LaMonte MJ, Lutsey PL, Klein BE, et al. Adequate vitamin D status is associated with the reduced odds of prevalent diabetic retinopathy in African Americans and Caucasians. Cardiovasc Diabetol. 2016;15(1):128.
126. Wong M, Man R, Fenwick EK, Gupta P, Li LJ, van Dam RM, Lamoureux EL, et al. Dietary intake and diabetic retinopathy: a systematic review. PLoS One. 2018;13(1):e0186582.
127. Chiu CJ, Taylor A. Dietary hyperglycemia, glycemic index and metabolic retinal diseases. Prog Retin Eye Res. 2011;30(1):18–53.
128. Blackwood AD, Salter J, Dettmar PW, Chaplin MF. Dietary fibre, physicochemical properties and their relationship to health. J R Soc Promot Health. 2000;120(4):242–7.
129. Ma Q, Shen JH, Shen SR, Das UN. Bioactive lipids in pathological retinopathy. Crit Rev Food Sci Nutr. 2014;54(1):1–16.
130. Das UN. Lipoxins, resolvins, and protectins in the prevention and treatment of diabetic macular edema and retinopathy. Nutrition. 2013;29(1):1–7.
131. Greenfield JR, Samaras K, Jenkins AB, Kelly PJ, Spector TD, Campbell LV. Moderate alcohol consumption, estrogen replacement therapy, and physical activity are associated with increased insulin sensitivity: is abdominal adiposity the mediator? Diabetes Care. 2003;26(10):2734–40.
132. Ma Q, Chen D, Sun HP, Yan N, Xu Y, Pan CW. Regular Chinese green tea consumption is protective for diabetic retinopathy: a clinic-based case-control study. J Diabetes Res. 2015;2015:231570.
133. Wang S, Wang JJ, Wong TY. Alcohol and eye diseases. Surv Ophthalmol. 2008;53(5):512–25.
134. Kumari N. Is coffee consumption associated with age-related macular degeneration and diabetic retinopathy? All Res J Biol. 2014;5(2):7–13.
135. American Diabetes Association. 3 foundations of care and comprehensive medical evaluation. Diabetes Care. 2016;39(1):S23–35.
136. Evert AB, Boucher JL, Cypress M, Dunbar SA, Franz MJ, Mayer-Davis EJ, et al. Nutrition therapy recommendations for the management of adults with diabetes. Diabetes Care. 2014;37(1):S120–43.
137. American Diabetes A. Standards of medical care in diabetes—2013. Diabetes Care. 2013;36(1):S11–66.

18 Quality of Life in Diabetic Macular Edema

Anupriya and Sandeep Saxena

18.1 Introduction

Diabetes mellitus is the major systemic cause of blindness in the World [1]. The major risk factor for severe reduction of vision in diabetic patients is macular edema resulting from increased vascular permeability and leakage of fluid into the retinal tissue of the macula. Diabetic retinopathy can affect an individual and society at various levels. On an individual level, this condition can cause visual loss and functional impairment, as measured through the loss of ability to perform specific tasks. Additionally, diabetic retinopathy can affect health-related quality of life (HRQoL) both in those who require insulin and in those who do not [2, 3]. This can be due to its effects on both vision-specific domains as well as ones that are labeled as vision non-specific ones, such as social functioning and emotional well-being.

A progressive decline in visual function may impact a patient's ability to complete daily routine activities, which can impact the psychological state. Therefore, in addition to measuring the functional outcome of therapeutic intervention, it is also important to measure a treatment's impact on vision-related QoL [4].

WHO defines Quality of Life (QoL) as an individual's perception of their position in life in the context of the culture and value systems in which they live and in relation to their goals, expectations, standards, and concerns [5]. The HRQoL refers to the effect of a disease on the way a person enjoys life, including the way illness affects a person's ability to live free of pain, work productively, and interact with loved ones. The HRQoL score is a valuation of a life lived in a particular health state. Although it is an end in itself, HRQoL valuation can also be used in the measurement of cost-effectiveness (i.e., cost per vision year saved) and cost-utility.

Diabetic retinopathy (DR) is a common microvascular complication of diabetes. In its early non-proliferative stages, there are few visual symptoms; however, as the disease progresses to vision-threatening stages (severe non-proliferative DR [NPDR] and proliferative DR [PDR]), significant vision loss can occur. Diabetic macular edema (DME), which can occur at any stage, affects central visual acuity.

The impact of DR on health-related quality of life (QoL) is substantial, especially at the vision-threatening stages. As compared to NPDR, patients with PDR have poorer QoL. Novel therapies such as anti-VEGF intravitreal injections have shown promising results for improving vision loss and QoL, particularly for DME [6].

Chronic hyperglycemia-related accumulation of advanced glycated end products (AGEs) causes disruption of the blood–retinal barrier (BRB) and an altered vitreoretinal interface. Altered BRB leads to interstitial fluid accumulation within the retina especially around the perifoveal retina leading to macular edema and diminution of vision [7]. Focal/grid lasers and intravitreal anti-VEGF therapy have been used to cure this condition. Both the modalities lead to improvement in visual acuity as well as quality of life. However, studies have shown that intravitreal therapy leads to more significant improvement in both the parameters than laser treatment [8].

18.2 Scales for Assessment of QoL

HRQoL measures functioning and well-being in physical, mental, and social health realms of life and reflects the influence of broad range of health conditions simultaneously. Because of the response burden and impact on participation rates it is imperative that HRQoL measures be as short as feasible. Various scales have been developed over the years to assess the quality of life (Table 18.1). Few of them are enlisted as follows.

Anupriya (✉) · S. Saxena
Department of Ophthalmology, King George's Medical University, Lucknow, India

S. Saxena et al. (eds.), *Diabetic Macular Edema*, https://doi.org/10.1007/978-981-19-7307-9_18

Table 18.1 Various scores for assessment of QoL

Score	Uses
VFQ-25	Vision-specific questionnaire, measures both vision-specific tasks and broader dimensions of HRQoL
VF-14	Measures vision-specific tasks
SF-36	Generic questionnaire, not specific to small changes in vision
RetDQol	Specifically designed for diabetic retinopathy, scores weighted by important to patient

18.2.1 EQ-5D

The EQ-5D is a standardized measure of health-related quality of life developed by the EuroQol Group [9]. EQ-5D is the most widely used health-related quality of life questionnaire in health economic evaluations. It is a descriptive system that covers five dimensions of self-reported health: mobility, self-care, usual activity, pain/discomfort, and anxiety/depression. Each dimension has three response categories: no problems, some problems, and extreme problems. The number of levels in these dimensions differ in the EQ-5D-3L (three levels) and the EQ-5D-5L (five levels). The EQ-5D-Y has the same five dimensions, but they are worded more appropriately for young people. EQ-5D-5L descriptive system uses the same five dimensions as the EQ-5D-3L but has two extra levels of severity in each dimension. The EQ-5D version (EQ-5D-Y) more suitable questionnaire for children and adolescents. It is based on the EQ-5D-3L, but the wording has been simplified for the younger people. The second part of the questionnaire in all three versions of EQ-5D comprises a standard vertical 20-cm VAS that is calibrated from "the worst health you can imagine" (scored 0) at its base to "the best health you can imagine" (scored 100) at its apex. Respondents are asked to "mark an X on the scale to indicate how your health is TODAY" and to write the number in an adjoining box [10].

18.2.2 NEI VFQ-25

National Eye Institute Visual Function Questionnaire (NEI VFQ-25) is a visual function specific QoL assessment tool measures the dimensions of self-reported vision-targeted health status that are most important for persons who have chronic eye diseases. The survey measures the influence of visual disability and visual symptoms on generic health domains such as emotional well-being and social functioning, in addition to task-oriented domains related to daily visual functioning. Questions included in the VFQ25 represent the content identified during a series of condition-specific focus groups with patients who had diabetic retinopathy, age-related cataracts, glaucoma, age-related macular degeneration or CMV retinitis.

The VFQ-25 is the product of an item-reduction analysis of the longer field test version of the survey called the 51-item National Eye Institute Vision Function Questionnaire (NEI-VFQ). The longer version contains 51 questions which represent 13 different subscales. The NEIVFQ Field Test Study collected the data needed to examine the reliability and validity of the survey across all of the above-mentioned ocular diseases [11].

This score has been vividly used in a number of clinical studies.

The VFQ-25 consists of a base set of 25 vision-targeted questions representing 11 vision-related constructs, plus an additional single-item general health rating question. The VFQ-25 also includes an appendix of additional items from the 51-item version that researchers can use to expand the scales up to 39 total items. The VFQ-25 takes approximately 10 mins on average to administer in the interviewer format.

The VFQ25 generates the following vision-targeted subscales: global vision rating (1), difficulty with near vision activities (3), difficulty with distance vision activities (3), limitations in social functioning due to vision (2), role limitations due to vision (2), dependency on others due to vision (3), mental health symptoms due to vision (4), driving difficulties (3), limitations with peripheral (1) and color vision (1), and ocular pain (2). Additionally, the VFQ-25 contains the single general health rating question which has been shown to be a robust predictor of future health and mortality in population-based studies. It is also sensitive to the effect of different therapeutic interventions such as anti-vascular endothelial growth factor (VEGF) therapy [3].

18.2.3 RetDQoL

The RetDQoL is an individualized measure of the impact of diabetic retinopathy on quality of life taking account of the relevance and importance of different aspects of life for quality of life of individuals as well as the individual's view of the impact of diabetic retinopathy on each aspect of life of relevance to them. The RetDQoL is written in large font with a layout designed to facilitate reading by those with visual impairment. The measure starts with two overview items. Overview item I ("present QoL") asks participants to complete the statement "In general, my present quality of life is:" using a seven-point scale from "excellent," scored as 3 through "neither good nor bad," scored as 0 to "extremely bad," scored as −3. Overview item II ("retinopathy-specific QoL") asks how QoL is affected by diabetic eye problems: "If I did not have diabetic eye problems, my quality of life would be:" with the response options: "very much better" (scored −3), "much better" (−2), "better" (−1), "the same" (0), "worse" (1) [12].

18.3 Impact of QOL After Treatment

18.3.1 Laser Therapy

The presence of diabetic retinopathy and macular edema, visual acuity impairment, and patient comorbidities lead to significant impairment of both the physical and mental components of health-related QoL [13]. Grid laser therapy for macular edema and pan retinal photocoagulation for proliferative diabetic retinopathy have been found beneficial in improving vision in sight threating scenarios. Studies over the years have concluded that laser therapy leads to positive impact on quality of life of the patients [14].

18.3.2 Anti-VEGF Therapy

VEGF is a pluripotent growth factor which is involved in the initiation of retinal vascular leakage and non-perfusion in diabetes. VEGF are crucial regulators of vascular development during vasculogenesis and angiogenesis. Anti-VEGF have revolutionized the treatment regimen of diabetic retinopathy. Various study trials have shown that increase in visual acuity after intravitreal anti-VEGF have led to enhancement of quality of life. Moreover, this therapy stands superior to the laser therapy for DME [15, 16].

The AQUA study conducted by Garweg et al. [17], was a multicenter, open-label, single-arm, phase 4 study. In total 553 patients were enrolled in this study and they received intravitreal aflibercept 2 mg every 8 weeks for 52 weeks, after 5 initial doses every 4 weeks. The change in 25-item National Eye Institute Visual Function Questionnaire (NEI VFQ-25) total score from baseline to week 52 was assessed after the intravitreal aflibercept. The AQUA trial demonstrated that intravitreal aflibercept was associated with clinically meaningful improvements in NEI VFQ-25 total score over 52 weeks in patients with DME and these were even more pronounced for near than for distant activities.

A prospective study by Turkoglu et al. [18] in which 70 patients with clinically significant macular edema (CSME) were randomized to undergo IVR injection ($n = 35$) and focal/grid laser ($n = 35$). Apart from Distance and near visual acuities, central retinal thickness (CRT), 25-item Visual Function Questionnaire (VFQ-25) was used to measure the effectiveness of treatments and VR-QoL before and after 6 months following IVR or laser treatment. In both groups, the VFQ-25 composite score tended to improve from baseline to 6 months. And at sixth month, the changes in composite score were significantly higher in IVR group than in laser group.

18.4 Conclusion

Diabetic patients need a holistic approach involving various body systems including psychiatric evaluation. Various treatment regimen targeted for DME have led to recuperation of patient's quality of vision and life as well. This could be assessed with the help of the scales described previously.

Not only these scales help us to assess the patient QoL but also helps in monitoring the effectiveness of treatment regimen. Moreover, these scores help clinicians to provide patients with optimized medical treatment, further increasing treatment adherence and persistence.

References

1. Aiello LM. Perspectives on diabetic retinopathy. Am J Ophthalmol. 2003;136:122–35.
2. Lloyd AJ, Loftus J, Turner M, et al. Psychometric validation of macular edema. Health Qual Life Outcomes. 2013;11:10.
3. Mangione CM, Lee PP, Gutierrez PR, Spritzer K, Berry S, Hays RD, National Eye Institute Visual Function Questionnaire Field Test Investigators. Development of the 25-item National eye Institute visual function questionnaire. Arch Ophthalmol. 2001;119:1050–8.
4. Brown GC, Brown MM, Sharma S. Value-based medicine: evidence-based medicine and beyond. Ocul Immunol Inflamm. 2003;11(3):157–70.
5. Skevington SM, Lotfy M, O'Connell KA. The World Health Organisation's WHOQOL-BREF quality of life assessment: psychometric properties and results of the international field trial. A report from the WHO QOL group. Qual Life Res. 2004;13:299–31.
6. Antcliff RJ, Marshall J. The pathogenesis of edema in diabetic maculopathy. Semin Ophthalmol. 1999;14:223–32.
7. Hariprasad SM, Mieler WF, Grassi M, Green JL, Jager RD, Miller L. Vision-related quality of life in patients with diabetic macular oedema. Br J Ophthalmol. 2008;92:89–92.
8. Fenwick EK, Pesudovs K, Khadka J, Dirani M, Rees G, Wong TY, Lamoureux EL. The impact of diabetic retinopathy on quality of life: qualitative findings from an item bank development project. Qual Life Res. 2012;21:1771–82.
9. Brooks R, Boye KS, Slaap B. EQ-5D: a plea for accurate nomenclature. J Patient Rep Outcomes. 2020;4:52.
10. EuroQol, Group. EuroQol—a new facility for the measurement of health-related quality of life. Health Policy. 1990;16:199–208.
11. Mangione CM, Berry S, Spritzer K, Janz NK, Klein R, Owsley C, Lee PP. Identifying the content area for the 51-item National eye Institute visual function questionnaire: results from focus groups with visually impaired persons. Arch Ophthalmol. 1998;116:227–33.
12. Brose LS, Bradley C. Psychometric development of the individualized retinopathy-dependent quality of life questionnaire (RetDQoL). Value Health. 2010;13:119–27.
13. Lee CM, Olk RJ. Modified grid laser photocoagulation for diffuse diabetic macular oedema. Long-term visual results. Ophthalmology. 1991;98:1594–602.
14. Tranos PG, Topouzis F, Stangos NT, Dimitrakos S, Economidis P, Harris M, Coleman AL. Effect of laser photocoagulation treatment for diabetic macular oedema on patient's vision-related quality of life. Curr Eye Res. 2004;29:41–9.

15. Granström T, Forsman H, Leksell J, Jani S, Raghib AM, Granstam E. Visual functioning and health-related quality of life in diabetic patients about to undergo anti-vascular endothelial growth factor treatment for sight-threatening macular edema. J Diabetes Complications. 2015;29:1183–90.
16. Korobelnik JF, Do DV, Schmidt-Erfurth U, Boyer DS, Holz FG, Heier JS, Midena E, Kaiser PK, Terasaki H, Marcus DM, Nguyen QD, Jaffe GJ, Slakter JS, Simader C, Soo Y, Schmelter T, Yancopoulos GD, Stahl N, Vitti R, Berliner AJ, Zeitz O, Metzig C, Brown DM. Intravitreal aflibercept for diabetic macular edema. Ophthalmology. 2014;121:2247–54.
17. Garweg JG, Stefanickova J, Hoyng C, Schmelter T, Niesen T, Sowade O, Sivaprasad S, AQUA Investigators. Vision-related quality of life in patients with diabetic macular edema treated with intravitreal aflibercept: the AQUA study. Ophthalmol Retina. 2019;3:567–75.
18. Turkoglu EB, Celık E, Aksoy N, Bursalı O, Ucak T, Alagoz G. Changes in vision related quality of life in patients with diabetic macular edema: ranibizumab or laser treatment? J Diabetes Complications. 2015;29(4):540–3.

19 Diabetic Macular Edema in Young Adults

Shivani Sinha

19.1 Introduction

According to the National Health and Nutrition Examination Survey, the prevalence of diabetes has increased significantly from 9.8% in 1999–2000 to 14.3% in 2017–2018 [1]. The prevalence of type 1 diabetes among those 19 years or younger has increased significantly from 1.48 to 2.15 per 1000 youths through 2001 to 2017 signifying a 45.1% relative increase [2]. For type 2 diabetes, in youth aged 10–19 years the prevalence has increased from 0.34 to 0.67 per 1000 youths signifying a 95.3% relative increase over 16 years [2]. Diabetic retinopathy (DR) accounts for 1.1% world blindness burden [3]. Diabetic eye disease also impacts visual functioning, limits daily activities, and also negatively impacts psychological well-being [4].

DR in early onset type 2 diabetes mellitus (T2DM) has been reported between 4% and 40% [5–11]. In a study on Asian individual, 15% had retinopathy when onset of T2DM was less than 30 years of age, compared to 8% in patient with onset after 30 years [12]. The duration of diabetes was 11 and 6 years in early onset and late onset, respectively. In patients with early onset T2DM significant DR has been shown to increase from 5.7% to 26.6% when the duration of follow-up increased from 10 years to 20 years [13]. In Wisconsin Epidemiologic Study of Diabetic Retinopathy (WESDR) cohort, Klein et al. have reported an overall prevalence of proliferative diabetic retinopathy (PDR) at 41% [14]. In an Indian study on young onset DM, DR was present in 53.3% people with T1DM and 52.7% with T2DM [15]. Raman et al. have reported that prevalence of DR was significantly higher in early onset diabetes at 33.3% compared to 15.6% in those with late onset [16]. India Retinal Disease Study group reported significantly higher prevalence of PDR with high-risk characteristics in diabetics with age of onset (AOD) <25 group at baseline and at 12-month follow-up compared to diabetics with AOD>25 group [17].

The leading cause for vision loss in diabetic patients is diabetic macular edema (DME). It has been estimated that over a 25-year study period, of the 515,000–1.3 million Americans thought to have type 1 diabetes at present, approximately 149,000–377,000 will develop macular edema (ME) and 88,000–21,000 will develop clinically significant macular edema (CSME) [18].

19.2 Diabetic Macular Edema

19.2.1 Epidemiology

Wang et al. have reported 39.3% prevalence of DME in the patients with early onset diabetes compared to 14.4% in late onset DM and was significantly higher [19]. Also moderate non-proliferative diabetic retinopathy (NPDR), severe NPDR, PDR, and CSME were consistently higher in early onset diabetes patients [19]. In another study, prevalence of CSME was 5.9% and 7.5% for the younger onset type 1 and type 2 DM groups, respectively [20]. In type 1 DM the 10-year incidence of any DR and DME was 35.90% and 11.07%, respectively [21]. Klein et al. have reported 25-year cumulative incidence of ME and CSME in type 1 DM as 29% and 17%, respectively [18]. In the same study the annualized incidences of ME were reported as 2.3%, 2.1%, 2.3%, and 0.9% in the first, second, third, and fourth follow-up periods, respectively. In WESDR cohort of type 1 DM patients, Klein et al. have reported the estimated prevalence of PDR as 41.0% per person visit and 23.8% for macular edema [14]. The estimated incidence of PDR was reported as 1.21% and 0.77% for macular edema in the same study [14]. In an Indian study (young onset DM), DME was present in 10% of T1DM patients and 12.7% of T2DM patients [15]. India Retinal Disease Study group reported severe DME in 23% of people with AOD above 25 compared to 15% in people with AOD under 25 [17]. Table 19.1 depicts the prevalence/incidence of DME in early onset diabetes.

S. Sinha (✉)
Regional Institute of Ophthalmology, Indira Gandhi Institute of Medical Sciences, Patna, Bihar, India

S. Saxena et al. (eds.), *Diabetic Macular Edema*, https://doi.org/10.1007/978-981-19-7307-9_19

Table 19.1 Table showing prevalence/incidence of diabetic macular edema in young onset diabetes

Sl. no	Study	Type of diabetes mellitus	Prevalence of diabetic macular edema
1.	Wang et al. [19]	Early onset DM	39.3% (DME)
2.	Klein et al. [14]	Type 1 DM	Prevalence: 23.8% (ME) Incidence:0.77% (ME)
3.	Rajlakshmi [15]	Type 1 DM Type 2 DM	10% 12.7%
4.	Romero-Aroca et al. [21]	Type 1 DM	11.07% (DME)
5.	Klein et al. [18]	Type 1 DM	25 year cumulative incidence ME:29% CSME: 17%
6.	Romero et al. [22]	Type 1 DM	20.5% (ME)
7.	Hirai et al. [20]	Type 1 DM	5.9% (CSME)

CSME clinically significant macular edema, *DME* diabetic macular edema, *DM* diabetes mellitus, *ME* macular edema

The exact mechanisms of the higher prevalence of DR and DME among young-onset diabetic patients are yet to be unravelled. The plausible mechanisms include: more active expression of the vascular endothelial growth factor in younger patients, metabolic memory or irreversible vascular damage after a prolonged uncontrolled hyperglycemia among young patients along with higher level of psychological pressure among young- and middle-aged working people [23–28].

19.2.2 Risk Factors

19.2.2.1 Glycemic Control

Hyperglycemia has been strongly associated with the incidence of ME.

Type 1 DM: Klein et al. have reported that lower levels of glycosylated hemoglobin were associated with lower incidence of ME irrespective of duration of diabetes [18]. In the study an increase of 1% in the glycosylated hemoglobin between baseline and follow-up was associated with an increase of 22% in 21-year cumulative incidence of ME [18]. Similarly 1% decrease in the glycosylated hemoglobin level from baseline to 4-year follow-up would lead to 24% decrease in the 14-year incidence of macular edema [29]. Intensive glycemic control was associated with 46% reduction in incidence of ME in type 1 diabetes compared to conventional group in Diabetes Control and Complications Trial [30]. Increased duration of diabetes and high levels of HbA1c have been reported as risk factors for DME in type 1 DM [21, 22]. Insulin use was associated with DME in both early and late onset DM patients [19].

19.2.2.2 Hypertension

Incidence of ME was associated with increased systolic blood pressure [18]. Various studies have reported inconsistent association between prevalence and incidence of ME with blood pressure in persons with type 1 diabetes [21, 22, 31–33].

19.2.2.3 Diabetic Nephropathy

Overt nephropathy has been associated with the development of DME in type 1 DM [21]. Proteinuria was found to be marginally associated with the incidence of ME in WESDR cohort [18]. Microalbuminuria has also been significantly associated with DME [19]. Furthermore, the presence of ESRD was reported as a stronger correlate for DME than serum lipids, HbA1c or duration of DM [14].

19.2.2.4 Lipid Profile

There are several studies with conflicting results regarding association of serum lipids and DME. In type 1 DM, TC/HDL-C and ApoB/ApoA1 ratio have been found to positively correlate with the incidence of DME [21]. High levels of triglycerides and LDL cholesterol also have been associated with the development of DME in type 1 DM [22]. In the WESDR cohort in type 1 DM, no association was reported between total serum cholesterol or HDL and incidence of DME [14].

19.2.3 Other Risk Factors

Smoking and body mass index have not been found to be associated with DME of young [14].

19.3 Diagnosis

Optical coherence tomography (OCT) helps in classification and characterization of DME.

19.3.1 Central Subfoveal Thickness

A decrease in central subfoveal thickness (CST) on OCT is a reliable objective measure of anatomical response in the treatment of DME. It is also considered the most common secondary anatomical outcome measure used to substantiate primary visual outcomes in treatment of DME but is not definitive predictor of visual outcome [34]. CST of similar thickness may have varying neuronal atrophy and Müller cell dysfunction that may relate better to visual outcomes. CST reduction has to be qualified with other morphological OCT features to predict visual outcome [34].

19.3.2 Morphological Phenotypes

There are several OCT morphological phenotypes of DME. The most common classification used by clinician are: diffuse thickening type (sponge like diffuse retinal thickening), cystoid macular edema type, serous retinal detachment (SRD), and mixed type [35] (Figs. 19.1, 19.2, 19.3, 19.4). In patients with type 1 DM, 56.52 had CME, 34.78 had spongiform edema and rest were mixed [22]. In a recent study in patients with early onset DM, CME was the most common pattern followed by NSD and spongiform edema [36]. Hard exudates and hyperreflective foci were frequently seen on OCT at presentation. The presence of intracystic retinal hyperreflective material, disorganization of retinal inner layers, and external limiting membrane disruption were not routinely seen at presentation in these patients [34]. Also in the same study, 5% of the eyes were reported to have tractional diabetic maculopathy. The individuals with CME, NSD, or a

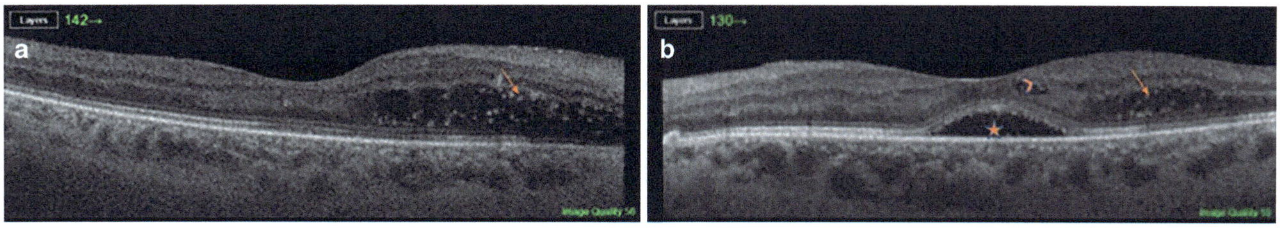

Fig. 19.1 OCT macula of a young 35-year-old early onset type 2 DM patient depicting DME. (**a**) OCT macula shows spongiform edema with hyper reflective foci (arrow). (**b**) OCT macula shows mixed macular edema with subretinal fluid (asterisk) and spongiform edema. Intracystic hyperreflective material is depicted by arrowhead

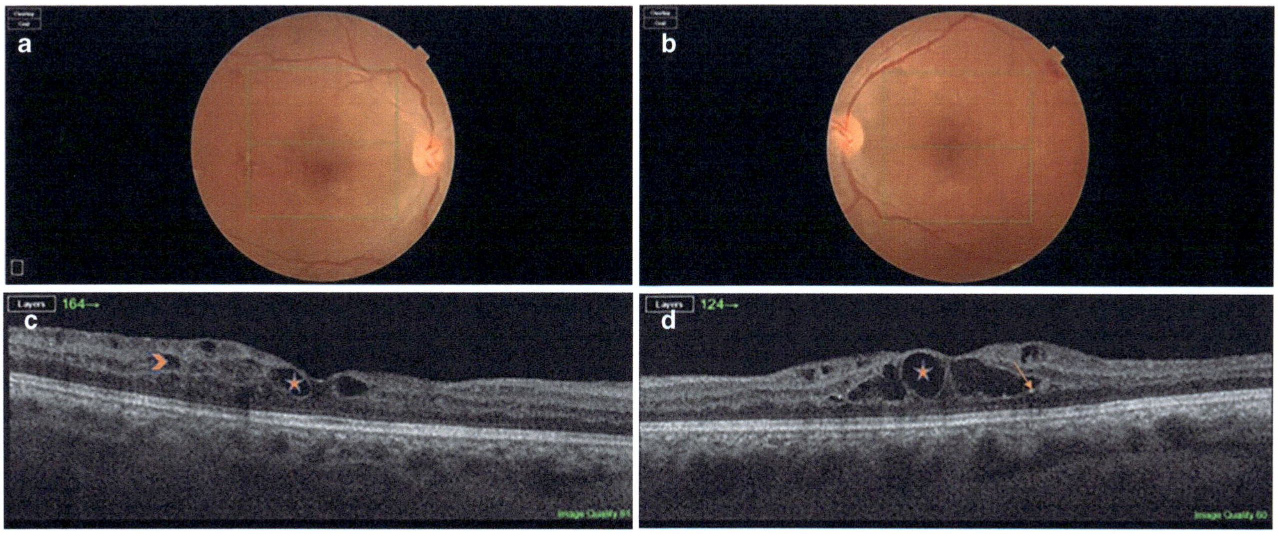

Fig. 19.2 (**a**, **b**) Fundus photo of a 19-year-old type 1 DM girl showing moderate nonproliferative diabetic retinopathy with DME. (**c**) OCT macula of right eye shows mixed DME phenotypic pattern with intact outer retinal layers, asterisk denoting cystoid macular edema and arrowhead pointing towards spongiform edema. (**d**) OCT macula of left eye depicts mixed DME phenotypic pattern with asterisk denoting cystoid macular edema and arrow signifying hyperreflective foci

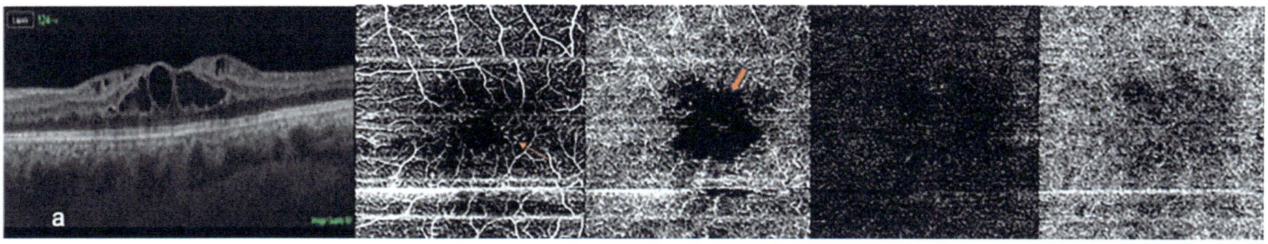

Fig. 19.3 OCT macula and OCT angiography of the same 19-year-old type 1 DM. The enface image of superficial capillary plexus shows distorted foveal avascular zone (FAZ) with arrow denoting microaneurysm with increased intercapillary distance. The enface image of deep capillary plexus shows an enlarged and distorted (FAZ)

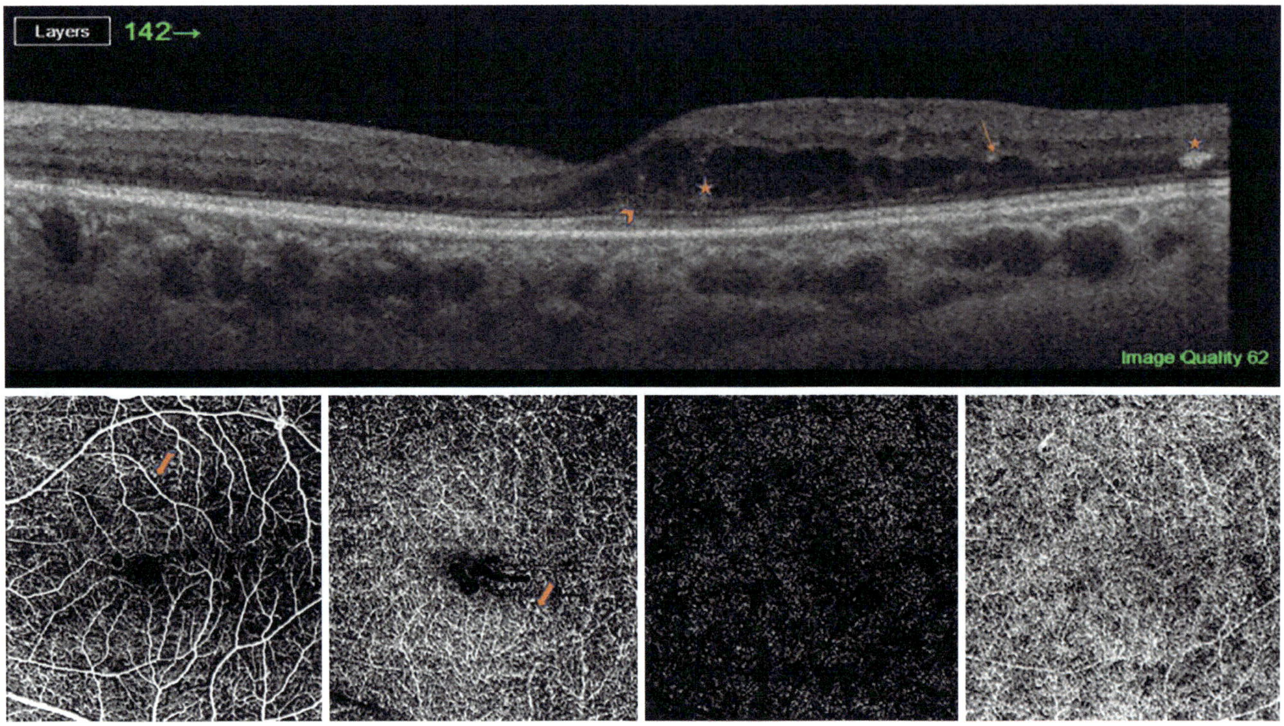

Fig. 19.4 OCT macula showing mixed diabetic macular edema with disruption of external limiting membrane (arrowhead), hyperreflective foci with no backshadowing (arrow), and hard exudate with backshadowing (asterisk). On OCTA: The enface image of superficial capillary plexus and deep capillary plexus shows distorted foveal avascular zone (FAZ) with arrow denoting microaneurysm with increased intercapillary distance

combination of both had poor vision and increased central retinal thickness (CRT) compared with patients with spongiform DME [34].

19.3.3 Hyperreflective Foci

Hyperreflective foci (HRF) were first described by Bolz et al. [37]. They are small, well-circumscribed deposits with high reflectance on OCT (Figs. 19.1, 19.2, 19.4). It has been hypothesized that HRF are cells involved in the inflammatory response like aggregations of activated microglia [38, 39]. Another hypothesis suggests that HRF could represent migrating retinal pigment epithelium cells or degenerated photoreceptor cells as they are associated with disruption of the photoreceptor layer [40, 41]. In a study in type 1 DM patients, significantly higher numbers of HRF were present in all stages of DME versus patients without DME and was independently associated with loss in visual acuity [42].

They can be used in combination with other OCT biomarkers to optimize monitoring and predict treatment strategy. The clinical relevance has also been demonstrated as a predictor for treatment response to intravitreal anti-vascular endothelial growth factor or corticosteroid therapy in DME [43, 44].

19.3.4 Angiographic Manifestations in DME

Fluorescein angiography (FA) can distinguish nonleaking from leaking microaneurysms (MA), identify IRMA, also delineates areas of capillary nonperfusion and foveal avascular zone (FAZ) in the macular retina. FA can identify areas of peripheral retinal ischemia and also macular ischemia. DME has also been correlated with peripheral retinal ischemia. A direct correlation between peripheral retinal ischemia with DME has been reported [45, 46]. FFA helps to differentiate between focal leak and diffuse capillary bed leak in cases of DME and plays an important role in focal or grid laser [47, 48].

19.3.4.1 OCT Angiography

OCT angiography (OCTA) helps in the evaluation of the perifoveal vascular network at different levels that are superficial capillary plexus (SCP), deep capillary plexus (DCP), and choriocapillaries [49]. It also helps to identify early changes such as capillary dilatation, FAZ enlargement, impaired capillary perfusion in paramacular areas, or presence of microaneurysms in a noninvasive way [50, 51]. OCT-A in patients with both type 1 diabetes with retinopathy reveals deterioration in FAZ and vessel density in the SCP and DCP with DR progression [52]. In type 1 DM, early DCP vascular alteration was found even before the diagnosis of clinically detectable DR [53, 54]. In diabetic macular ischemia nonperfusion of DCP is associated with photoreceptor disruption [55]. Poor response to anti-VEGF agents in DME has been associated with damage to the integrity of the DCP irrespective of SCP [56]. OCTA features have been described in Figs. 19.3, 19.4.

19.4 Treatment

19.4.1 Laser Therapy

Laser treatment was standard of care for DME for more than three decades. Currently, the relative indications are laser application in vasogenic subform of DME characterized by focally grouped MA and leaking capillaries [57]. Also eyes with DME with CRT less than 300 µm or eyes with persisting vitreomacular adhesion can be considered for laser therapy as comparable results have been achieved by laser photocoagulation or anti-VEGF injections [58]. Subthreshold grid laser treatment can be considered in eyes with higher visual acuity affected by early diffuse DME as a less expensive option with less chorioretinal damage [57].

DME has been correlated with peripheral retinal ischemia as ischemia leads to increased VEGF production [45, 46]. Targeted retinal photocoagulation with anti-VEGF therapy leads to better response in these patients. It has been reported that mean decrease in central macular thickness is correlated inversely with ischemic index as measured on ultra-widefield FA [46].

19.4.2 Steroids

Anti-VEGF agents are considered as a first-line option for DME, but dexamethasone (DEX) implant can also be used in patients with naive DME and not only for refractory cases [59]. Steroids can be used as the first-line therapy in patients who have a history of a major cardiovascular event and also in patients who are not willing for monthly injections [57]. DEX implant should be considered early in patients not responding to monthly anti-VEGF injections to allow optimal treatment outcomes. Fluocinolone acetonide implant should be considered in cases with chronic DME not responsive to other treatment after they have been proven to be nonsteroid responders [57, 59]. TA causes more increase in IOP and cataract and needs to be reinjected frequently and hence should be considered in cases who cannot receive the approved agents [57, 59].

19.4.3 Anti-VEGF Therapy

The anti-VEGF remains the preferred modality for treatment of DME. DME in the young people with diabetes was observed more commonly with proliferative disease. Also the development of DME from increased VEGF secretion favors treatment with intravitreal anti-VEGF injections [57]. Intraocular steroids are avoided because of the risk of cataract and glaucoma in young patients. In an Indian study, mean number of intravitreal injections were comparable between diabetics with AOD <25 and more than 25 years group [17].

19.4.4 Surgery

DME surgery should be considered based on the evaluation of the vitreous and retinal status. The following are indications for pars plana vitrectomy (PPV) in eyes with DME: presence of anterior–posterior traction and tangential traction due to an epiretinal or hyaloid membrane. In case of tangential traction PPV should be considered only when the response to anti-VEGF or dexamethasone implants is incomplete. In cases with no evidence of traction there is no consensus regarding the advantages of PPV [57].

19.5 Systemic Diabetic Disease and Management

19.5.1 The Role of Metabolic Control

Diabetes mellitus is a systemic disease with microvascular and macrovascular complications. Therefore, the role of metabolic control should be evaluated in treatment of diabetic retinopathy and DME. Hypertension also worsens DME and needs to be managed through systemic approach. Early ocular intervention is very important and systemic work up should not delay the retinal intervention. A communication between diabetologist and retinologist is important as tightness of glycemic control and fluctuations in this regimen influences the progression of diabetic retinopathy [57].

19.6 Conclusion

The burden of diabetes and diabetic macular edema in young patients is increasing. Intravitreal anti VEGF agents are effective modality of treatment but requires multiple injections per year. This contributes to treatment burden for both patients and healthcare system. Increase of 1% in the glycosylated hemoglobin between baseline and follow-up was associated with an increase of 22% in 21-year cumulative incidence of ME. Therefore, a collaborative effort involving patient, the primary care provider and the ophthalmologist is necessary to lower the health care burden and optimize clinical outcomes for this sight-threatening complication of diabetes.

References

1. Wang L, Li X, Wang Z, et al. Trends in prevalence of diabetes and control of risk factors in diabetes among US adults, 1999-2018. JAMA. 2021;326(8):704–16. https://doi.org/10.1001/jama.2021.9883.
2. Lawrence JM, Divers J, Isom S, et al. Trends in prevalence of type 1 and type 2 diabetes in children and adolescents in the US, 2001-2017. JAMA. 2021;326(8):717–27. https://doi.org/10.1001/jama.2021.11165.
3. Bourne RR, Jonas JB, Bron AM, Cicinelli MV, Das A, Flaxman SR, Friedman DS, Keeffe JE, Kempen JH, Leasher J, Limburg H. Prevalence and causes of vision loss in high-income countries and in eastern and Central Europe in 2015: magnitude, temporal trends and projections. Br J Ophthalmol. 2018;102(5):575–85.
4. Cooper OA, Taylor DJ, Crabb DP, Sim DA, McBain H. Psychological, social and everyday visual impact of diabetic macular oedema and diabetic retinopathy: a systematic review. Diabet Med. 2020;37(6):924–33.
5. Eppens MC, Craig ME, Cusumano J, Hing S, Chan AK, Howard NJ, Silink M, Donaghue KC. Prevalence of diabetes complications in adolescents with type 2 compared with type 1 diabetes. Diabetes Care. 2006;29(6):1300–6.
6. Krakoff J, Lindsay RS, Looker HC, Nelson RG, Hanson RL, Knowler WC. Incidence of retinopathy and nephropathy in youth-onset compared with adult-onset type 2 diabetes. Diabetes Care. 2003;26(1):76–81.
7. Okudaira M, Yokoyama H, Otani T, Uchigata Y, Iwamoto Y. Slightly elevated blood pressure as well as poor metabolic control are risk factors for the progression of retinopathy in early-onset Japanese type 2 diabetes. J Diabetes Complications. 2000;14(5):281–7.
8. Pavkov ME, Bennett PH, Knowler WC, Krakoff J, Sievers ML, Nelson RG. Effect of youth-onset type 2 diabetes mellitus on incidence of end-stage renal disease and mortality in young and middle-aged Pima Indians. JAMA. 2006;296(4):421–6.
9. Scott A, Toomath R, Bouchier D, Bruce R, Crook N, Carroll D, Cutfield R, Dixon P, Doran J, Dunn P, Hotu C. First national audit of the outcomes of care in young people with diabetes in New Zealand: high prevalence of nephropathy in Māori and Pacific islanders. N Z Med J. 2006;119(1235):U2015.
10. Yokoyama H, Okudaira M, Otani T, Watanabe C, Takaike H, Miuira J, Yamada H, Mutou K, Satou A, Uchigata Y, Iwamoto Y. High incidence of diabetic nephropathy in early-onset Japanese NIDDM patients: risk analysis. Diabetes Care. 1998;21(7):1080–5.
11. TODAY Study Group. Retinopathy in youth with type 2 diabetes participating in the TODAY clinical trial. Diabetes Care. 2013;36(6):1772–4.
12. Chuang LM, Soegondo S, Soewondo P, Young-Seol K, Mohamed M, Dalisay E, Go R, Lee W, Tong-Yuan T, Tandhanand S, Nitiyanant W. Comparisons of the outcomes on control, type of management and complications status in early onset and late onset type 2 diabetes in Asia. Diabetes Res Clin Pract. 2006;71(2):146–55.
13. Song SH, Gray TA. Early-onset type 2 diabetes: high risk for premature diabetic retinopathy. Diabetes Res Clin Pract. 2011;94(2):207–11.
14. Klein BE, Myers CE, Howard KP, Klein R. Serum lipids and proliferative diabetic retinopathy and macular edema in persons with long-term type 1 diabetes mellitus: the Wisconsin epidemiologic study of diabetic retinopathy. JAMA ophthalmol. 2015;133(5):503–10.
15. Rajalakshmi R, Amutha A, Ranjani H, Ali MK, Unnikrishnan R, Anjana RM, Narayan KV, Mohan V. Prevalence and risk factors for diabetic retinopathy in Asian Indians with young onset type 1 and type 2 diabetes. J Diabetes Complications. 2014;28(3):291–7.
16. Raman R, Vaitheeswaran K, Vinita K, Sharma T. Is prevalence of retinopathy related to the age of onset of diabetes? Sankara Nethralaya diabetic retinopathy epidemiology and molecular genetic report no. 5. Ophthalmic Res. 2011;45:36–41.
17. Parameswarappa DC, Rajalakshmi R, Mohamed A, Kavya S, Munirathnam H, Manayath G, Kumar MA, Raman R, Vignesh TP, Ramasamy K, Mani S, Muralidhar A, Agarwal M, Anantharaman G, Bijlani N, Chawla G, Sen A, Kulkarni S, Behera UC, Sivaprasad S, Das T, Rani PK. Severity of diabetic retinopathy and its relationship with age at onset of diabetes mellitus in India: a multicentric study. Indian J Ophthalmol. 2021;69(11):3255–61. . PMID: 34708783; PMCID: PMC8725142. https://doi.org/10.4103/ijo.IJO_1459_21.
18. Klein R, Knudtson MD, Lee KE, Gangnon R, Klein BE. The Wisconsin epidemiologic study of diabetic retinopathy XXIII: the twenty-five-year incidence of macular edema in persons with type 1 diabetes. Ophthalmology. 2009;116(3):497–503.
19. Wang Y, Lin Z, Zhai G, Ding XX, Wen L, Li D, Zou B, Feng KM, Liang YB, Xie C. Prevalence of and risk factors for diabetic retinopathy and diabetic macular edema in patients with early and late onset diabetes mellitus. Ophthalmic Res. 2020;65(3):293–9.
20. Hirai FE, Knudtson MD, Klein BE, Klein R. Clinically significant macular edema and survival in type 1 and type 2 diabetes. Am J Ophthalmol. 2008;145(4):700–6.
21. Romero-Aroca P, Baget-Bernaldiz M, Fernandez-Ballart J, Plana-Gil N, Soler-Lluis N, Mendez-Marin I, Bautista-Perez A. Ten-year incidence of diabetic retinopathy and macular edema. Risk factors in a sample of people with type 1 diabetes. Diabetes Res Clin Pract. 2011;94(1):126–32.
22. Romero P, Baget M, Mendez I, Fernández J, Salvat M, Martinez I. Diabetic macular edema and its relationship to renal microangiopathy: a sample of type I diabetes mellitus patients in a 15-year follow-up study. J Diabetes Complications. 2007;21(3):172–80.
23. Chiarelli F, Spagnoli A, Basciani F, Tumini S, Mezzetti A, Cipollone F, Cuccurullo F, Morgese G, Verrotti A. Vascular endothelial growth factor (VEGF) in children, adolescents and young adults with type 1 diabetes mellitus: relation to glycaemic control and microvascular complications. Diabet Med. 2000;17:650–6.
24. Zhong Q, Kowluru RA. Epigenetic modification of sod2 in the development of diabetic retinopathy and in the metabolic memory: role of histone methylation. Invest Ophthalmol Vis Sci. 2013;54:244–50.
25. Kowluru RA. Mitochondria damage in the pathogenesis of diabetic retinopathy and in the metabolic memory associated with its continued progression. Curr Med Chem. 2013;20:3226–33.
26. Reddy MA, Zhang E, Natarajan R. Epigenetic mechanisms in diabetic complications and metabolic memory. Diabetologia. 2015;58:443–55.
27. Fenwick E, Rees G, Pesudovs K, Dirani M, Kawasaki R, Wong TY, Lamoureux E. Social and emotional impact of diabetic retinopathy: a review. Clin Experiment Ophthalmol. 2012;40:27–38.
28. Kalantari S, Jafarinezhad A, Zohrevand B. Association of depression with type 2 diabetes and relevant factors. Adv Biomed Res. 2014;3:244.

29. Klein R, Klein BE, Moss SE, Cruickshanks KJ. The Wisconsin epidemiologic study of diabetic retinopathy: XVII: the 14-year incidence and progression of diabetic retinopathy and associated risk factors in type 1 diabetes. Ophthalmology. 1998;105(10):1801–15.
30. Diabetes control and complications trial/epidemiology of diabetes interventions and complications research group. Retinopathy and nephropathy in patients with type 1 diabetes four years after a trial of intensive therapy. N Engl J Med. 2000;342(6):381–9.
31. Vitale S, Maguire MG, Murphy RP, et al. Clinically significant macular edema in type I diabetes: incidence and risk factors. Ophthalmology. 1995;102:1170–6.
32. Aroca PR, Salvat M, Fernández J, Méndez I. Risk factors for diffuse and focal macular edema. J Diabetes Complications. 2004;18(4):211–5.
33. Roy MS, Affouf M. Six-year progression of retinopathy and associated risk factors in African American patients with type 1 diabetes mellitus: the New Jersey 725. Arch Ophthalmol. 2006;124(9):1297–306.
34. Sen S, Ramasamy K, Sivaprasad S. Indicators of visual prognosis in diabetic macular Oedema. J Pers Med. 2021;11(6):449.
35. Otani T, Kishi S, Maruyama Y. Patterns of diabetic macular edema with optical coherence tomography. Am J Ophthalmol. 1999;127(6):688–93.
36. Reddy NG, Venkatesh R, Jayadev C, Gadde SGK, Agrawal S, Mishra P, Yadav NK, Chhablani J. Diabetic retinopathy and diabetic macular edema in people with early-onset diabetes. Clin Diabetes. 2022;40:cd210110. (in press). https://doi.org/10.2337/cd21-0110.
37. Bolz M, Schmidt-Erfurth U, Deak G, Mylonas G, Kriechbaum K, Scholda C, Diabetic Retinopathy Research Group Vienna. Optical coherence tomographic hyperreflective foci: a morphologic sign of lipid extravasation in diabetic macular edema. Ophthalmology. 2009;116(5):914–20.
38. Coscas G, De Benedetto U, Coscas F, et al. Hyperreflective dots: a new spectral-domain optical coherence tomography entity for follow-up and prognosis in exudative age-related macular degeneration. Ophthalmologica. 2013;229:32–7.
39. Framme C, Schweizer P, Imesch M, Wolf S, Wolf-Schnurrbusch U. Behavior of SD-OCT–detected hyperreflective foci in the retina of anti-VEGF–treated patients with diabetic macular edema. Invest Ophthalmol Vis Sci. 2012;53(9):5814–8.
40. Uji A, Murakami T, Nishijima K, Akagi T, Horii T, Arakawa N, Muraoka Y, Ellabban AA, Yoshimura N. Association between hyperreflective foci in the outer retina, status of photoreceptor layer, and visual acuity in diabetic macular edema. Am J Ophthalmol. 2012;153(4):710–7.
41. Framme C, Wolf S, Wolf-Schnurrbusch U. Small dense particles in the retina observable by spectral-domain optical coherence tomography in age-related macular degeneration. Invest Ophthalmol Vis Sci. 2010;51(11):5965–9.
42. Schreur V, de Breuk A, Venhuizen FG, Sánchez CI, Tack CJ, Klevering BJ, de Jong EK, Hoyng CB. Retinal hyperreflective foci in type 1 diabetes mellitus. Retina. 2020;40(8):1565.
43. Schreur V, Altay L, van Asten F, Groenewoud JM, Fauser S, Klevering BJ, Hoyng CB, de Jong EK. Hyperreflective foci on optical coherence tomography associate with treatment outcome for anti-VEGF in patients with diabetic macular edema. PLoS One. 2018;13(10):e0206482.
44. Hwang HS, Chae JB, Kim JY, Kim DY. Association between hyperreflective dots on spectral-domain optical coherence tomography in macular edema and response to treatment. Invest Ophthalmol Vis Sci. 2017;58(13):5958–67.
45. Wessel MM, Nair N, Aaker GD, Ehrlich JR, D'Amico DJ, Kiss S. Peripheral retinal ischaemia, as evaluated by ultra-widefield fluorescein angiography, is associated with diabetic macular oedema. Br J Ophthalmol. 2012;96(5):694–8.
46. Patel RD, Messner LV, Teitelbaum B, Michel KA, Hariprasad SM. Characterization of ischemic index using ultra-widefield fluorescein angiography in patients with focal and diffuse recalcitrant diabetic macular edema. Am J Ophthalmol. 2013;155(6):1038–44.
47. Photocoagulation for diabetic macular edema. Early treatment diabetic retinopathy study report number 1. Arch Ophthalmol. 1985;103:1796–806.
48. Kylstra JA, Brown JC, Jaffe GJ, et al. The importance of fluorescein angiography in planning laser treatment of diabetic macular edema. Ophthalmology. 1999;106:2068–73.
49. Spaide RF, Klancnik JM, Cooney MJ. Retinal vascular layers imaged by fluorescein angiography and optical coherence tomography angiography. JAMA ophthalmol. 2015;133(1):45–50. https://doi.org/10.1001/jamaophthalmol.2014.3616.
50. Jia Y, Bailey ST, Hwang TS, McClintic SM, Gao SS, Pennesi ME, Flaxel CJ, Lauer AK, Wilson DJ, Hornegger J, Fujimoto JG. Quantitative optical coherence tomography angiography of vascular abnormalities in the living human eye. Proc Natl Acad Sci. 2015;112(18):E2395–402.
51. Ishibazawa A, Nagaoka T, Takahashi A, Omae T, Tani T, Sogawa K, Yokota H, Yoshida A. Optical coherence tomography angiography in diabetic retinopathy: a prospective pilot study. Am J Ophthalmol. 2015;160(1):35–44.
52. Um T, Seo EJ, Kim YJ, Yoon YH. Optical coherence tomography angiography findings of type 1 diabetic patients with diabetic retinopathy, in comparison with type 2 patients. Graefes Arch Clin Exp Ophthalmol. 2020;258(2):281–8.
53. Carnevali A, Sacconi R, Corbelli E, Tomasso L, Querques L, Zerbini G, Scorcia V, Bandello F, Querques G. Optical coherence tomography angiography analysis of retinal vascular plexuses and choriocapillaris in patients with type 1 diabetes without diabetic retinopathy. Acta Diabetol. 2017;54(7):695–702.
54. Inanc M, Tekin K, Kiziltoprak H, Ozalkak S, Doguizi S, Aycan Z. Changes in retinal microcirculation precede the clinical onset of diabetic retinopathy in children with type 1 diabetes mellitus. Am J Ophthalmol. 2019;207:37–44. https://doi.org/10.1016/j.ajo.2019.04.011.
55. Scarinci F, Nesper PL, Fawzi AA. Deep retinal capillary nonperfusion is associated with photoreceptor disruption in diabetic macular ischemia. Am J Ophthalmol. 2016;168:129–38. https://doi.org/10.1016/j.ajo.2016.05.002.
56. Lee J, Moon BG, Cho AR, Yoon YH. Optical coherence tomography angiography of DME and its association with antiVEGF treatment response. Ophthalmology. 2016;123(11):2368–75. https://doi.org/10.1016/j.ophtha.2016.07.010.
57. Schmidt-Erfurth U, Garcia-Arumi J, Bandello F, Berg K, Chakravarthy U, Gerendas BS, Jonas J, Larsen M, Tadayoni R, Loewenstein A. Guidelines for the management of diabetic macular edema by the European Society of Retina Specialists (EURETINA). Ophthalmologica. 2017;237(4):185–222.
58. Mitchell P, Bandello F, Schmidt-Erfurth U, Lang GE, Massin P, Schlingemann RO, Sutter F, Simader C, Burian G, Gerstner O, Weichselberger A. The RESTORE study: ranibizumab monotherapy or combined with laser versus laser monotherapy for diabetic macular edema. Ophthalmology. 2011;118:615–25.
59. Zur D, Iglicki M, Loewenstein A. The role of steroids in the management of diabetic macular edema. Ophthalmic Res. 2019;62(4):231–6. https://doi.org/10.1159/000499540.

Diabetic Retinopathy and Diabetic Macular Edema: Fighting the Emerging Global Burden

20

Harsha Bhattacharjee, Manabjyoti Barman, and Mohit Garg

20.1 Introduction

Type 2 diabetes mellitus (DM) is preventable in the population through change in dietary quality, modification of physical activity, mitigation of the risk factors and control of obesity [1–4]. At the same time regular screening can detect diabetes early and screening for diabetic complications through well-organised programme can reduce chronic morbidity, complication and improve the quality and expectancy of life. Proper diet, regular medication, good glycaemic control and elimination of risk factors can modify the disease and break the cycle of its chronic pathogenesis [5–7]. The fact is that globally burden of diabetic microvascular complications including diabetic retinopathy (DR), diabetic macular oedema (DME) and related blindness and other morbidities are increasing. In reality, the diabetic health burden is apprehended to reach epidemic proportion in near future [8]. The impact will be not only in personal life but also on the social community and will adversely affect economy of the country due to missed production opportunity and rising healthcare expenditure. Increase in the burden of DME also indicates the mass people are missing the opportunity of evidence based preventive and curative eye care and healthcare as well, particularly in the low-income countries where public health spending is less and mostly eye care and health care as a whole is an out of pocket expenditure of the affective individual [9–11]. While public spending for control of diabetes can prove to be a burden in short term, it can be paid off in the long run by gain in productivity and increase in quality of life [5, 9, 12–16].

H. Bhattacharjee · M. Barman · M. Garg (✉)
Sri Sankaradeva Nethralaya, Guwahati, Assam, India

20.2 Understanding the Disease Burden

Diabetes, its complications and their impact, are a huge public health concern. According to WHO, the number of people with diabetes rose from 108 million in 1980 to 422 million in 2014. The International diabetes federation (IDF) estimated the global population with DM to be 463 million in 2019 and 700 million in 2045. 80% of people suffering from diabetes resides in low- and middle-income countries [17]. Diabetic retinopathy is one of the leading causes of vision loss and has a huge impact on the quality of life, social well-being and financial health of the affected individual. Apprehended global impact and cost will grow substantially and will effect mostly in the lower and middle class income countries, and economically marginalised people of high-income countries [18–20]. It is estimated that 1 in 3 patients with diabetes suffer from DR and 1 in 10 suffer from vision threatening diabetic eye disease [21]. DME is one of the main causes of visual impairment in patients suffering from diabetic retinopathy. A 2015–2018 Global prevalence of diabetes related retinopathy study reported prevalence of DR in 27% including 25.2% Non-Proliferative Diabetic Retinopathy (NPDR), 1.4% Proliferative Diabetic Retinopathy (PDR) and 4.6% of DME amongst diabetic population across the world and there was considerable regional variation of prevalence and incidences [22]. The presence of DME leads to a greater financial burden, higher utilisation of healthcare services and a deterioration of quality of life, which is more significant than those suffering from DR without DME [10].

With the projected increase in the incidence of diabetes due to rapid urbanisation, ageing population and changing food habits, the burden of diabetic retinopathy is also expected to increase in the future [23]. Also with high rate of increase in the burden of the disease, increasing urbanisation and sedentary lifestyle we run the risk of the burden surpassing the health system's capacity, especially in the developing and underdeveloped countries.

In order to address the public health burden due to diabetic retinopathy, we have to develop a thorough understand-

S. Saxena et al. (eds.), *Diabetic Macular Edema*, https://doi.org/10.1007/978-981-19-7307-9_20

ing of the epidemiology of the disease. The distribution of the disease in various ethnic and racial groups has been studied extensively but is not yet conclusive [24, 25]. Environmental factors leading to the development and progression of DR have also been studied in various studies [21, 26, 27]. Many risk factors such as the duration of diabetes, glycaemic control, hypertension, dyslipidaemia, etc. have been identified. But these risk factors have not been able to satisfactorily explain the risk susceptibility. For instance, in some patients despite of good glycaemic control and shorter duration of disease DR is present while in some despite of poor glycaemic control and longer disease duration no evidence of DR is present [28, 29]. Similar discrepancies have been observed with other risk factors also. This suggests that certain other, yet to be identified, risk factors also play a significant role in the development of diabetic retinopathy. One such possibility is genetic susceptibility. Genetics may play an essential role potentially explaining various aspects of DR like incidence, pathogenesis, hereditability and progression of the disease. However, accumulated evidences and different candidate studies that have tried to identify genetic loci for DR susceptibility have not been able to come to a conclusion due to discrepancy in the results and the level of inheritance could not be ascertained [30, 31]. Studies have observed differences in DR heritability and differences in response to anti-VEGF therapy in different individuals. This suggests that further research is required to completely understand the genetics of diabetic retinopathy [31].

DR can lead to DME leading to significant visual loss. Newer investigative modalities such as OCT and treatment options like anti-VEGF molecules have improved diagnosis and treatment outcomes. But still we have a large number of patients who are either refractory to treatment or develop a chronic disease. Also studies have identified the fact that therapeutic response depends on clinical and demographic patient characteristics. This points to the fact that our understanding of the disease and factors affecting its progression is not yet complete and further research is required.

Even though the epidemiological understanding of the disease is not yet complete, we have obtained some consistent findings across studies. A uniform, up to date and population oriented strategy focused on the control of these identified risk factors has to be formulated and implemented. Also, a continuous and patient inquiry into the causation and risk stratification of the disease has to go on by the means of quality peer-reviewed scientific population based research.

20.3 Strategies for Disease Prevention

Diabetic retinopathy has scaled to an alarming level and is expected to further increase in prevalence in the future. Tackling this challenge requires a broad population based planning and intervention aimed at decreasing the disease burden at an affordable cost. This requires a coordinated and synchronised approach with participation of government and non-governmental organisations and healthcare institutions to develop scientific guidelines for prevention of disease, outline norms and standards for diagnosis, build awareness and conduct population based surveys.

Disease prevention, as defined by WHO, includes population based and individual based interventions for primary and secondary (early detection) prevention, aiming to minimise the burden of diseases and associated risk factors.

Primordial prevention focussing on risk factor prevention is done in order to prevent healthy people from developing diabetes mellitus. Measures such as diabetes awareness building, promoting healthy diet and exercise, mobilising people at risk to attend diabetes screening camp, etc. can be undertaken with the help of telecommunication services, health care workers and community workers.

Primary prevention aims at preventing or delaying the onset of DR in people diagnosed with diabetes. Measures include good control of glycaemic status, blood pressure, serum lipids, etc. with the use of pharmacological therapies, lifestyle modification and behavioural change. The access to healthcare services has to be improved for people to be screened and diagnosed early. Mass communication and individual counselling has to be done for each diagnosed case of diabetes about the risks and complications of the disease and the means to prevent them.

Secondary prevention aims at early diagnosis of subclinical cases and preventing the progression of the disease state. For DR, this would translate to early diagnosis and treatment of the disease targeted at preventing it from progressing to a vision threatening stage. Measures include strengthening DR screening programmes with a hierarchical referral structure in order to diagnose early and treat appropriately. This requires a sensitisation of primary health care workers, optometrists, pharmacists, physicians, endocrinologists and ophthalmologists regarding the importance of screening for DR. Any opportunistic encounter with a patient at a risk of developing DR must be utilised to identify and diagnose cases of DR at all levels of healthcare system [32].

While secondary prevention aims at preventing the onset of the disease, tertiary prevention aims at reducing the impact of the disease once it has been diagnosed in an individual. It is implemented in symptomatic patients to reduce severity and prevent sequalae of the disease. Measures include laser photocoagulation for DR, anti-VEGF injections for DME and proliferative diabetic retinopathy (PDR), vitrectomy and visual rehabilitation in patients with severe vision loss.

A greater amount of focus and resources has been dedicated to tertiary prevention than primary and secondary prevention. In order to effectively fight the global burden of DR and DME, a paradigm shift in policy has to be under-

Table 20.1 Barriers to access of diabetic retinopathy screening survices and suggested approaches to overcome them

Barrier	Suggested Approach
Lack of knowledge and awareness amongst patients and physicians	Use of health education material in printed and digital format along with repeated inputs by the treating physician and ophthalmologists. The patients must be made aware about potential risks of DR and its complications and the impact it can have over the quality of life Sensitisation camps and seminars must be undertaken for primary healthcare workers, physicians and diabetologists regarding the importance of regular eye screening. They must be motivated to refer each patient at risk for eye screening and proper channels of communication must be operational between ophthalmologists and referring doctor
Lack of human resources	Training programmes for doctors, optometrists and community workers must be undertaken to sensitise them on identifiers of at risk patients. A uniform region and population specific guideline must be formulated based on evidence based medicine for early screening of patients at risk
Accessibility	Use of tele-ophthalmology with support of skilled optometrists Artificial intelligence platforms with capability to screen patients with DR Expansion of ophthalmology services with infrastructure upgradation
Financial constraints	Health and general Well-being promotion can help decrease the financial burden of treatment by preventing or delaying the onset Health insurance expansion with inclusion of procedures required for DR in the coverage Collaborated approach of government and non-governmental not for profit health organisations
Lack of motivation amongst patients for lifestyle modification	Health awareness campaigns using different medias such as print, social media etc Empowerment of patients by imparting knowledge about the disease and ways to self-monitor and improve efficacy of treatment Individualised plan for each patients to be formulated by a team of health workers such as of physician, ophthalmologist, dietician etc Increasing patient participation in healthcare decision making by involving them actively while formulating their treatment plan

[2, 3, 33]

taken. But implementation of such prevention strategies is quite complicated and presents with new challenges in different income and geographical settings. A systematic review on barriers and enablers for access to diabetic retinopathy screening services in different income settings has identified some of the barriers. Lack of knowledge, lack of awareness, low educational attainment and poor literacy, asymptomatic nature of DR, financial barriers and time and priority issues emerged as the major barriers at the recipient level of the healthcare intervention. Similarly, at the provider level accessibility issues, lack of human resources, lack of knowledge and awareness among the providers, lack of screening infrastructure, cost of services and deficiencies in educating the users reported as major barriers. A few suggestions to overcome some of these barriers are enumerated in Table 20.1.

20.4 Role of National Screening Programmes for DR and DME

Diabetes and diabetic retinopathy have grown to epidemic proportions and requires intervention at a mass level. Some countries have established national screening programmes for screening of diabetic retinopathy and are making good progress too [34–36]. But the cost of case finding in a screening programme has to balance with the possible expenditure on the medical care as a whole. Hence, in countries which are not resource rich such programmes are hindered by lack or resources or a lack of uptake by the population. Diabetic eye disease screening is mostly done as opportunistic screening when the patient is being investigated for other ailments. But these screenings are being done only in a localised defined population. A nationwide population based screening, even though complex and challenging, can be successful as demonstrated in some locations.

A national plan for screening of DR and DME has to be equitable and widespread. It has to be supplemented by a robust referral system and a trained set of health care workers well equipped with required armamentarium. Patient education, registry maintenance and population based study has to be made an integral part of the programme. In countries with resource constraint, government must partner with local and global not for profit organisations in order to successfully organise and implement such a national plan.

We also have to keep in mind that diabetic eye disease screening is just a part of the whole process of reducing the burden of visual loss due to diabetes. If done in isolation, from the treatment of diabetes, patient empowerment and inclusion in decision making and lifestyle modifications, it is bound to fail.

20.5 Role of Public Health Policy for Diabetic Retinopathy

The growing prevalence of diabetes has contributed to realisation of its public health importance and of its complications, including diabetic retinopathy (DR). The epidemic proportions that diabetic retinopathy is forecasted to achieve in the future is a serious public health concern and mandates the formulation of a public health policy centred on DR and its complications [8]. Such a policy has to clearly enumerate the guidelines for screening, diagnosis, management, follow-ups and rehabilitation of affected individuals. Provisions and targets for infrastructural and logistical support, equipment, human resource management, capacity building and public outreach have to be there. The policy has to be based on the principle of evidence based medicine and the working of the policy to be regularly monitored and the data to be used to regularly update the policy provisions. Such a policy has to have a uniform framework globally with regional variations as per special needs of the targeted population. A people centric policy focussing on collaborative care and based upon evidence based medicine and implemented with genuine political will can help us overcome the challenge of diabetes related blindness as demonstrated in some high-income countries [37, 38].

20.6 Newer Advances and Future Prospects

The current available treatment modalities and recent advances for management of DR and DME have been covered in great detail in the previous chapters. Technological advancement and scientific research has led to development of newer treatment modalities and screening tools.

20.6.1 Diagnosis and Screening

With the advent of non-mydriatic ultra-widefield fundus cameras the rate of detection of DR and referable DR has become more effective [39]. Handheld devices can help increase the accessibility of fundus imaging and screening to a widespread area and can be more cost effective. The use of artificial intelligence based models for analysis of these fundus photos is an upcoming field with promising research outcomes. Deep mind based models for diabetic retinopathy screening from fundus photos has achieved a significantly high sensitivity and specificity [40]. Use of such models can help us overcome the deficiency of skilled healthcare workers and reduce the cost burden of patient screening by automating the process.

Recently, a non-invasive imaging device was developed to measure retinal flavoprotein fluorescence (FPF) which are oxidised and reduced within the mitochondria. The study revealed a significant difference in between diabetic eyes and age matched control. A statistically significant difference was also noted between diabetic eyes with DR and diabetic eyes without DR [41]. This presents as a novel metabolic tool to assess the retinal status in diabetic patients.

20.6.2 Predictive Medicine

Predictive medicine relies on detecting a disease before its manifestation in an individual [42]. It is based upon identification of risk factors based upon population based cross sectional studies and bell curve distribution and the application of this knowledge along with the clinical acumen. Big data revolution in healthcare by the use of electronic medical records has led to development of large health information databases. Learning systems for predicting the risk of developing DR can be designed to assimilate and aggregate these databases [43]. These systems can help us design predictive models to assist ophthalmologists, develop personalised treatment plans for people at risk and generate better treatment outcomes.

20.6.3 Pharmacotherapy

In order to effectively combat the global burden of DR and DME we have to equip ourselves with the best treatment options. With the understanding of the role of VEGF (vascular endothelial growth factor) in the pathogenesis of DME and diabetic eye disease newer pharmacological treatments came to light. These anti-VEGF molecules such as ranibizumab, bevacizumab, pegaptanib, VEGF-Trap fusion molecule have been tried and tested under formal clinical trials. Significant vision improvement was seen in DME patients in trials such as the RIDE/RISE (ranibizumab versus sham injection) and VIVID/VISTA (aflibercept versus laser) studies. Out of these drugs in DME patients, the use of intravitreal ranibizumab and aflibercept has been approved by the Food and Drug Administration (FDA), but intravitreal bevacizumab still remains an off-label drug.

As monthly injection remains a burden in the use of these anti-VEGF molecules, port delivery systems are under trial. A ranibizumab port delivery system under study is a refillable, sustained delivery implant that can be placed in the pars plana using standard vitreoretinal surgical techniques without scleral sutures. It has completed phase I clinical study in wet AMD patients, and a phase II trial (LADDER, ClinicalTrials.gov NCT02510794) has been started.

But despite impressive advancements in treating diabetic retinopathy over the past two decades with anti-vascular endothelial growth factor (anti-VEGF-A) therapy, there is a great need to reduce the treatment burden from frequent injections and to improve visual outcomes. Newer pathways are being investigated for intervention in DME. Studies indicate that Rho-associated kinase (Rho-kinase/ROCK) is an essential molecule in the pathogenesis of DME and evaluation of its role in management of DME is being investigated [44]. Another pathway that is being studied is the plasma kallikrein pathway. Early studies indicate some improvement in visual acuity but limited improvement in macular oedema occurred by modulation of this pathway [45]. Further studies are warranted to ascertain whether this can be explored as a treatment option by altering dose, delivery method, etc. Similarly, small molecule integrin antagonist THR-687 is under investigation as a promising drug candidate for treatment of vision threatening DR [46]. We do not, yet, have the perfect pharmacological agent for treatment of DR and DME, but recent progress by scientific research bears great hope for the future.

20.6.4 Genetics and Epigenetics

Role of genetics in understanding the disease process and finding new treatment modalities is becoming ever more relevant. Gene therapy is designed to introduce genetic material into the cells of patients to compensate faulty genes or deliver therapeutic transgenes. Current investigations into gene therapy for DR are utilising two approaches according to disease pathophysiology: target existing neovascularization and vascular hyperpermeability, and second to protect retinal blood vessels and neurons from damage. But these research are still in their infancy due to a number of constraints such as limited understanding of the complex disease pathophysiology, safety and efficacy of vectors, patient selection and standardisation of outcome measures [47].

The science of epigenetics is ever growing and providing new insights in disease pathophysiology. Epigenetic term has evolved to include any change in the gene activity without any structural change in the DNA [48]. Recent research demonstrates that a diabetic environment may lead to a number of epigenetic changes in genes involved in pathogenesis of diabetic retinopathy. The use of inhibitors and mimics to target this epigenetic change can prove to be a useful treatment modality [49].

Recent research such as use of azo based probes for evaluating retinal hypoxia [50], molecular probes for retinal ischaemia [51], ROS-responsive microspheres for on demand antioxidant therapy [52], use of hydrogels [53] and nanoparticles [54] for sustained delivery of anti-VEGFs have brought to light many prospects in diagnosis and management of diabetic retinopathy.

20.7 Conclusion

To combat the impending epidemic of DR, DME and diabetic blindness an integrated global approach is needed. It will start with the prevention of diabetes and delaying the onset of diabetic retinopathy. Increased networking and collaborative effort will be needed where clinician, basic scientist, industry, regulatory agency, policy makers and politician will work together with one objective combating blindness learning the lesson and success of other programmes like HIV [55] control and resolution 74.4 of World Health Assembly by reducing the burden of diabetes and other non-communicable disease through set targets prioritisation and stimulus for action, and integration of programme implementation at the global level where no one will be left behind [56]. It is estimated that there will be more than half a billion-diabetic people in the world by 2040. To meet the target of once-a-year eye screening approximately 2000 eyes have to examined per minutes. Moreover, to reach people of remote rural as well as in urban area particularly in middle- and low-income countries will be an immense challenge [8]. Therefore, to prioritise the development of matrix and target level a careful and evidence based scientific approach will be needed to combat diabetes related blindness.

References

1. Galaviz KI, Weber MB, Straus A, Haw JS, Narayan KMV, Ali MK. Global diabetes prevention interventions: a systematic review and network meta-analysis of the real-world impact on incidence, weight, and glucose. Diabetes Care. 2018;41(7):1526–34.
2. Haw JS, Galaviz KI, Straus AN, Kowalski AJ, Magee MJ, Weber MB, et al. Long-term sustainability of diabetes prevention approaches: a systematic review and meta-analysis of randomized clinical trials. JAMA Intern Med. 2017;177(12):1808–17.
3. Gillies CL, Abrams KR, Lambert PC, Cooper NJ, Sutton AJ, Hsu RT, et al. Pharmacological and lifestyle interventions to prevent or delay type 2 diabetes in people with impaired glucose tolerance: systematic review and meta-analysis. BMJ. 2007;334(7588):299.
4. Balk EM, Earley A, Raman G, Avendano EA, Pittas AG, Remington PL. Combined diet and physical activity promotion programs to prevent type 2 diabetes among people at increased risk: a systematic review for the community preventive services task force. Ann Intern Med. 2015;163(6):437–51.
5. Chan JCN, Lim L-L, Wareham NJ, Shaw JE, Orchard TJ, Zhang P, et al. The lancet commission on diabetes: using data to transform diabetes care and patient lives. Lancet. 2021;396(10267):2019–82.
6. Jonas DE, Crotty K, Yun JDY, Middleton JC, Feltner C, Taylor-Phillips S, et al. Screening for prediabetes and type 2 diabetes mellitus: an evidence review for the U.S. Preventive services task force [Internet]. Rockville, MD: Agency for Healthcare Research and Quality (US); 2021. http://www.ncbi.nlm.nih.gov/books/NBK574057/. Accessed 12 Feb 2022.
7. Intensive blood-glucose control with sulphonylureas or insulin compared with conventional treatment and risk of complications in patients with type 2 diabetes (UKPDS 33). UK prospective diabetes study (UKPDS) group. Lancet. 1998;352(9131):837–53.
8. Das A. Diabetic retinopathy: battling the global epidemic. Invest Ophthalmol Vis Sci. 2016;57(15):6669–82. https://doi.org/10.1167/iovs.16-21031. https://iovs.arvojournals.org/article.aspx?articleid=2593012. Accessed 12 Feb 2022.
9. Ng CS, Lee JYC, Toh MP, Ko Y. Cost-of-illness studies of diabetes mellitus: a systematic review. Diabetes Res Clin Pract. 2014;105(2):151–63.
10. Gonder JR, Walker VM, Barbeau M, Zaour N, Zachau BH, Hartje JR, et al. Costs and quality of life in diabetic macular edema: Canadian burden of diabetic macular edema observational study (C-REALITY). J Ophthalmol. 2014;2014:e939315.

11. Magliano DJ, Martin VJ, Owen AJ, Zomer E, Liew D. The productivity burden of diabetes at a population level. Diabetes Care. 2018;41(5):979–84.
12. Fang M, Wang D, Coresh J, Selvin E. Trends in diabetes treatment and control in U.S. adults, 1999–2018. N Engl J Med. 2021;384(23):2219–28. https://doi.org/10.1056/NEJMsa2032271. https://pubmed.ncbi.nlm.nih.gov/34107181/. Accessed 12 Feb 2022.
13. Manne-Goehler J, Geldsetzer P, Agoudavi K, Andall-Brereton G, Aryal KK, Bicaba BW, et al. Health system performance for people with diabetes in 28 low- and middle-income countries: a cross-sectional study of nationally representative surveys. PLoS Med. 2019;16(3):e1002751.
14. Ali MK, Bullard KM, Gregg EW. Achievement of goals in U.S. diabetes care, 1999-2010. N Engl J Med. 2013;369(3):287–8.
15. Ali MK, Chwastiak L, Poongothai S, KMF E-F, Patel SA, Anjana RM, Sagar R, Shankar R, Sridhar GR, Kosuri M, Sosale AR, Sosale B, Rao D, Tandon N, KMV N, Mohan V, INDEPENDENT Study Group. Effect of a collaborative care model on depressive symptoms and glycated hemoglobin, blood pressure, and serum cholesterol among patients with depression and diabetes in India: the INDEPENDENT randomized clinical trial. JAMA. 2020;324(7):651–62. https://doi.org/10.1001/jama.2020.11747. https://www.ncbi.nlm.nih.gov/pmc/articles/PMC7435347/. Accessed 12 Feb 2022.
16. Flood D, Hane J, Dunn M, Brown SJ, Wagenaar BH, Rogers EA, et al. Health system interventions for adults with type 2 diabetes in low- and middle-income countries: a systematic review and meta-analysis. PLoS Med. 2020;17(11):e1003434.
17. Home, Resources, Diabetes L with, Acknowledgement, FAQs, Contact, et al. IDF Diabetes Atlas. 10th ed. [Internet]. https://diabetesatlas.org/. Accessed 12 Feb 2022.
18. Williams R, Karuranga S, Malanda B, Saeedi P, Basit A, Besançon S, et al. Global and regional estimates and projections of diabetes-related health expenditure: results from the International Diabetes Federation Diabetes Atlas, 9th edition. Diabetes Res Clin Pract. 2020;162:108072.
19. Atun R, Davies JI, Gale EAM, Bärnighausen T, Beran D, Kengne AP, et al. Diabetes in sub-Saharan Africa: from clinical care to health policy. Lancet Diabetes Endocrinol. 2017;5(8):622–67.
20. NCD Risk Factor Collaboration (NCD-RisC). Worldwide trends in diabetes since 1980: a pooled analysis of 751 population-based studies with 4.4 million participants. Lancet. 2016;387(10027):1513–30.
21. Yau JWY, Rogers SL, Kawasaki R, Lamoureux EL, Kowalski JW, Bek T, et al. Global prevalence and major risk factors of diabetic retinopathy. Diabetes Care. 2012;35(3):556–64.
22. Thomas RL, Halim S, Gurudas S, Sivaprasad S, Owens DR. IDF diabetes atlas: a review of studies utilising retinal photography on the global prevalence of diabetes related retinopathy between 2015 and 2018. Diabetes Res Clin Pract. 2019;157:107840.
23. Rowley WR, Bezold C, Arikan Y, Byrne E, Krohe S. Diabetes 2030: insights from yesterday, today, and future trends. Popul Health Manag. 2017;20(1):6–12.
24. Thomas CG, Channa R, Prichett L, Liu TYA, Abramoff MD, Wolf RM. Racial/ethnic disparities and barriers to diabetic retinopathy screening in youths. JAMA Ophthalmol. 2021;139(7):791–5.
25. Sivaprasad S, Gupta B, Crosby-Nwaobi R, Evans J. Prevalence of diabetic retinopathy in various ethnic groups: a worldwide perspective. Surv Ophthalmol. 2012;57(4):347–70.
26. Diabetes Control and Complications Trial Research Group, Nathan DM, Genuth S, Lachin J, Cleary P, Crofford O, et al. The effect of intensive treatment of diabetes on the development and progression of long-term complications in insulin-dependent diabetes mellitus. N Engl J Med. 1993;329(14):977–86.
27. King P, Peacock I, Donnelly R. The UK prospective diabetes study (UKPDS): clinical and therapeutic implications for type 2 diabetes. Br J Clin Pharmacol. 1999;48(5):643–8.
28. Sun JK, Keenan HA, Cavallerano JD, Asztalos BF, Schaefer EJ, Sell DR, et al. Protection from retinopathy and other complications in patients with type 1 diabetes of extreme duration. Diabetes Care. 2011;34(4):968–74.
29. Ipp E, Kumar M. A clinical conundrum: intensifying glycemic control in the presence of advanced diabetic retinopathy. Diabetes Care. 2021;44(10):2192–3.
30. Kuo JZ, Wong TY, Rotter JI. Challenges in elucidating the genetics of diabetic retinopathy. JAMA Ophthalmol. 2014;132(1):96–107.
31. Bhatwadekar AD, Shughoury A, Belamkar A, Ciulla TA. Genetics of diabetic retinopathy, a leading cause of irreversible blindness in the industrialized world. Genes (Basel). 2021;12(8):1200.
32. Vashist P, Singh S, Gupta N, Saxena R. Role of early screening for diabetic retinopathy in patients with diabetes mellitus: an overview. Indian J Commun Med. 2011;36(4):247–52.
33. Ali MK, Echouffo-Tcheugui J, Williamson DF. How effective were lifestyle interventions in real-world settings that were modeled on the diabetes prevention program? Health Aff (Millwood). 2012;31(1):67–75.
34. Pandey R, Morgan MM, Murphy C, Kavanagh H, Acheson R, Cahill M, et al. Irish National diabetic retinascreen programme: report on five rounds of retinopathy screening and screen-positive referrals. (INDEAR study report no. 1). Br J Ophthalmol. 2020;106(3):409–14. https://bjo.bmj.com/content/early/2020/12/16/bjophthalmol-2020-317508. Accessed 12 Feb 2022.
35. Scanlon PH. The English National Screening Programme for diabetic retinopathy 2003-2016. Acta Diabetol. 2017;54(6):515–25.
36. Danielsen R, Jónasson F, Helgason T. Prevalence of retinopathy and proteinuria in type 1 diabetics in Iceland. Acta Med Scand. 1982;212(5):277–80.
37. Gaiha SM, Shukla R, Gilbert CE, Anchala R, Gudlavalleti MVS. Is India's policy framework geared for effective action on avoidable blindness from diabetes? Indian J Endocrinol Metab. 2016;20(Suppl 1):S42–50.
38. Wong TY, Sabanayagam C. Strategies to tackle the global burden of diabetic retinopathy: from epidemiology to artificial intelligence. Ophthalmologica. 2020;243(1):9–20.
39. Silva PS, Horton MB, Clary D, Lewis DG, Sun JK, Cavallerano JD, et al. Identification of diabetic retinopathy and ungradable image rate with ultrawide field imaging in a National Teleophthalmology Program. Ophthalmology. 2016;123(6):1360–7.
40. Wong TY, Bressler NM. Artificial intelligence with deep learning technology looks into diabetic retinopathy screening. JAMA. 2016;316(22):2366–7.
41. Chen AX, Conti TF, Hom GL, Greenlee TE, Raimondi R, Briskin IN, et al. Functional imaging of mitochondria in retinal diseases using flavoprotein fluorescence. Eye. 2021;35(1):74–92.
42. Yan W, He M. Predictive medicine in ophthalmology. Ophthalmology. 2017;124(4):420–1.
43. Celi LA, Hinske Christian L, Alterovitz G, Szolovits P. An artificial intelligence tool to predict fluid requirement in the intensive care unit: a proof-of-concept study. Crit Care. 2008;12(6):R151.
44. Mateos-Olivares M, García-Onrubia L, Valentín-Bravo FJ, González-Sarmiento R, Lopez-Galvez M, Pastor JC, et al. Rho-kinase inhibitors for the treatment of refractory diabetic macular oedema. Cell. 2021;10(7):1683.
45. Bhatwadekar AD, Kansara VS, Ciulla TA. Investigational plasma kallikrein inhibitors for the treatment of diabetic macular edema: an expert assessment. Expert Opin Investig Drugs. 2020;29(3):237–44.
46. Hu T-T, Vanhove M, Porcu M, Van Hove I, Van Bergen T, Jonckx B, et al. The potent small molecule integrin antagonist THR-687 is a promising next-generation therapy for retinal vascular disorders. Exp Eye Res. 2019;180:43–52.

47. Wang J-H, Roberts GE, Liu G-S. Updates on gene therapy for diabetic retinopathy. Curr Diab Rep. 2020;20(7):22.
48. Weinhold B. Epigenetics: the science of change. Environ Health Perspect. 2006;114(3):A160–7.
49. Kowluru RA, Santos JM, Mishra M. Epigenetic modifications and diabetic retinopathy. Biomed Res Int. 2013;2013:e635284.
50. Uddin MI, Evans SM, Craft JR, Marnett LJ, Uddin MJ, Jayagopal A. Applications of azo-based probes for imaging retinal hypoxia. ACS Med Chem Lett. 2015;6(4):445–9. https://pubs.acs.org/doi/10.1021/ml5005206. Accessed 12 Feb 2022. https://doi.org/10.1021/ml5005206.
51. Evans SM, Kim K, Moore CE, Uddin MI, Capozzi ME, Craft JR, Sulikowski GA, Jayagopal A. Molecular probes for imaging of hypoxia in the retina. Bioconjug Chem. 2014;25(11):2030–7. https://pubs.acs.org/doi/10.1021/bc500400z. Accessed 12 Feb 2022. https://doi.org/10.1021/bc500400z.
52. Poole KM, Nelson CE, Joshi RV, Martin JR, Gupta MK, Haws SC, et al. ROS-responsive microspheres for on demand antioxidant therapy in a model of diabetic peripheral arterial disease. Biomaterials. 2015;41:166–75.
53. Yu Y, Lau LC, Lo AC, Chau Y. Injectable chemically crosslinked hydrogel for the controlled release of bevacizumab in vitreous: a 6-month in vivo study. Transl Vis Sci Technol. 2015;4(2):5. https://tvst.arvojournals.org/article.aspx?articleid=2212994. Accessed 12 Feb 2022. https://doi.org/10.1167/tvst.4.2.5.
54. Yandrapu SK, Upadhyay AK, Petrash JM, Kompella UB. Nanoparticles in porous microparticles prepared by supercritical infusion and pressure quench technology for sustained delivery of bevacizumab. Mol Pharm. 2013;10(12):4676–86.
55. Medlock J, Pandey A, Parpia AS, Tang A, Skrip LA, Galvani AP. Effectiveness of UNAIDS targets and HIV vaccination across 127 countries. Proc Natl Acad Sci U S A. 2017;114(15):4017–22.
56. Improving health outcomes of people with diabetes mellitus [Internet]. https://www.who.int/publications/m/item/improving-health-outcomes-of-people-with-diabetes-mellitus. Accessed 12 Feb 2022.

GPSR Compliance

The European Union's (EU) General Product Safety Regulation (GPSR) is a set of rules that requires consumer products to be safe and our obligations to ensure this.

If you have any concerns about our products, you can contact us on ProductSafety@springernature.com

In case Publisher is established outside the EU, the EU authorized representative is:

Springer Nature Customer Service Center GmbH
Europaplatz 3
69115 Heidelberg, Germany

Batch number: 10731528

Printed by Printforce, the Netherlands